Clinical nutrition

Clinical nutrition

Victoria F. Thiele, Ph.D., R.D.

Professor of Human Nutrition, Director
of Coordinated Undergraduate Program-Clinical
Nutrition Specialists, College for Human
Development, Syracuse University,
Syracuse, New York

SECOND EDITION

with 30 *illustrations*

The C. V. Mosby Company

ST. LOUIS • TORONTO • LONDON   1980

SECOND EDITION

Copyright © 1980 by The C. V. Mosby Company

All rights reserved. No part of this book may be reproduced in any manner without written permission of the publisher.

Previous edition copyrighted 1976

Printed in the United States of America

The C. V. Mosby Company
11830 Westline Industrial Drive, St. Louis, Missouri 63141

Library of Congress Cataloging in Publication Data

Thiele, Victoria F   1933-
    Clinical nutrition.

    Includes bibliographical references and index.
    1.   Diet therapy.   I.   Title.
RM216.T33   1980   615.8'54   80-13265
ISBN 0-8016-4901-3

AC/M/M   9   8   7   6   5   4   3   2   1   03/D/336

To
my mother
Frances Victor Thiele
with deep appreciation

Preface

Clinical Nutrition discusses the rationale for the dietary treatment of a wide spectrum of disorders such as obesity, gastrointestinal disorders, liver and gallbladder disease, renal disease, diabetes mellitus, cardiovascular disease, inborn errors of metabolism, and cancer. A biochemical and medical background of these diseases is presented where appropriate to aid in a better understanding of diet therapy. Some of the past dietary practices are included as an aid to understanding current dietary treatment. An appreciation of the medical and dietary treatment of the patient is essential to the dietitian or nutritionist on the health care team, since the nutritional care plan for the patient's medical treatment must provide an optimum nutritional status.

This book is intended to serve as a text for undergraduate and graduate dietetic and nutrition students both in diet therapy and clinical dietetics courses. It should be useful to students in coordinated undergraduate programs that incorporate clinical experience into the undergraduate curriculum and to internship students majoring in therapeutic nutrition. The contents should also be useful to physicians, nurses, and other members of the health professions.

The omission of basic nutrition information allows for more in-depth coverage of clinical nutrition. Current research is cited in order to serve as an impetus for the student to continue perusal of the literature upon becoming a practitioner. It is important that as new knowledge and insights into dietary treatment are developed they be incorporated into current practice more quickly than they have been in the past.

Specific diets are not included in the text, since they can be found in hospital diet manuals. Food habits differ from one part of the country to the other, so it is difficult to cite specific diets. It is important that such diets serve only as guidelines. The diet must be planned to the preferences of the individual within the restrictions of the dietary prescription. People do not adhere to diets in standard printed diet sheets or booklets that differ from their own normal patterns; therefore, individualization and careful diet instruction are necessary. The old and new exchange lists for diabetic diets are included in Appendixes B and C. Once the student masters the use of these lists, the same principles can be applied to exchange lists dealing with nutrients whose intake must be carefully controlled.

I am indebted to my students who provided the inspiration for this book. I would like to thank them for their criticism and comments. I would also like to express my appreciation to my mother for her contribution above and beyond the call of motherly love and duty, for her support, for her encouragement, and especially for her diligent proofreading.

Victoria F. Thiele

Contents

1 Nutrition and disease

To maintain optimal nutrition an individual must consume a diet that contains a variety of foods so that an adequate supply of the nutrients needed to promote a state of well-being is received. The amounts of nutrients are important because an excess, deficiency, or imbalance can result in malnutrition. An excess of energy intake leads to obesity and excessive intakes of vitamins A and D are toxic, due in part to the ability of the body to conserve these fat-soluble vitamins. A deficiency of protein can result in kwashiorkor, a disease found in many parts of the world where food is in short supply and protein calorie malnutrition is rampant. Thousands face death by starvation. Infants who do survive never reach their full physical and mental potential. Others who consume inadequate intakes of food develop vitamin and mineral deficiency diseases. The classic vitamin deficiency states—scurvy, beri-beri, pellagra, rickets, night blindness, and anemia—are still evident in many parts of the world.

In the United States, although severe nutritional deficiency diseases are found infrequently, many individuals suffer from marginal intakes. They have no clinically well-defined symptoms, yet they are not in the best of health. For the most part, however, the greatest nutritional problem is not undernutrition but overnutrition. The incidence of obesity is increasing even though it predisposes the individual to various illnesses and shortens his life span. Millions of dollars are spent by people who attempt to lose weight by methods other than those of decreasing caloric intake or increasing physical activity.

Since individuals are different, their nutrient requirements are also different and cannot be determined by a nutritional status survey of a large group of people. Therefore allowances have been established that include a safety factor to account for individual variation. However, the allowance for energy does not include a safety factor, since any excess will lead to weight gain. The 1980 Revised Recommended Daily Dietary Allowances (RDA) include allowances for kilocalories, protein, vitamins (A, D, E, K, ascorbic acid, niacin, folacin, thiamine, riboflavin, pyridoxine, B_{12}, biotin, and pantothenic acid), minerals (calcium, phosphorus, iron, iodine, zinc, and magnesium), trace elements (copper, manganese, fluoride, chromium, selenium, and molybdenum), and electrolytes (sodium and potassium). See Appendix A. The RDA can be used as guidelines for establishing regular diets for hospital patients to ensure an adequate intake of nutrients.

When the diet must be modified because of illness, the objective is to maintain the patient in optimal nutrition. The patient's food habits must be considered in planning the diet. A meal plan that meets the dietary prescription but is not acceptable to the patient will accomplish little. However, poor dietary practices must be corrected. This is difficult especially during illness or hospitalization. An attempt to change food habits at this time may not be beneficial, but may create stress and frustration for the patient. If the diet is drastically different and restrictive, the patient may totally reject it. Therefore it is essential that the rationale for the diet be carefully explained.

The feeding of a hospital patient is a difficult task. The patient is in an unfamiliar environment and subject to all sorts of stresses. Mealtimes may be different from what the patient is accustomed to as well as the method of food preparation. Meals are especially important to patients in intensive care units where mealtime comes at regular intervals and may be the patient's only indication of the time of day. It may also be the only pleasant part of the day.

Many complaints are registered about hospital food perhaps because this is the only avenue open to the patient to register unhappiness without serious repercussions. The patient is afraid to complain to the physician or nurse since he is dependent on them and cannot afford to lose their services should they become annoyed. However, no matter how many complaints are registered about the food, he knows he will still be fed. Since in the hospital situation the patient loses his freedom and must follow the dictates of the hospital staff taking care of him, by expressing an opinion about one aspect of his care, he can still feel he has some control over his life.

NUTRIENT REQUIREMENTS IN DISEASE

Illness may have several different effects on nutrition. Nutrient requirements may either decrease or increase because of changes in metabolism. Nutrient intake is often diminished because of anorexia, vomiting, or pain. The patient may be unconscious or unable to take food by mouth; tube or parenteral feeding can be used to maintain the patient in these instances. Malabsorption, which may result from malabsorptive syndromes (cystic fibrosis, celiac disease or nontropical sprue), diarrhea, or after surgery on the gastrointestinal tract, also leads to a diminished intake of nutrients. In certain situations, such as during fever and after surgery or burns, nutrient needs are increased. In particular, burn patients have such excessive requirements that enough food cannot be taken orally, so tube or parenteral feeding may be indicated.

In certain metabolic disorders or diseases there is an inability to use nutrients. For example, in phenylketonuria the amino acid phenylalanine cannot be metabolized; in galactosemia, galactose cannot be utilized; and in diabetes mellitus, glucose tolerance is impaired. Therefore the offending nutrient must either be excluded from the diet or, in cases where it is an essential nutrient, provided in small quantities. Protein must be restricted in liver disease since ammonia cannot be converted to urea. In kidney disease urea is not removed from the circulation, so again protein must be restricted. Sodium may also need to be restricted in liver and renal disease.

Many illnesses result in a catabolic state. After surgery, even though adequate nutrients are provided, negative nitrogen balance occurs. Bed rest and immobilization lead to negative nitrogen and calcium balance. This state can also occur without illness; the same effect was observed in astronauts who were confined to space capsules.

The therapy instituted for the management of the illness may contribute to the deficiency state. Cancer patients subject to radiation or chemotherapy become anorexic and unable to eat. Drug-induced nutritional deficiencies occur and are more severe in the patient whose nutritional intake is inadequate. Drugs such as phenolphthalein, colchicine, methotrexate, para-aminosalicylic acid, cholestyramine, and neomycin interfere with absorption of nutrients from the small intestine.[1] Other drugs complex with vitamins and minerals. A vitamin B_6 deficiency can develop when isonicotinic acid hydrazide, hydralazine, penicillamine, and l-dopa are administered. Methotrexate, pyrimethamine, and aminopterin act as vitamin antagonists. Multiple vitamin deficiencies can result from taking anticonvulsants or oral contraceptive agents. Thus the nutritional status of a patient on drug therapy must be closely monitored.

MODIFICATION OF THE NORMAL DIET

A modified diet is based on a normal intake but is altered to meet the specific requirement of a disease or metabolic disorder. Prior nutritional deficiencies should be corrected. The ideal weight of the patient should be attained either by an increase or decrease in calories. The latter is not attempted when the patient is seriously ill. A diet may be high in a nutrient and thus provide more than is normally required, or conversely it may be low in a nutrient. However, these terms are not specific and cannot be interpreted in terms of definite amounts. A free diet is one that does not contain either a specific nutrient or food; for example, a galactose-free diet does not contain galactose in any form, whereas a milk-free diet would not contain any milk or milk products. The term "free diet" has also been used in connection with diabetes mellitus to denote a diet that does not have any restrictions. The term "restricted" indicates that a nutrient is prescribed in amounts that are lower than in the usual normal diet. A controlled diet is one in which a nutrient or nutrients are regulated from day to day; for example, a fat-controlled diet is regulated as to the amount and type of fat included. In some instances the diet is modified so as to provide physiologic rest for an organ. Diets are restricted to allow for recovery from ulcers and heart, liver, and kidney disease.

Normal diets may be modified in consistency, texture, flavor, energy value, nutrient levels, types of food, or combinations of these factors. Liquid diets are prescribed after acute vomiting, diarrhea, or surgery. This modification is followed for only a short period of time since it is nutritionally inadequate. A full fluid diet consists of liquids and foods that liquefy at body temperature and follows a liquid diet or is used for acute infections, fever, gastrointestinal upsets, and for patients who cannot chew. Tube feeding is used when the patient is unconscious or paralyzed, after oral or gastric surgery, or if there is an obstruction in the gastrointestinal tract.

Mechanical soft diets are composed of soft foods and are used primarily with people who have difficulty in chewing. Soft diets are low in fiber content and connective tissue, soft in consistency, and bland in flavor and are used for surgical patients who have progressed from the full fluid diet in acute infections, fevers, or gastrointestinal disturbances. A bland diet contains foods that are mild in flavor. It has also been interpreted as a diet exclusive of foods high in fiber. However, the term "bland fiber-restricted diet" should then be used.[2] This diet was previously prescribed for various gastrointestinal disorders such as peptic ulcer, ulcerative colitis, and diverticulosis. But current practice does not advocate bland low-fiber diets for peptic ulcer therapy. High-fiber diets have been found to be more useful for diverticulosis.

Confusion also exists over the terminology "fiber" and "residue." Fiber has been defined as indigestible plant material,[3] and when it is used with therapeutic diets, it includes both indigestible plant and animal tissue.[4] When fiber content is modified, the amount of fruits, vegetables, and cereals are either increased or decreased. Low-residue diets exclude both fiber and milk, since the latter is thought to increase the residue in the colon. The low-residue diet is prescribed prior to surgery on the intestinal tract to reduce the amount of residue in the colon and after surgery to allow for healing and also for acute diarrhea, regional enteritis, and colitis.

High-calorie diets are prescribed for weight loss that accompanies a long illness. When nausea is diminished and appetite is regained, then a high-calorie diet is useful. In fever and hyperthyroidism, metabolism increases and there is need for additional calories. Burn patients need to replace nutrients lost from the exudate at the burn site and also for the synthesis of new tissue; therefore calorie requirements are extremely high. On the other hand, low-calorie diets are prescribed for weight reduction. Fasting or semistarvation diets may be employed for patients who need to lose weight rapidly.

High-protein diets of from 100 to 125 g per day may be prescribed for a variety of conditions. Certain individuals, for example, the elderly, indigent, or alcoholics, may have low intakes of protein and thus need additional protein to replace that which has been lost from the body. Extra protein is needed when protein catabolism is high such as in fevers and hyperthyroidism. Protein is lost from the body of patients with burns, nephrotic syndrome, hemorrhaging, or after surgery. Diarrhea, ulcerative colitis, sprue, celiac disease, and cystic fibrosis all decrease amino acid absorption so that more protein must be provided to compensate for this defect.

Protein requirements for liver patients are dependent upon the condition of the patient. High amounts may be needed to promote protein biosynthesis and the regeneration of hepatocytes. Yet, if the protein cannot be used for synthesis, the amino acids are catabolized and the excess ammonia cannot be converted to urea for excretion and the patient develops hepatic coma. In this situation, protein levels must be decreased or completely restricted for a few days. Patients with kidney disease, such as acute and chronic glomeruloneprhitis, nephrosclerosis, and acute and chronic renal failure, require low-protein diets since the kidney cannot excrete nitrogenous wastes. Diets containing 18 to 22 g of high biological value protein may be needed for the chronic uremic patient who is not being dialyzed. Low-protein diets are also prescribed for patients with inborn errors of metabolism that result from a lack of enzymes of the urea cycle. In gluten-induced enteropathy (celiac disease) the protein gluten in wheat and rye brings out a metabolic defect in the intestinal mucosal cells. The protein gluten is composed of two fractions—glutenin and gliadin. The latter protein causes the difficulty. Treatment involves the removal of this protein from the diet (gliadin-free diet).

The amino acid composition of the diet may need to be modified in cases of an inborn error of metabolism in which the amino acid cannot be metabolized normally and as a result other metabolites are formed that in most instances are toxic. Most often the amount of the amino acid in the diet is decreased, such as phenylalanine in phenylketonuria, methionine in homocystinuria, and valine in hypervalinemia. The treatment of maple syrup urine disease is difficult since the amounts of three essential amino acids must be regulated, namely, valine, leucine, and isoleucine.

For several years low-carbohydrate diets were prescribed for diabetes. However, since high-carbohydrate diets have not impaired glucose tolerance, severe carbohydrate restriction is not necessary. Simple sugars are prohibited as they are rapidly absorbed and cause hyperglycemic peaks.

Galactose is restricted in the inborn error of metabolism, galactosemia. In disaccharidase deficiencies the sugars are not digested because of the inactivity of the digestive enzymes; therefore the disaccharide must be omitted from the diet. For example, in lactase deficiency, lactose, the sugar in milk, cannot be digested. All milk and milk products with this sugar must be excluded from the diet. In the inherited disorder glucose-galactose malabsorption the amounts of both of these sugars must be restricted.

The average American diet provides about 45% of calories from fat. Since steatorrhea occurs in gallbladder disease and certain malabsorptive syndromes such as nontropical sprue or celiac disease and cystic fibrosis, the amount of fat in the diet is decreased. Medium-chain triglycerides are useful for individuals with these disorders that result in the impairment of fat digestion or absorption. Fat-controlled diets regulate the amount and type of fat allowed. The calories from fat should provide about 30% to 35% of the total calories with 10% from saturated fat and 12% to 14% from polyunsaturated fats. The remainder of the calories come from monounsaturated fats. Cholesterol is also decreased from the average daily intake of 600 to 300 mg. These diets are prescribed for atherosclerosis, myocardial infarction, and stroke. Some groups have advocated the use of these diets for individuals at risk with hyperlipidemia. Others do not agree and are of the opinion that there is presently not enough evidence to indicate that a dietary change would be beneficial.

The mineral content of the diet may also be altered. Four levels of sodium restriction are most often used—250, 500, 1000, and 2400 to 4500 mg. The first diet is a severe restriction that excludes salty foods and salt in cooking and at the table. This diet is used both to prevent and treat edema; therefore it is prescribed for congestive heart failure, hypertension, toxemia of pregnancy, and liver and renal disease. Some renal patients may not be able to regulate sodium excretion and become hyponatremic. Then sodium must be added back by means of the diet. In renal patients with chronic uremia it may be necessary to also restrict potassium and phosphorus. Patients who have had extensive hemorrhaging, anemia, or chronic uremia may need an iron supplement.

Therapeutic vitamins are prescribed for patients who are unable to consume an adequate amount of food because of illness or whose requirements are excessively high, such as after surgery and for burn patients. Patients on dialysis lose vitamins into the dialyzing solution, so supplements must be provided. When drugs that are vitamin antagonists are administered, larger amounts of the vitamin are needed. Certain inborn errors of metabolism have been treated by giving extremely large doses of vitamins. A variant form of maple syrup urine disease responds to a high intake of thiamine. Large doses of vitamin B_6 are needed in homocystinuria, cystathioninuria, and the vitamin B_6 dependency syndrome.

The diet therapy for obesity, gastrointestinal disorders, liver disease, gallbladder disease, renal disease, cardiovascular disease, and diabetes mellitus is discussed in greater detail in later chapters.

TEST DIETS

Prior to some diagnostic procedures it is necessary to prescribe a test diet. Before a glucose tolerance test can be performed, a 150 g carbohydrate diet should be ingested for 3 days. When fecal fat determinations are to be made, 100 g of fat should be ingested. On the day before a cholecystogram is performed, the noon meal contains 60 g of fat while the evening meal is fat free.

A low-calcium diet containing 7 mEq calcium is used for 3 days as an aid in diagnosing hypercalciuria. A low sodium diet (230 mg or 10 mEq) is used to detect the clinical conditions that cause hypertension resulting from abnormal renin synthesis. To test for food allergies, all the common foods known to cause reactions are excluded for 2 weeks. Foods are added back for 3 days at a time until the offending food is found.

The vanillylmandelic acid test diet is used to detect a pheochromocytoma. Vanilla and vanilla-containing products and caffeine are omitted prior to the test. However, with a new chemical method for measuring vanillylmandelic acid, dietary restrictions are no longer necessary. The 5-hydroxyindoleacetic acid diet, which is used to test for carcinoid tumors, restricts foods that contain serotonin, such as walnuts, bananas, and avocados, for 72 hours prior to the test.

Tyramine-restricted diets are prescribed for patients on monoamine oxidase (MAO) inhibitor drug therapy who develop hypertension when tyramine or 3,4-

dihydroxyphenylalanine is ingested. Therefore the following foods must be avoided: aged cheese; alcoholic beverages such as ale, beer, and certain wines; herring; cod; yogurt; and liver.

Other diets that may be ordered are acid ash, alkaline ash, hypoglycemic, keto-genic, restricted purine, low copper, low leucine, and low oxalate.

RESEARCH DIETS

De St. Jeor and Bryan described the clinical research diets as proposed by the National Conference of General Clinical Research Dietitians in 1970.[5] Five diet classifications were proposed: estimated, weighed, controlled nutrient, constant, and metabolic balance (Table 1-1). The estimated diet is the fastest means of getting an indication of an individual's intake. Equivalency lists or tables of averages are used to calculate the intakes. This method does not provide accurate information since the food intake is not weighed; however, it can provide information to indicate what future studies might be needed. More information is gained from the weighed clini-cal research diet. The food is weighed before intake and after the completion of a meal to determine waste. Standard tables are used to calculate the nutrient intake. This then provides a more accurate indication of the patient's nutrient intake.

In some research studies the intake of one nutrient is controlled. The amount of food served is weighed. If some of the food is refused, it is weighed and the amount of the nutrient under study is calculated. This amount may then be served to the patient in other foods. Standard tables or laboratory analyses are used to calculate the intake. The constant diet is similar to the controlled diet except that more rigid conditions are followed. The subject is discouraged from refusing food, and if this is impossible, an attempt is made to replace the foods that are refused.

The most sensitive and detailed studies are those done to determine metabolic balance. Foods must be analyzed in the laboratory, or data from the manufacturer is used. For the duration of the study, food is supplied from a constant source and lot. For example, the same brand of canned products must be used, and meat is obtained from one cut if at all possible. All food must be carefully weighed, and again the food refused must be kept to a minimum. In addition, all body excretions, such as urine, feces, and in some cases perspiration, must be collected and analyzed. Some re-searchers use liquid formula diets on metabolic balance studies since it is easier to regulate nutrient intake by this method. The metabolic balance study provides the most reliable data; however, a metabolic unit with properly trained personnel is needed. Patients must be motivated since rigid adherence to the dietary protocol is necessary. It is sometimes difficult to maintain subjects on this regimen for long periods of time. For nitrogen balance studies a period of adaptation is necessary prior to the initiation of the diet to be tested. It becomes especially difficult if several different diets of varying composition are to be tested on the same individual. The greatest problem often is patient adherence to the rigid conditions for the time necessary to collect meaningful data.

Table 1-1. Clinical research diets—definition of terms*

Classification	Intake calculated	Measurement of diet	Food source	Water source	Food preparation procedures
Estimated	Daily (after intake charted), using equivalency lists or tables of averages	Estimated in household measures	Varied	Varied	Varied
Weighed	Daily (charted sometimes before and always after intake), using standard tables	Weighed (gram scale) portions (usual or calculated)	Varied	Varied	Varied or controlled
Controlled nutrient	Daily (before and after serving to patient), using standard tables, special references, or laboratory analyses	Weighed (torsion balance), controlled portions	Varied	Controlled or varied	Controlled or varied
Constant	Before study, using analyzed laboratory data, reliable manufacturers' data, USDA Handbook No. 8, or other tables and references	Weighed (torsion balance), controlled portions	Constant	Controlled or constant	Constant
Metabolic balance	Before study, using analyzed laboratory data, reliable manufacturers' data, USDA Handbook No. 8, or other tables and references	Weighed (torsion balance), controlled portions	Constant	Constant	Constant

*From De St. Jeor, S. T., and Bryan, G. T.: Clinical research diets: definition of terms, J. Am. Diet.

Food refusals	Laboratory analysis of diet	Advantages	Disadvantages	Application
Estimated	No	Closest to "free diet"; ease and speed of estimation; most accurate observational data	Least reliable nutritive data; biased by change to hospital setting, different foods, etc.	Estimate of patient's preferred intake; data to supplement dietary history
Weighed	No	Minimal inconvenience to patient; more reliable nutritive data	Increased work with some increase in accuracy of data	More accurate idea of patient's preferred intake; more reliable observational data; general test diets
Weighed, calculated, and perhaps replaced	Rarely	Flexible, food variety; offers some variety and flexibility to patient	Expensive (dietitian's time) unless computer available; constant monitoring for replacements	Diets with focus on desired maximum or minimum quantity or quality of nutrients; investigative diets
Discouraged, replaced if possible, otherwise, weighed, calculated, and perhaps analyzed	Occasionally	Highly accurate; dietitian's time used more efficiently; minimal calculations	Lack of variety and flexibility; requires a research kitchen, properly trained personnel, and standardized food preparation procedures; requires trial period for acceptability	Diagnostic diets, research diets
Discouraged, replaced if possible; otherwise, weighed, calculated, and analyzed	2-3 Times per menu	Most reliable data; supported by actual laboratory analyses; dietitian's time used most efficiently; minimal calculations	Requires analyses of all intake and excreta; only as accurate as collections and laboratory analyses; lack of variety and flexibility; requires research kitchen, properly trained personnel, and standardized food preparation procedures; requires trial period for acceptability	Metabolic balance studies only

HOSPITAL MALNUTRITION

Much concern has been expressed within recent years of the increasing incidence of malnutrition in hospitals. Hospital employees (51), patients with mild reversible illnesses (144), and more severely ill patients (351) were evaluated for nutritional status.[6] Serum protein, extractable protein hair roots (measure of protein stores), hemoglobin, hematocrit, and vitamins A, E, and C were measured. The hospital employees were found to have less than the reported lower limits of normal for ascorbic acid, hemoglobin, and protein (hair root values). Approximately one fifth of the patients with mild illnesses were deficient in each nutrient studied. Of the seriously ill patients, the diabetics exhibited the best nutritional state, whereas the patients with alcoholic liver disease showed the most evidence of malnutrition. Low ascorbic acid levels (42%) were found in ulcer patients. This is surprising since vitamin C is needed for wound healing, and yet it was not routinely prescribed. From 17% to 45% of the severely ill patients and 12% to 24% of the patients with mild illnesses were below normal levels for each nutritional parameter when compared with the hospital employees.

Evidence of malnutrition in a Boston hospital has also been reported.[7,8] Protein status was determined by measuring triceps skinfold, mid-arm circumference, and in some instances serum albumin levels and height and weight. On the basis of arm muscle circumference, which is a measure of protein stores, protein calorie malnutrition (PCM) appeared in 48% of the patients. Results from triceps skinfold measurements were similar in that 56% of the patients had PCM. Low levels of serum albumin were found in 30 of the 56 patients surveyed. This level correlated with both skinfold and mid-arm circumference measurements. Since height-weight data are not good predictions of PCM, in many instances heights and weights were not recorded. The PCM could be reversed by oral and total parenteral nutrition, so it was not a result of illness but caused by dietary inadequacy. Since PCM results in a loss of cellular immunity, the patient is more susceptible to infection, and the rate of wound healing is decreased.

In another study, Bistrian et al. used weight/height, triceps skinfold, arm muscle circumference, serum albumin, and hematocrit to assess the nutritional status of medical patients in a teaching hospital.[9] The incidence of PCM by the criteria used were weight/height, 45%; triceps skinfold, 76%; arm muscle circumference, 55%; serum albumin, 44%; and hematocrit, 48%. Medical patients were more depleted calorically but had better protein nutriture than did surgical patients.

In a study by Butterworth the charts of 80 patients hospitalized for 2 weeks were reviewed.[10] Height (in 56% of the patients) and weight (in 23% of the patients) were not recorded. An average weight loss of 6 kg was reported in 22 patients. The oral ingestion of food was not allowed for 3.1 days. Hypoalbuminemia was present in 37% of the cases, yet therapy was instituted in only 15 instances. Anemia was found in 37% of the patients on admission, and it developed in still another 16% after hospitalization. It was felt that this was in part a result of the taking of frequent blood samples. Supplements were not given to 14 patients who had signs of poor vitamin nutriture. During 1 year 128,000 units of intravenous 5% or 10% glucose solutions were used. If each unit represents a meal, it was calculated that this represented a deficit of 2600 kcal weekly for each patient.

Tobias and Van Itallie evaluated patients' hospital charts at two teaching hospitals for evidence of malnutrition.[11] Four categories were used: overt, probable, likely possible, and no malnutrition. The criteria used to assess the patients' nutritional status were chronic alcoholism, endentulism, emaciated appearance, obese appearance, premature coronary heart disease, and a history of previous gastrointestinal disorders. If the patient had one of these problems, then he was considered to have actual or potential malnutrition. Of the 67 patients studied 91% fell into this category. In the physical examination, patients were assessed as "well nourished" or "well developed." Yet there are no objective standards to define these terms.

The data from the medical history and examination indicated the need for a diet history in 89.6% of the patients. This was done in 10.4% of the cases but not by a dietitian. Generally heights and weights were not recorded. Nutritional problems indicated on the initial medical record were often not treated. For example, 20 patients had lost weight, yet attempts to promote weight gain were seen in only four patients. Sixteen patients were obese, yet weight reduction diets were ordered for five. An analysis of diet modifications prescribed by the physician indicated that they were appropriate in 31 cases, incomplete for 32 patients, and inappropriate in four cases. Prescription of nutritional supplements and drugs was appropriate in 46.3% of the cases and incomplete for the remainder. Forty-six patients needed vitamin and mineral supplements, yet only 18 received them. When the oral ingestion of food was limited, no attempt was made to assess the caloric intake. Sixty-one percent of the patients were at nutritional risk, yet no dietitian obtained a dietary history or provided nutritional counseling. The authors concluded that the roles of the physician and the dietitian in providing nutritional care for the patients were not clearly defined. Physicians, dietitians, and nurses do not give adequate care because of insufficient knowledge of nutritional problems, a lack of goals for assessment and management of patients' nutritional problems; and a misunderstanding of team members and their specific responsibilities.

Weinsier et al. assessed the nutritional status of 134 patients in a teaching hospital.[12] The parameters evaluated were serum folate, serum ascorbic acid, triceps skinfold, arm muscle circumference, weight/height, lymphocytes, serum albumin, and hematocrit. A scoring system was based on these parameters. There were three categories of malnutrition: major, intermediate, and minor. Points were assigned to each parameter so that the likelihood of malnutrition (LOM) could be calculated. Folate and ascorbic acid were chosen as indicators of vitamin nutriture, while a decrease in the number of lymphocytes is associated with impaired cell-mediated immunity and an increased susceptibility to infection. A deficiency of several nutrients lowers hematocrit values.

A high LOM was found in slightly less than 50% of the patients on hospital admission. Low-serum folate levels were found most often. After 2 weeks of hospitalization or longer 69% of the patients had a high LOM. These patients lost subcutaneous fat, weight, and muscle mass, and serum folate, serum albumin, and hematocrit values fell. Thus nutritional status became worse during hospitalization.

Many standard hospital practices contribute to the malnutrition of the patient according to Butterworth.[10] The staff of the hospital is rotated rather frequently, and so the patient is not attended by one physician for the duration of the hospital stay. Even residents are permitted to change orders without the approval of the attending physician. Therefore the patient may not receive the best treatment while an attempt is made to educate the medical student.[13] This matter is complicated by the fact that patient care is divided among many individuals. Intravenous saline and glucose solutions that cannot meet the nutritional needs of any individual are used for long periods of time.[10] Tube feedings do not provide an adequate nutrient intake because of improper composition, preparation under unsanitary conditions, and too rapid feeding. Patients often do not get meals because diagnostic tests are to be performed. Increased nutrient requirements occur during infection, severe illness, or after surgery, and many times these needs are not met. Incorrect vitamin mixtures may be prescribed. On the other hand, additional nutrients may be ordered only when the patient is severely debilitated, and thus the hospital stay is prolonged needlessly. Laboratory tests to detect marginal nutritional deficiency are rarely performed.

Another problem Butterworth stated was the lack of communication between the physician and the dietitian.[10] Enloe indicated that dietitians should be more assertive, since they have the most knowledge about the nutritional needs of the patients.[14] The physician receives little nutrition education in medical school and yet is responsible for the diet prescription. The dietitian should be a member of the health care team that provides the total care for the patient and be allowed to participate in hospital rounds. This occurs for the most part infrequently and in most cases only in teaching hospitals. The dietitian must not only be assertive but must be knowledgeable in dietetics and understand the biochemical and medical aspects of the disease and how it relates to nutrition. Physicians must also recognize the expertise of dietitians and use them to provide the optimal nutritional care of patients.

The hospital food delivery system has also contributed to hospital malnutrition.[13] Of the many people who are involved in food delivery and preparation, the patient has the least input. Meals may not be prepared to the patient's tastes and are served at times appropriate to hospital routine and may not be the times the patient is accustomed to eating. Usually no one checks to see if the meal has been eaten. Indeed the patient may have difficulty feeding himself.

Concern about the incidence of malnutrition in hospitals is growing. Additional surveys will further document this as a problem that must be dealt with by changing current practices. A greater emphasis must be placed on monitoring the nutritional status of the hospitalized patient. Dietary, clinical, anthropometric, and biochemical information must be collected on patients even though this procedure becomes time consuming and expensive. Physicians must be made more aware of the role of nutrition both in the prevention and treatment of disease. Study of nutrition is important in the curriculum of the medical student, who must recognize the role of the dietitian in contributing to the total care of the patient. The dietitian must keep up with current dietary practice and become a functioning member of the health care team. Along with good medical care the patient is entitled to good nutritional care. This will not only hasten recovery but also reduce the complications of illness. A shortened hospital stay will also reduce medical expenses.

EVALUATION OF NUTRITIONAL STATUS[15]

The nutritional status of an individual or group may be determined by clinical, anthropometric, biochemical, or dietary methods. A combination of two or more of these methods is generally used since nutritional status is dependent upon intake and body metabolism. In extensive surveys of large population groups all the methods may be utilized but not on the total sample population since the collection of such data would be both lengthy and expensive.

Clinical tests

The clinical assessment involves a medical history to detect any prior illnesses that may have affected nutritional status. A trained physician conducts a physical examination of hair, skin, eyes, eyelids, lips, mouth, tongue, teeth, gums, thyroid, parotid gland, liver, and neuromuscular, skeletal, and cardiovascular systems. The general appearance of the individual is also noted. Classic deficiency diseases such as pellagra, scurvy, beri-beri, and rickets are easily detected. Today, these are relatively rare in the United States. Most abnormal signs that occur are nonspecific. For example, dermatitis is associated with a deficiency of several vitamins. The clinical assessment is dependent to a certain extent on the judgment of the observer.

Anthropometric tests

Anthropometric data are useful in determining the growth and development of children. Malnutrition is generally evidenced by a retardation of the growth rate. The measures used most often are height, weight, and skinfold thickness. Head, chest, and arm circumference measurements can be used with children. X-ray examinations of bones such as the wrist are frequently used in nutritional status surveys. Subcutaneous fat in various parts of the body can be measured by the use of x-ray films.

Biochemical analyses

Many biochemical tests can be performed. Most often blood and urine samples are collected. The following hematologic determinations have been used: red and white cell count, hemoglobin, hematocrit, serum vitamin A, serum carotene, serum vitamin C, serum folate, red-cell folate, total serum protein, serum albumin, serum iron, total iron-binding capacity, serum magnesium, and serum cholesterol.

Serum enzyme levels have also been used to reflect the status of vitamin nutriture. Enzyme activity is dependent on the presence of a coenzyme that has a part of its structure a vitamin; therefore, if the vitamin is lacking, enzyme activity will decrease. Transketolase levels are used to determine thiamine status; transaminase levels reflect vitamin B_6 status; and erythrocyte glutathione reductase levels are decreased in a riboflavin deficiency. Alkaline phosphatase levels increase in vitamin D and protein deficiency.

During surveys, timed urine collections cannot be obtained; casual urine samples are collected. Urinary creatinine levels are measured, and urinary thiamine, riboflavin, and iodine levels are reported in terms of a gram of creatinine. Reagent strips can be used to measure the urinary pH and to detect the presence of blood, albumin, and glucose. The measurement of urinary metabolites can be used as an indicator of nutritional status. The hydroxyproline index (concentration of urinary hydroxyproline and creatinine per kilogram of body weight) is related to the amount of growth. Urinary n-methylnicotinamide has been used to evaluate niacin status, but it has not proved satisfactory. Levels of urinary 4-pyridoxic acid are used to ascertain vitamin B_6 nutriture.

The extractable protein in hair roots has been used to measure tissue protein stores.[16] Chemical analysis of hair for mineral content such as zinc also provides useful information.

Saturation and load tests can be used to determine the status of certain nutrients. An excess of a nutrient is administered to an individual, and then the amount excreted in the urine is measured. A subject whose tissues are saturated will excrete large amounts in the urine, whereas the deleted individual will retain most of the dose. A tryptophan load test is used to detect vitamin B_6 deficiency. In folate deficiency when a histidine load is given, increased amounts of formiminoglutamic acid (FIGLU) appear in the urine.

Dietary analysis

One method employed for dietary analysis is the 24-hour recall. The subject recalls all the food eaten for the past day. Food models, measuring devices, and pictures may be used as aids. This is the easiest way to collect data, but the results are qualitative rather than quantitative. A food record can be kept usually for 3 to 7 days. The individual is asked to keep a day-by-day record of all the food he consumes. The accuracy is dependent on the ability of the subject to record the food eaten in correct amounts.

The diet history is utilized to gain information about food habits and practices over a longer period of time. The subject is interviewed about past practices regarding the number of meals eaten, food likes, dislikes, allergies, and typical meal patterns according to the four food groups. A 24-hour recall is also taken, and it then can be ascertained whether this is a normal intake.

The most accurate data are obtained by a weighed intake. The food is weighed before serving and after the meal so that the waste is recorded. Samples of food may be taken for laboratory analysis of the nutrient content. However, this method is time-consuming and expensive.

Dietary data may be analyzed in several different ways. The most rapid analysis is a scoring system based on the amounts of the four food groups. This system can be used by the lay person to evaluate dietary intake. Food composition tables such as the United States Department of Agriculture Handbook No. 456[17] and Home and Garden Bulletin No. 72, Nutritive Value of Foods,[18] are used to calculate the nutrient content of the diet. The information in Handbook No. 456 and the Home and Garden Bulletin are available on punched cards or magnetic tape for computer analysis. Additional publications are available or in preparation that include additional nutrient and food data.[19] The Nutrient Data Research Center is in the process of developing a nutrient data bank. Current food composition data will be supplemented by additional research and information from the food industry as to the composition of its products. Data on variety, breed, stage of maturity, season pro-

Table 1-2. Dietary standards used by the U.S. Public Health Service in evaluating dietary intake in the National Nutritional Survey, 1970

Age	Energy (kcal/kg)	Protein (g/kg)	Cal-cium (mg)	Iron (mg)	Thiamine	Riboflavin	Vitamin A (IU)	Ascorbic acid (mg)
6-7 years	82	1.3	450	10	0.4 mg/1000 kcal	0.55 mg/1000 kcal	2500	30
10-12 years								
Male	68	1.2	650	10	0.4 mg/1000 kcal	0.55 mg/1000 kcal	2500	30
Female	64	1.2	650	18	0.4 mg/1000 kcal	0.55 mg/1000 kcal	2500	30
17-19 years								
Male	44	1.1	550	18	0.4 mg/1000 kcal	0.55 mg/1000 kcal	3500	30
Female	35	1.1	550	18	0.4 mg/1000 kcal	0.55 mg/1000 kcal	3500	30
Adults								
Male	38	1.0	400	10	0.4 mg/1000 kcal	0.55 mg/1000 kcal	3500	30
Female	38	1.0		18	0.4 mg/1000 kcal	0.55 mg/1000 kcal		
Pregnant	+200	+20	800	18	0.4 mg/1000 kcal	0.55 mg/1000 kcal	3500	30
Lactating	+1000	+25	900	18	0.4 mg/1000 kcal	0.55 mg/1000 kcal	4500	30

Table 1-3. Standards for evaluation of daily dietary intake used in the Health and Nutrition Examination Survey (HANES), United States, 1971-1974

Age and sex	Calories (per kg)	Protein (g/kg)	Calcium (mg)	Iron (mg)	Vitamin A* (IU)	Vitamin C (mg)
1-5 years						
12-23 months, male and female	90	1.9	450	15	2000	40
24-47 months, male and female	86	1.7	450	15	2000	40
48-71 months, male and female	82	1.5	450	10	2000	40
6-7 years, male and female	82	1.3	450	10	2500	40
8-9 years, male and female	82	1.3	450	10	2500	40
10-12 years						
Male	68	1.2	650	10	2500	40
Female	64	1.2	650	18	2500	40
13-16 years						
Male	60	1.2	650	18	3500	50
Female	48	1.2	650	18	3500	50
17-19 years						
Male	44	1.1	550	18	3500	55
Female	35	1.1	550	18	3500	50
20-29 years						
Male	40	1.0	400	10	3500	60
Female	35	1.0	600	18	3500	55
30-39 years						
Male	38	1.0	400	10	3500	60
Female	33	1.0	600	18	3500	55
40-49 years						
Male	37	1.0	400	10	3500	60
Female	31	1.0	600	18	3500	55
50-54 years						
Male	36	1.0	400	10	3500	60
Female	30	1.0	600	18	3500	55
55-59 years						
Male	36	1.0	400	10	3500	60
Female	30	1.0	600	10	3500	55
60-69 years						
Male	34	1.0	400	10	3500	60
Female	29	1.0	600	10	3500	55
70 years and over						
Male	34	1.0	400	10	3500	60
Female	29	1.0	600	10	3500	55
Pregnancy (fifth month and beyond), add to basic standard	200	20	200		1000	5†
Lactating, add to basic standard	1000	25	500		1000	5

	B vitamins (mg/1000 kcal)		
All ages, male and female	Thiamine	Riboflavin	Niacin
	0.4	0.55	6.6

*Assumed 70% carotene, 30% retinol.
†For all pregnant women.

duced, geographic location, and method of processing will be included. The information will be available for use with a computer.

In the United States the recommended daily dietary allowances (RDA) as prepared by the Food and Nutrition Board, National Academy of Sciences-National Research Council Washington, D.C. (see Appendix A) are used to evaluate dietary data. However, the results must be interpreted carefully, since (except in the case of caloric intake) a safety factor has been added. If an individual's intake is less than the RDA, it does not necessarily indicate a deficiency state. The RDA were based on the average individual, so additional information must be collected to ascertain whether the individual is truly deficient. Different dietary standards were established by the United States Public Health Service for use in evaluating the dietary intake of the National Nutrition Survey of 1970 (Table 1-2). Similar standards are being used by the Health and Nutrition Examination Survey (HANES) that is now being conducted in the United States (Table 1-3).

NUTRITIONAL STATUS OF HOSPITALIZED PATIENTS

The assessment of nutritional status of hospitalized patients is not very detailed. For the most part a diet history, height, weight, and some biochemical analyses such as cell counts, hemoglobin, hematocrit and serum albumin are performed. However, in some instances some of these data are not collected.

Due to the high incidence of hospital malnutrition, much concern has recently been expressed about the initial nutritional assessment and monitoring of the patient during his hospital stay. The stress of disease and the reduced intake of protein and calories are the major factors contributing to the development of protein calorie malnutrition.[20] In this PCM state the calories must be provided by fat, skeletal muscle, and viscera of the body. Therefore to determine the degree of depletion of body fat and protein stores, the following measurements have been used: triceps skinfold, body fat; arm muscle circumference and the creatinine height index, skeletal protein; secretory proteins albumin and transferrin, visceral protein; and height/weight, total body status. The two types of malnutrition seen in hospitalized patients are similar to marasmus and kwashiorkor that have been described in children. In the cachectic adult with marasmus weight/height and triceps skinfold, arm muscle circumference and creatinine height index are depressed. The kwashiorkor-like syndrome is characterized by a decrease in serum transferrin and albumin and a depression of cellular immunity. Surgical patients commonly develop the kwashiorkor type of malnutrition, while marasmus is associated with illness.

After the initial nutritional assessment the patient's nutritional status should be monitored periodically. Four parameters have been found useful: percent weight loss, skin test responsiveness, nitrogen balance, and serum albumin and transferrin levels.[21] A weight loss greater than 10% is cause for concern, while a loss of 20% to 30% can be fatal. Nitrogen balance is measured by calculating the protein intake and measuring urinary urea nitrogen. The procedures for nutritional assessment are described in detail in a manual prepared by Blackburn and his co-workers.[21]

Young and Hill studied surgical patients in an attempt to determine methods that could be used to assess marginal PCM.[22] The parameters measured were transferrin, prealbumin, albumin, retinol binding protein, complement C3, ceruloplasmin, weight loss, arm muscle circumference, hemoglobin, and total lymphocytes. Nineteen normal subjects and 54 surgical patients were studied prior to 1 week, less than 1 week, and more than 1 week after surgery. Preoperatively all values were normal except those for prealbumin, retinol binding protein, and arm muscle circumference. After surgery there was a decrease in the anthropometric measures, hemoglobin, total lymphocytes, and in all plasma proteins except ceruloplasmin and complement C3. On the basis of this study the indices found to be most useful in assessing PCM in surgical patients were plasma prealbumin, transferrin, arm muscle circumference, percentage weight loss, and hemoglobin.

Recent surveys have shown that 25% of hospitalized patients are malnourished and that 10% develop additional complications due to PCM.[23] Medical audits have revealed that height, weight, serum albumin, iron binding capacity, and total lymphocyte counts are not routinely measured. Malnutrition generally contributes to a longer hospital stay and more complications for the patient. New techniques such as total parenteral nutrition, defined-formula diet, and protein-sparing therapy are available for the nutritional support of the patient.[20] Thus to provide the best optimal nutritional care for the patient, a nutritional assessment should be performed, and the appropriate nutritional support should then be prescribed. Adequate nutritional care can help to contribute toward lowering increasing medical costs.

DIETARY GOALS FOR THE UNITED STATES

The Senate Select Committee on Nutrition and Human Needs published the Dietary Goals for the United States in 1977.[24] Information presented at the hearings indicated that the composition of the average diet has changed during the past 70 years. The consumption of fruit, vegetables, and grain products has decreased, while the consumption of fats and sugar has increased. It was stated that "The overconsumption of fat, generally, and saturated fat in particular, as well as cholesterol, sugar, salt and alcohol have been related to six of the 10 leading causes of death: heart disease, cancer, cerebrovascular disease, diabetes, arteriosclerosis and cirrhosis of the liver." The stated goals were as follows:

1. Increase carbohydrate consumption to account for 55% to 60% of the energy (caloric) intake.
2. Reduce overall fat consumption from approximately 40% to 30% of energy intake.
3. Reduce saturated fat consumption to account for about 10% of total energy intake and balance that with polyunsaturated and monounsaturated fats, which should account for about 10% of energy intake each.
4. Reduce cholesterol consumption to about 300 mg a day.
5. Reduce sugar consumption by about 40% to account for about 15% of total energy intake.

6. Reduce salt consumption by about 50% to 85% to approximately 3 g a day.

After the release of the first edition of the dietary goals, eight more hearings were held, and then the second edition of the dietary goals was published:[25]

1. To avoid overweight, consume only as much energy (calories) as is expended; if overweight, decrease energy intake and increase energy expenditure.
2. Increase the consumption of complex carbohydrates and "naturally occurring" sugars from about 28% of energy intake to about 48% of energy intake.
3. Reduce the consumption of refined and processed sugars by about 45% to account for about 10% of total energy intake.
4. Reduce overall fat consumption from approximately 40% to about 30% of energy intake.
5. Reduce saturated fat consumption to account for about 10% of total energy intake and balance that with polyunsaturated and monounsaturated fats, which should account for about 10% of energy intake each.
6. Reduce cholesterol consumption to about 300 mg a day.
7. Limit the intake of sodium by reducing the intake of salt to about 5 g a day.

To implement these goals the committee made the following suggestions for changes in food selection and preparation:

1. Increase consumption of fruits and vegetables and whole grains.
2. Decrease consumption of refined and other processed sugars and foods high in such sugars.
3. Decrease consumption of foods high in total fat and partially replace saturated fats, whether obtained from animal or vegetable sources, with polyunsaturated fats.
4. Decrease consumption of animal fat and choose meats, poultry, and fish that will reduce saturated fat intake.
5. Except for young children, substitute low-fat and nonfat milk for whole milk and low-fat dairy products for high-fat dairy products.
6. Decrease consumption of butterfat, eggs, and other high cholesterol sources. Some consideration should be given to easing the cholesterol goal for premenopausal women, young children, and the elderly in order to obtain the nutritional benefits of eggs in the diet.
7. Decrease consumption of salt and foods high in salt content.

Fig. 1-1 compares the caloric distribution of the current diet versus the diet proposed by the goals.

The committee stated that it is not known whether the suggested dietary changes can reduce the leading causes of death, but the goals do increase the probability of protection. The publication of the dietary goals resulted in much controversy. Some researchers supported the goals; others made additional recommendations; and other investigators stated that at the present time there is insufficient evidence to support these changes.[26-35]

Peterkin, Shore, and Kerr of the U.S. Department of Agriculture have translated the goals into diets that also meet the Recommended Daily Dietary Allowances.[36,37]

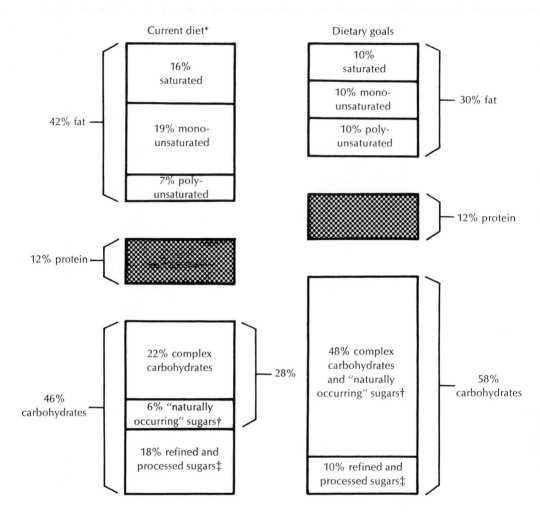

*These percentages are based on calories from food and nonalcoholic beverages. Alcohol adds approximately another 210 calories per day to the average diet of drinking-age Americans.

†"Naturally occurring": Sugars that are indigenous to a food, as opposed to refined (cane and beet) and processed (corn sugar, syrups, molasses, and honey) sugars, that may be added to a food product.

‡In many ways alcoholic beverages affect the diet in the same way as refined and other processed sugars. Both add calories (energy) to the total diet but contribute little or no vitamins or minerals.

Fig. 1-1. Caloric distribution of the current diet and of the dietary goals. Sources for current diet: Friend, B.: Changes in nutrients in the U.S. diet caused by alterations in food intake patterns, Washington, D.C., 1974, Agricultural Research Service, U.S. Department of Agriculture. Proportions of saturated versus unsaturated fats based on unpublished Agricultural Research Service data. (From Select Committee on Nutrition and Human Needs: U.S. Senate dietary goals for the United States, ed. 2, Washington, D.C., Dec., 1977, U.S. Government Printing Office.)

The changes needed to meet the goals are an increase of grain products, vegetables, fruits, legumes, nuts, and milk and a decrease in fats, oils, meat, poultry, fish, eggs, refined sugars, and sweets. Much research is still needed on human nutritional requirements, food composition, and dietary and nutritional status of the United States population. In addition, food production and processing methods need to be altered to provide foods suggested by the goals. A massive nutrition education program is needed to enable the public to choose diets that meet the dietary goals.

REFERENCES

1. Roe, D. A.: Nutritional side effects of drugs, Food Nutr. News **45(1)**:1, 1973.
2. Robinson, C. H.: Updating clinical dietetics: terminology, J. Am. Diet. Assoc. **62**:645, 1973.
3. Cummings, J. H.: Dietary fiber, Gut **14**:69, 1973.
4. Turner, D.: Handbook of diet therapy, Chicago, 1970, The University of Chicago Press.
5. De St. Jeor, S. T., and Bryan, G. T.: Clinical research diets: definition of terms, J. Am. Diet. Assoc. **62**:47, 1973.
6. Bollet, A. J., and Owens, S.: Evaluation of nutritional status of selected hospitalized patients, Am. J. Clin. Nutr. **26**:931, 1973.
7. Bistrian, B. R., et al.: Protein status of general surgical patients, J.A.M.A. **230**:858, 1974.
8. Blackburn, G. L., and Bistrian, B.: A report from Boston, Nutr. Today **9(3)**:30, 1974.
9. Bistrian, B. R., et al.: Prevalence of malnutrition in general medical patients, J.A.M.A. **235**:1567, 1976.
10. Butterworth, C. E., Jr.: The skeleton in the hospital closet, Nutr. Today **9(2)**:4, 1974.
11. Tobias, A. L., and Van Itallie, T. B.: Nutritional problems of hospitalized patients, J. Am. Diet. Assoc. **71**:253, 1977.
12. Weinsier, R. L., et al.: Hospital malnutrition: a prospective evaluation of general medical patients during the course of hospitalization, Am. J. Clin. Nutr. **32**:418, 1979.
13. Meiling, R. L.: The institutional system, Nutr. Today **9(4)**:34, 1974.
14. Enloe, C. F., Jr.: "Dietitians' lib" (editorial), Nutr. Today **9(3)**:14, 1974.
15. Sandstead, H. H., and Pearson, W. N.: Clinical evaluation of nutritional status. In Goodhart, R. S., and Shils, M. E., editors: Modern nutrition in health and disease, ed. 5, Philadelphia, 1973, Lea & Febiger.
16. Crounse, R. G., Bollet, A. J., and Owens, S. L.: Tissue assay of human protein malnutrition using scalp hair roots, Trans. Assoc. Am. Physicians **83**:185, 1970.
17. Adams, C. F.: Nutritive value of American foods in common units, U.S. Department of Agriculture, Handbook No. 456, 1975.
18. Consumer and Food Economics Research Division: Nutritive value of foods, U.S. Department of Agriculture Home and Garden Bulletin 72, revised 1970, slightly revised 1971.
19. Murphy, E. W., Watt, B. K., and Rizek, R. L.: Tables of food composition: availability, uses, and limitations, Food Tech. **27**:40, 1973.
20. Bistrian, B. R.: Nutritional assessment and therapy of protein-calorie malnutrition in the hospital, J. Am. Diet. Assoc. **71**:393, 1977.
21. Blackburn, G. L., et al.: Manual for nutritional metabolic assessment of the hospitalized patient, Boston New England Deaconess Hospital, Harvard Medical School, 1976.
22. Young, G. A., and Hill, G. L.: Assessment of protein-calorie malnutrition in surgical patients from plasma proteins and anthropometric measurements, Am. J. Clin. Nutr. **31**:429, 1978.
23. Blackburn, G. L.: Hospital malnutrition—a diagnostic challenge, Arch. Intern. Med. **139**:278, 1978.
24. Select Committee on Nutrition and Human Needs, U.S. Senate: Dietary goals for the United States, Washington, D.C., Feb. 1977, U.S. Government Printing Office.
25. Select Committee on Nutrition and Human Needs, U.S. Senate: Dietary goals for the United States, ed. 2, Washington, D.C., Dec. 1977, U.S. Government Printing Office.
26. Twenty commentaries: The McGovern dietary goals for the U.S. are examined by 20 correspondents, Nutr. Today **12(6)**:11, 1977.
27. Statement of American Medical Association to Select Committee on Nutrition and Human Needs, U.S. Senate: Dietary goals for the

United States, Supplementary News, Washington, D.C., April 1977, U.S. Government Printing Office.

28. Harper, A. E.: Dietary goals—a skeptical view, Am. J. Clin. Nutr. **31:**310, 1978.

29. Harper, A. E.: What are appropriate dietary guidelines? Food Technology **32:**48, 1978.

30. Hegsted, D. M.: Dietary goals—a progressive view, Am. J. Clin. Nutr. **31:**1504, 1978.

31. McNutt, K. W.: An analysis of dietary goals for the United States, ed. 2, J. Nutr. Ed. **10:**61, 1978.

32. Dietary goals: A statement by the American Dietetic Association, J. Am. Diet. Assoc. **71:**227, 1977.

33. Dietary goals for the United States, ed. 2—a reaction statement by the American Dietetic Association, J. Am. Diet. Assoc. **74:**529, 1979.

34. Simopoulos, A. P.: The scientific basis of the "goals": What can be done now? J. Am. Diet. Assoc. **74:**539, 1979.

35. Olson, R. E.: Are professionals jumping the gun in the fight against chronic diseases? J. Am. Diet. Assoc. **74:**543, 1979.

36. Peterkin, B. B., Kerr, R. L., and Shore, C. J.: Diets that meet the dietary goals, J. Nutr. Ed. **10:**15, 1978.

37. Peterkin, B. B., Shore, C. J., and Kerr, R. L.: Some diets that meet the dietary goals, J. Am. Diet. Assoc. **74:**423, 1979.

2 Laboratory diagnosis

Much information can be ascertained about the state of the body by the analysis of body fluids such as blood and urine. Certain disease states produce alterations in levels of one or more normal constituents. In addition, in some pathological conditions certain abnormal substances appear in the urine. Recently the measurement of serum enzyme levels has proved to be a valuable diagnostic aid. An analysis of blood or urine samples thus is useful both in a diagnosis of disease and for following the progress of the disorder.

Normal blood and urine values can be found in Appendixes F and G. Specific diagnostic tests that are used to detect a disorder of a certain organ, for example, kidney disease, are discussed in the chapter pertaining to that organ.

URINALYSIS[1-6]
Physical properties

Volume. For some determinations a casual urine sample may be collected. In determining the amount of certain vitamins excreted in the urine, the values are reported per gram of creatine. Since urinary creatinine excretion is relatively constant in adults, comparisons can be made regardless of the amount of sample collected. In other instances it is necessary to collect a 24-hour specimen since the constituents vary throughout the day. The volume of urine may also be indicative of disease. The normal adult puts out from 600 to 2500 ml per day but a large intake of fluid, coffee, or alcohol can result in an increased excretion. In disease states such as diabetes mellitus, diabetes insipidus, and nephritis, large volumes are voided. During the later stages of kidney failure there is a decrease in urine volume (oliguria) followed by no output of urine (anuria). Dehydration, fever, or heart failure may also contribute to oliguria.

Color. The amber yellow color of urine is caused by a mixture of pigments. The main pigment is urochrome, which is composed of urobilin or urobilinogen and a peptide. The color may be changed because of the excretion of large amounts of coproporphyrin and uroporphyrin or by hemoglobin, urobilin, bile pigments, and melanins. In alkaptonuria, an inborn error of metabolism, homogentisic acid is excreted. On standing, this compound is oxidized to a black pigment.

pH. The pH of urine ranges from 5 to 8, but it is generally slightly acidic with an average pH of 6. The pH is dependent on the time of sampling and the food that is ingested. Immediately after a meal the urine becomes alkaline. Because of the large amount of hydrogen ions secreted in gastric juice the kidney excretes alkaline ions to prevent the pH of the blood from increasing. The urine also becomes alkaline when a large quantity of fruits and vegetables is consumed. Acidic urine results from the ingestion of proteins. The sulfur-containing amino acids give rise to sulfuric acid, while the phosphoproteins, phospholipids, and nucleic acids contribute phosphate groups, which are converted to phosphoric acid.

Specific gravity. The specific gravity of the urine falls between 1.008 to 1.030. In the normal individual it varies throughout the day. A constant specific gravity is an indication of abnormal kidney function. The kidneys are able to adjust to variations in the intake of food and fluids by either increasing or decreasing the output of urine. In renal disease this is no longer possible, and thus the concentration of substances in the urine remains relatively constant. This is the basis for the Mosenthal test in which urine is collected every 2 hours from an individual on a fixed intake of food and water. In the absence of disease there are fluctuations in the specific gravity. However, other conditions can also alter the specific gravity of urine. Low values are found in diabetes insipidus. High values are found in fevers because of the decrease in volume excreted and in diabetes mellitus as a result of the presence of large amounts of glucose.

Microscopic examination. A microscopic examination of urine may reveal the presence of crystals of the following: ammonium or magnesium phosphate, calcium oxalate, calcium phosphate, calcium carbonate, uric acid, sodium urate, ammonium urate, hippuric acid, cystine, leucine, or tyrosine. In pathological conditions pus and protein are excreted and indicate the presence of inflammation in the genitourinary tract. Casts denote the presence of renal disease.

Normal constituents

The major components of urine can be divided into three categories, namely, water, inorganic salts, and organic compounds. The major inorganic ions excreted are the cations—sodium, potassium, calcium, magnesium, and ammonium—and the anions—chloride, phosphate, and sulfate. The nitrogenous organic compounds excreted in the urine are the waste products of metabolism such as urea, uric acid and other purines, creatinine, creatine, hippuric acid, indican, and peptides. The nonnitrogenous organic substances found are glucuronic acid, cholesterol, ketone bodies, oxalate, and salts of other organic acids. Water-soluble vitamins and their metabolites may be excreted in the urine. The amount is dependent on how much of the vitamin was consumed.

Abnormal constituents

Amylase. Amylase, which is synthesized by the salivary glands and pancreas, is secreted in the urine during acute pancreatitis, obstruction of the pancreatic duct, mumps, diabetic acidosis, and when the pancreas is inflamed as a result of a perforating ulcer. In renal insufficiency, serum levels are elevated but urinary excretion may not be increased. Urinary amylase levels are used to follow the recovery from pancreatic disease since urinary levels remain elevated for up to 7 days after blood amylase levels return to normal.

Glucosuria. When the renal threshold of 180 mg/dl of blood for glucose is exceeded, it is excreted in the urine. This occurs in diabetes mellitus, hyperthyroidism, hyperadrenalism, hyperpituitarism, asphyxia, and acidosis. It most commonly occurs in diabetes mellitus. Glucose can be tested by using Benedict's reagent, which is positive for reducing sugars, or by test-paper strips impregnated with glucose oxidase. The latter test is specific for glucose.

Pentosuria. A temporary excretion of pentoses in the urine can occur after the ingestion of large amounts of fruit and fruit juices. The chronic excretion of *l*-xylulose occurs in the inborn error of metabolism known as pentosuria. It is caused by the lack of the enzyme *l*-xylulose dehydrogenase. The individual suffers no apparent ill effects.

Galactosuria. Galactose appears in the urine of infants with galactosemia, an inborn error of metabolism and also in individuals with hepatic disease.

Fructosuria. Fructose may be excreted in the urine of severe diabetics. In the inborn error of metabolism called essential fructosuria or levulosuria a lack of the enzyme fructokinase or fructose-1-phosphate aldolase results in the excretion of fructose. No other symptoms appear.

Lactosuria. Lactose appears frequently in the urine of lactating women.

Lipuria. Lipuria appears after the ingestion of large amounts of fat, in lipemia associated with diabetes mellitus and lipoid nephrosis, fractures of the long bone, injuries to subcutaneous layers of fat, pyelitis, pyonephrosis, and in alcohol and phosphorus poisoning. After the urine is allowed to stand, a creamy layer appears on top.

Chyluria. The urine appears milky because of the presence of chyle. This is the fluid taken up in the lacteals in the small intestine and consists of emulsified fat and lymph. Chyluria occurs when there is an obstruction to the thoracic duct. The lymph vessels in the urinary tract rupture as a result of this blockage, and lymph is voided with urine.

Ketonuria. The ketone bodies—acetone, acetoacetic acid, and β-hydroxybutyric acid—are excreted in the urine when the renal threshold is exceeded. This occurs in the acidosis of diabetes mellitus, starvation, pregnancy, alkalosis, and after ether anesthesia.

Bile. If the bile duct is obstructed, bile pigments and salts enter the bloodstream and appear in the urine. The bile pigments can be measured. In obstructive jaundice, large amounts of bilirubin diglucuronide are present, while none is found with hemolytic and toxic jaundice. Urobilinogen appears in the urine in hemolytic and toxic jaundice but not in obstructive jaundice.

Proteinuria. Urinary protein can be found in cardiac disease, abdominal tumors, accumulation of abdominal fluid, fever, convulsions, anemia, diseases of the liver, collagen disease, and inflammatory disease. Proteinuria occurs in kidney diseases such as acute glomerulonephritis, nephrosclerosis, nephrosis, and sometimes in tuberculosis and carcinoma of the kidney. Bence Jones protein is excreted in the urine of individuals with multiple myeloma, diseases of the bone marrow, and occasionally in leukemia.

Aminoaciduria. Aminoaciduria is commonly found in many of the inborn errors of metabolism.

Hematuria. Blood may be voided in the urine because of neoplasms of the kidney or urinary tract, injury to the kidney, infections of the urinary tract, ingestion of drugs such as salicylates, barbiturates, and anticoagulants, allergic reactions, or low prothrombin levels.

Urinary calculi. Substances that are not very soluble in urine may precipitate out and form stones. (See Chapter 6, Renal Disease.)

Inborn errors of metabolism. Various metabolites are found in the urine of individuals with an inborn error of metabolism. (See Chapter 10, Inborn Errors of Metabolism.)

5-Hydroxyindoleacetic acid (5-HIAA). Argentaffinomas (carcinoid tumors) cause the excretion of elevated levels of 5-HIAA, a metabolite of serotonin in the urine. These tumors appear in the intestinal tract. For 72 hours before the collection of urine, foods that contain serotonin, such as walnuts, bananas, and avocados, should not be consumed.

Vanillylmandelic acid (VMA). Urinary levels of catecholamines and VMA increase in pheochromocytoma. This disease is caused by a tumor most often in the medulla of the adrenal glands and infrequently along the sympathetic nervous system. As a result, norepinephrine or epinephrine is released into the circulation and causes hypertension. Previously, for 2 days prior to the test and during the collection of the urine sample, aspirin, coffee, tea, caffeine-containing beverages, fruit, fruit juices, nuts, chocolate, foods containing vanilla, and jellies and jams had to be avoided. However, this dietary restriction no longer is followed since newer test methods have eliminated the dietary and drug interference.

BLOOD[1-6]

The total volume of blood in a human is approximately 8% of body weight or 5 to 6 liters. The fluid remaining after the cellular elements have been removed from blood is called plasma. Serum is obtained by clotting the blood before the removal of cells; therefore the serum does not contain the protein fibrinogen. The pH of the blood is between 7.35 and 7.45. The buffer systems—carbonate, bicarbonate, sodium dihydrogen phosphate, disodium hydrogen phosphate, and protein—help to maintain the pH within this narrow range.

The blood performs a variety of functions. Nutrients absorbed after digestion are transported to the cells, and the waste products of metabolism such as urea and uric acid are brought to the kidney for excretion. Substances synthesized by the cells, such as hormones, are carried by the circulation to the site where they function. Oxygen and carbon dioxide are continually carried back and forth between the tissues and the lungs. Antibodies in the bloodstream protect the body from microorganisms. Heat regulation is a function of blood as is the maintenance of acid-base, electrolyte, and water balance. In the event of a severing of a blood vessel, excessive hemorrhaging is prevented by means of coagulation.

Either an increase or decrease in the cellular elements or constituents of the blood can be indicative of disease. Blood analysis is useful not only for diagnosis but also in following the course of a disease.

The blood tests are run in the laboratory according to standardized procedures. However, the instrument SMA-20 (Sequential Multiple Autoanalyzer, Technicon

Table 2-1. Normal values for blood analysis from the SMA-20*

Blood constituent	Normal range of values
Glucose	70-110 mg/dl
BUN	7-22 mg/dl
Creatinine	0.6-1.4 mg/dl
Sodium	135-145 mEq/L
Potassium	3.5-5.0 mEq/L
Chloride	100-110 mEq/L
Carbon dioxide	23-32 mEq/L
Uric acid	
Male	4.3-8.5 mg/dl
Female	2.8-6.8 mg/dl
Calcium	8.5-10.5 mg/dl
Phosphorus	2.6-4.2 mg/dl
Total protein	6.0-7.8 g/dl
Albumin	3.8-5.0 g/dl
Cholesterol	
>40 years	140-300 mg/dl
<40 years	120-260 mg/dl
Triglyceride	
>50 years	0-190 mg/dl
<50 years	0-150 mg/dl
Total bilirubin	0-1.4 mg/dl
Direct bilirubin	0-0.2 mg/dl
Serum glutamic oxaloacetic transaminase	0-41 U/L
Lactic dehydrogenase	100-225 U/L
Creatine phosphokinase	0-200 U/L
Aklaline phosphatase	20-90 U/L
Calculated Values	
BUN/creatinine	
Albumin/globulin	
Ion Balance (Na + K) − (Cl + CO_2)	

*Technicon Instruments Corporation, Tarrytown, N.Y.

Instruments Corporation, Tarrytown, New York) is able to analyze 2 ml of serum for 20 parameters. As many as 120 samples can be run per hour. The printout also includes the normal accepted ranges for each constituent. These values are shown in Table 2-1.

Hematology

Erythrocytes (RBC)—4.2 to 5.9 million/mm³. A decrease in the number of red blood cells is seen in anemia, hemorrhage, and chronic infectious diseases. Elevated levels are seen in dehydration and polycythemia.

Leukocytes (WBC)—4800 to 10,800/mm³. The number of white blood cells is decreased in leukopenia and elevated in acute infections and leukemias.

Hemoglobin (Hb)—males, 13 to 16 g/dl; females, 12 to 15 g/dl. Low levels of hemoglobin may occur in iron deficiency anemia, protein deficiency, or during excessive hemorrhaging. Elevated levels are seen in polycythemia and dehydration.

Hematocrit (packed cell volume—PCV)—males, 42% to 50%; females, 40% to 48%. The hematocrit is the percentage volume of packed red blood cells in whole blood. Low values are indicative of anemias resulting from inadequate dietary intake of iron. The PCV is elevated in polycythemia.

Mean corpuscular volume (MCV)—80 to 94 μm³

$$\text{MCV} = \frac{\text{PCV}}{\text{Number of RBC (in millions)}} \times 10$$

The MCV is the average volume of the erythrocytes expressed in cubic micrometers. In microcytic anemias the MCV is less than 80 μm³, whereas in macrocytic anemias it is greater than 94 μm³.

Mean corpuscular hemoglobin (MCH)—27 to 32 pg

$$\text{MCH} = \frac{\text{Hb}}{\text{Number of RBC (in millions)}} \times 10$$

The MCH is the weight of hemoglobin in the average erythrocyte expressed as picograms of hemoglobin.

Mean corpuscular hemoglobin concentration (MCHC)—33% to 38%

$$\text{MCHC} = \frac{\text{Hb}}{\text{PCV}} \times 100$$

The MCHC is the concentration of hemoglobin per unit volume of erythrocytes expressed as a percentage. In hemoglobin deficiency or hypochromic anemia the MCH is less than 27 and the MCHC is less than 32%. The MCH is greater than 32 and the MCHC is normal in cases of macrocytic anemia.

Blood constituents

Glucose (fasting)—70 to 100 mg/dl. A glucose tolerance test is indicated when the glucose value exceeds 120 mg/dl. Hyperglycemia can occur in diabetes mellitus, hypothyroidism, and hyperpituitarism (an adrenocortical hyperactivity). Hypoglycemia appears in hyperinsulinemia, hypopituitarism, adrenal and hepatic insufficiency, and tumors of the pancreas.

Ammonia—80 to 110 µg/dl. Ammonia is a product of amino acid metabolism and is also generated by intestinal bacteria. The liver converts ammonia to urea, which is then excreted by the kidneys; therefore in liver disease hyperammonemia results.

Blood urea nitrogen (BUN)—8 to 25 mg/dl. BUN levels vary directly with the amount of protein ingested in the diet. When the glomerular filtration rate of the kidney is diminished, BUN levels are increased. Impaired renal blood flow and gastrointestinal bleeding will increase the BUN. Low blood levels are found in hepatic failure, nephrosis, and cachexia. The term "serum urea nitrogen" (SUN) is used now.

Creatinine—0.7 to 1.5 mg/dl. Creatinine is filtered through the glomerulus and thus can be used to measure the renal filtration rate. However, early renal damage does not lead to elevated blood levels.

Albumin—4 to 5 g/dl. Albumin levels are elevated in dehydration and shock. Lower values are observed in malnutrition, malabsorptive syndromes, nephrosis, glomerulonephritis, hepatic insufficiency, and leukemia.

Globulin—2 to 3 g/dl. Increased globulin levels are seen in hepatic disease, infectious hepatitis, cirrhosis, hemochromatosis, and infectious diseases. In malnutrition, serum globulin levels are low.

Fibrinogen—0.15 to 0.35 g/dl. Fibrinogen is an inactive protein found in the circulation. During clotting it is converted to fibrin by the removal of a peptide. Glomerulonephritis, nephrosis, and infectious diseases elevate blood levels, whereas lower levels are found in hepatic insufficiency.

Uric acid—3 to 7 mg/dl. Uric acid is an end product of nucleic acid metabolism and is excreted via the kidneys. In gout an enzymatic defect leads to hyperuricemia and a deposition of uric acid in tissues. Elevated levels are also found in renal disease, toxemia of pregnancy, leukemia, polycythemia, and alcoholism. Hypouricemia occurs in acute hepatitis.

Bilirubin—direct (glucuronide), 0.4 mg/dl; indirect (unconjugated), 0.3 mg/dl. When erythrocytes are destroyed, hemoglobin is converted to bilirubin. In the liver it is conjugated with glucuronic acid and excreted in the bile. Elevated serum bilirubin occurs in liver disease, biliary obstruction, increased hemolysis, and in toxic reactions to drugs, chemicals, and toxins.

Cholesterol—150 to 280 mg/dl. Increased cholesterol levels are observed in lipid disorders, nephrotic syndrome, hypothyroidism, pancreatitis, diabetes mellitus, obstructive jaundice, pregnancy, chronic hepatitis, and biliary cirrhosis. Blood levels are depressed in acute hepatitis, Gaucher's disease, hyperthroidism, acute infections, anemia, and malnutrition.

Cholesterol esters—60 to 75% of total. Cholesterol is esterified with fatty acids in the intestinal mucosa and liver.

Triglycerides (fasting)—40 to 150 mg/dl. Increased triglyceride levels are found in coronary artery disease, diabetes mellitus, nephrotic syndrome, hypothyroidism, and hepatic disease.

Lipoproteins. The blood lipid profile can be determined by electrophoresis or ultracentrifugation. In electrophoresis an electric current is applied to a paper or agarose gel. Due to differences in the electrical charges of the protein moiety, the lipoproteins migrate at different rates. The alpha lipoproteins containing the most protein migrate the farthest distance from the origin followed by the prebeta and beta lipoproteins. The chylomicrons, with 1% to 2% protein, do not move very far from the origin.

Ultracentrifugation can also be used to separate the blood lipoproteins according to their densities. Chylomicrons are the least dense followed by the very-low-density (VLDL—prebeta), low-density (LDL—beta), and the high-density (HDL—alpha) lipoproteins.

The measurement of cholesterol levels and the blood lipid profile can be used to classify the various types of familial hyperlipoproteinemias. (See Chapter 8, Cardiovascular Disease.)

Ceruloplasmin—27 to 37 mg/dl; copper—100 to 200 µg/dl. A small amount of copper (5%) is loosely bound to the protein albumin. The remainder is found in ceruloplasmin. Elevated levels are found in pregnancy, hyperthyroidism, infections, acute leukemia, Hodgkin's disease, cirrhosis, and after the administration of oral contraceptives. In Wilson's disease a defect in copper metabolism leads to low blood levels of copper accompanied by increased urinary excretion.

Iodine—protein-bound iodine (PBI)— 4 to 8 µg/dl. The PBI is an indication of the amount of thyroid hormone bound to protein in the peripheral blood. It is elevated in hyperthyroidism, thyroiditis, hepatitis, pregnancy, and in individuals on estrogens or oral contraceptives. The PBI is decreased in hypothyroidism, chronic thyroiditis, nephrosis, chronic liver disease, and after the administration of androgens, anabolic steroids, and salicylates.

Iron—50 to 150 µg/dl. Iron concentration in the blood is regulated by absorption in the mucosal cells of the intestine. It can be stored in the intestine, liver, spleen, and bone marrow. Increased levels occur in hemochromatosis, hemosiderosis, hemolytic disease, pernicious anemia, and viral hepatitis. Inadequate dietary intakes of iron, nephrosis, renal disease, and active hematopoiesis lead to low blood levels.

Iron-binding capacity (IBC)—250 to 400 µg/dl. Iron is transported in the circulation bound to a globulin either as transferrin or siderophilin. Normally the transport protein carries only 30% to 40% of its capacity to bind with iron. The IBC is elevated when serum iron is low, in iron deficiency anemia, after blood loss, in hepatitis, in pregnancy, and in users of oral contraceptives. Low levels are found when serum iron is high, in hemochromatosis, hemosiderosis, hemolytic disease, pernicious anemia, cirrhosis, uremia, malignancy, and infections.

Bicarbonate—24 to 30 mEq/L. One of the buffer systems that maintain the normal pH of the blood is the carbonic acid–bicarbonate system. This test is used to measure the acid-base balance of the blood. Elevated values are seen in metabolic alkalosis, which can be a result of the ingestion of large amounts of sodium bicarbonate, excessive vomiting of gastric juice, or a potassium deficiency. Increased levels are also found in respiratory acidosis due to an inadequate removal of carbon dioxide in the lungs. This happens in pulmonary emphysema, heart failure with pulmonary involvement, and ventilatory failure caused by oversedation. Bicarbonate levels are decreased in metabolic acidosis, which can occur in diabetic ketosis, starvation, diarrhea of long duration, and renal insufficiency. This same situation exists in respiratory alkalosis caused by hyperventilation.

Calcium—8.5 to 10.5 mg/dl. Approximately half the calcium in the blood is ionized, and the remainder is bound to the protein albumin. An increase or decrease in serum protein is followed by either an increase or decrease in protein-bound calcium. Hypercalcemia is found in hyperparathyroidism, hypervitaminosis D, milk–alkali syndrome, bone disease, and following immobilization. Coma results if the values exceed 13 mg/dl. Hypocalcemia occurs in hypoparathyroidism, hypovitaminosis D, renal disease, hypoproteinemia, pancreatitis, and malabsorptive syndromes. Values below 7 mg/dl can be fatal.

Chloride—100 to 106 mEq/L. Chloride is the major anion found in extracellular fluid. It aids in the maintenance of acid-base balance. Alkalosis results from the loss of chloride, and acidosis is brought about by the retention of this ion. Elevated levels occur in dehydration, renal insufficiency, nephrosis, and renal tubular acidosis. Reduced values are observed in gastrointestinal disease with a loss of gastrointestinal fluid, renal insufficiency, emphysema, diabetic acidosis, excessive perspiration, adrenal insufficiency, hyperadrenocorticism, and metabolic acidosis.

Magnesium—1.5 to 2.5 mEq/L. Magnesium is found primarily inside the cell. Extracellularly it is involved in neuromuscular irritability and response. Low levels result in tetany, weakness, disorientation, and somnolence. This can be caused by chronic diarrhea, loss of intestinal fluid, starvation, hepatic insufficiency, chronic hepatitis, and alcoholism. Elevated levels may be caused by renal insufficiency or excessive administration of magnesium salts either intravenously or intramuscularly.

Phosphorus, inorganic—3 to 4.5 mg/dl. Phosphate levels are influenced by dietary intake, intestinal absorption, parathormone, renal function, and bone metabolism. Hyperphosphatemia occurs in hypoparathyroidism, hypervitaminosis D, and malabsorptive syndromes.

Potassium—3.5 to 5 mEq/L. Most of the potassium is found in the cell (90%), with 8% in bone and less than 1% in the circulation. Potassium ions are necessary for the maintenance of neuromuscular and muscular irritability. Changes in the concentration of this ion interfere with muscular contraction. Hyperkalemia appears in renal and adrenal insufficiency and untreated diabetes mellitus. After tissue damage such as occurs with surgery, accidents, or burns, potassium is released into the circulation. If renal failure also occurs, the ability to excrete potassium is diminished. Hypokalemia is the result of inadequate intake, malabsorption, or excessive losses through vomiting and diarrhea.

Sodium—135 to 145 mEq/L. Sodium is found extracellularly and is important in the maintenance of water balance. As sodium moves into the cell, the volume of extracellular fluid decreases. This disturbs the circulatory, renal, and and nervous systems. Hypernatremia occurs in dehydration, hyperadrenocorticism, uremia, and central nervous system disorders. Hyponatremia can result from a variety of conditions such as adrenal and renal insufficiency, trauma, burns, losses from the gastrointestinal tract, diarrhea, perspiration, untreated diabetes mellitus, and excessive use of diuretics.

Serum enzymes[6-9]

Enzymes are catalysts that are synthesized by cells specifically for the purpose of accelerating biologic reactions. They are found throughout the body and are present in all secretions except for bile and urine. Varying amounts of enzymes are found in organs such as the heart, liver, kidney, and brain, and muscle and bone. Some are found in high concentrations in a specific organ, while others may be absent. In

Table 2-2. Enzymes used in diagnosis

Class	Function	Enzymes

Transferase	Transfer of a group from one compound to another	Transaminases
		    Glutamic pyruvic
		    Glutamic oxaloacetic
		Kinases
		    Creatine phosphokinase

Oxidoreductase (dehydrogenase)	Removal or addition of hydrogen in oxidative processes	Lactic dehydrogenase α-Hydroxybutyric acid dehydrogenase Isocitric dehydrogenase Malic acid dehydrogenase
Hydrolase	Cleavage of a bond with the addition of water	Amylase Lipase Alkaline phosphatase Acid phosphatase 5'-Nucleotidase Leucine aminopeptidase
Lyase	Removal of a group without transfer to another compound	Aldolase
Isomerase	Conversion of compound from one structure to another intermolecular rearrangement	Phosphohexose isomerase
Ligase (synthetase)	Joining of two molecules with the breakdown of ATP	

healthy individuals blood enzyme levels are low; however, in certain diseases necrosis occurs in the organ, and the cellular enzymes are released into the blood.

The measurement of serum enzyme levels does not provide sufficient information to diagnose a disease, but the location and degree of disease can be ascertained. In some instances the measurement of enzyme levels is an aid in differential diagnosis. The course of a disease may be followed by monitoring enzyme levels.

There are thousands of enzymes in the human body. Enzymes are classified into six major categories—transferases, oxidoreductases, hydrolases, lyases, isomerases, and ligases (synthetases). Approximately 15 of these enzymes are being used for diagnostic purposes. These are illustrated in Table 2-2.

Some enzymes exist in multiple molecular forms called isoenzymes (isozymes). They catalyze the same reaction but have different physiochemical properties. As a result the isoenzymes can be separated by electrophoresis. One of the first enzymes to be studied was lactic dehydrogenase (LDH). Each isoenzyme is a tetramer made up of four polypeptide chains, of which two are different. The polypeptide isolated from heart muscle is designated as H, and the one from skeletal muscle is called M. Following are the five LDH isoenzymes:

LDH 1	H	H	H	H
LDH 2	H	H	H	M
LDH 3	H	H	M	M
LDH 4	H	M	M	M
LDH 5	M	M	M	M

In tissues concerned with aerobic metabolism (lactate → pyruvate) there are more H subunits, whereas in tissues involved in anaerobic metabolism (pyruvate → lactate) the M subunits predominate. LDH is widely distributed throughout the body tissues. The highest concentrations are found in the liver and skeletal muscle followed by the heart. Serum enzyme levels are low. After tissue injury the isoenzyme levels increase at different rates depending on where the damage occurred. For example, following a myocardial infarct there is a large increase in LDH 1 and a moderate increase in LDH 2 (Fig. 2-1). However, in liver damage LDH 5 increases dramatically (Fig. 2-1). Thus the electrophoretic pattern of the isoenzymes is a useful diagnostic aid.

Clinically the three isoenzymes of creatine phosphokinase-CPK have been used for diagnosis. The isoenzymes are dimers and exist in the muscle (MM-CPK 3), heart (MB-CPK 2), and the brain (BB-CPK 1). Serum levels will be elevated following injury to the muscle and heart but not the brain. A myocardial infarct will elevate CPK 2 serum levels, whereas skeletal muscle damage increases the CPK 3 isoenzyme.

The measurement of enzyme levels has been particularly useful in cases of myocardial infarction. In some instances the electrocardiogram will not indicate the presence of injured heart muscle, but serum enzyme levels will be elevated (Fig. 2-2). The patient's progress can also be followed by monitoring enzyme levels. Glu-

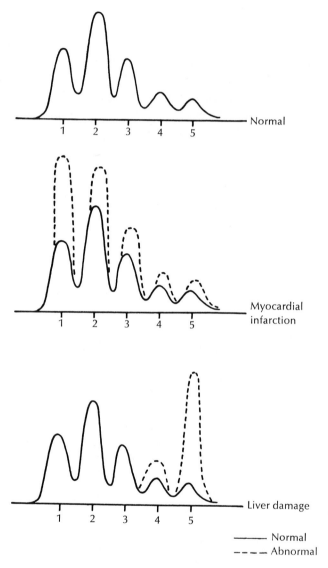

Fig. 2-1. LDH serum isoenzyme patterns.

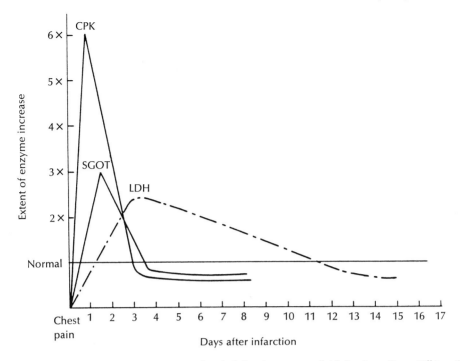

Fig. 2-2. Typical changes in serum enzyme levels following myocardial infarction. (From Tilkian, S. M., Conover, M. B., and Tilkian, A. G.: Clinical implications of laboratory tests, ed. 2, St. Louis, 1979, The C. V. Mosby Co., p. 81.)

tamic-oxaloacetic transaminase (GOT) is elevated within 6 to 8 hours of an attack and peaks at 24 hours. Normal levels are reached within 4 to 6 days. If there is a second infarction, GOT levels will remain elevated. This is useful because this would not be shown on an electrocardiogram. Creatine phosphokinase (CPK) levels are rapidly elevated within 3 to 4 hours and peak at 18 to 30 hours. The levels return to normal within 3 to 4 days. Lactic dehydrogenase (LDH) may be two to 10 times higher than normal, and peak values are attained within 2 to 3 days. The levels return to normal much more slowly, generally in 1 to 2 weeks. The enzyme α-hydroxybutyric acid dehydrogenase exhibits a pattern similar to that of LDH. The enzyme phosphohexose isomerase is elevated in 12 hours and remains high for 1 week. Thus these five enzymes provide useful information about a myocardial infarction.

There are many disorders that result in an elevation of serum enzymes. These are shown in Table 2-3.

• • •

The values for blood and urine constituents vary depending upon the laboratory performing the test and the method used. For additional blood and urine values see Appendixes F and G.

Table 2-3. Disorders in which serum enzymes are elevated

Enzyme	Origin	Reaction	Disorder
Aldolase	Muscle: skeletal, heart Liver RBC	Fructose 1,6 P→ Dihydroxyacetone P + Glyceraldehyde-3-P	Myocardial infarction Muscular dystrophies Hemolytic anemia Metastatic prostatic carcinoma Leukemia Acute pancreatitis Acute hepatitis

Amylase	Salivary glands
	Pancreas
		Starch → Dextrins →
		Maltose
			Acute pancreatitis
			Obstruction of pancreatic
			  duct
			Mumps
			Occasionally, renal
			  insufficiency; diabetic
			  acidosis
			Perforated peptic ulcer

Creatine phospho-kinase (CPK)	Muscle: skeletal, heart Brain	Creatine-P + ADP → Creatine + ATP	Skeletal muscle disease Myocardial infarction Cerebral infarction Hypothyroidism

CPK isozymes			Differentiate heart attack or
			  muscle fatigue
			Genetic counseling for
			  muscular dystrophy

Glutamic-oxaloacetic trans-aminase	Muscle: skeletal, heart Liver Kidney	Glutamate + Oxalo- acetate → α-Ketoglutarate + Aspartate	Myocardial infarction Hepatitis Infectious mononucleosis Cirrhosis Muscular dystrophy Obstructive jaundice
Glutamic-pyruvic trans-aminase	Liver	Glutamate + Pyruvate → α-Ketoglutarate + Alanine	Acute hepatic disease Infectious or toxic hepatitis Infectious mononucleosis Cirrhosis Obstructive jaundice Metastatic carcinoma
α-Hydroxy-butyric acid dehydro-genase	Heart	α-Ketobutyrate + NADH + H$^+$ → α-Hydroxybutyrate + NAD$^+$	Myocardial infarction Muscular dystrophy Megaloblastic anemia

Table 2-3. Disorders in which serum enzymes are elevated—cont'd

Enzyme	Origin	Reaction	Disorder
Isocitric dehy-drogenase	Liver Muscle: skeletal, heart	D-Isocitrate + NAD$^+$ → α-Ketoglutarate + CO_2 + NADH + H$^+$	Acute hepatitis Metastatic prostatic carcinoma Homologous serum jaundice Neoplastic disease with liver metastases Infectious mononucleosis
Leucine amino-peptidase	Pancreas Liver	Hydrolysis of peptides in which free amine group is leucine residue	Obstructive jaundice Carcinoma of pancreas Moderately elevated hepatic cirrhosis, cholecystitis, carcinomatic metastases of liver
Lactic acid dehydro-genase (LDH)	Heart Liver Kidney Muscle	Lactate + NAD$^+$ → Pyruvate + NADH + H$^+$	Hemolytic anemia B$_{12}$ + folate deficiency Polycythemia rubra vera Myocardial infarction Hepatitis Cirrhosis Metastatic involvement of liver Pulmonary embolism Muscular dystrophy Leukemia Destructive renal disease

LDH isozymes	Fast moving
	  Heart
	  RBC
	  Kidney cortex
	Slow moving
	  Liver
	  Skeletal muscle
			Myocardial infarction
			Renal cortex infarction
			Hemolytic anemia
			
			Acute hepatitis
			Acute muscle injury
			Muscular dystrophies
			Dermatomyositis

Lipase	Pancreas	Triglycerides → Fatty acids + Glycerol	Pancreatitis Obstruction of intestine and pancreatic duct Perforated ulcer Acute cholecystitis Bacterial peritonitis Opiates

Continued.

Table 2-3. Disorders in which serum enzymes are elevated—cont'd

Enzyme	Origin	Reaction	Disorder
5'-Nucleo-tidase	Liver	ATP → ADP + Pi	Infectious, infiltrative, nutritional, obstructive, and neoplastic liver disease
Phospho-hexose isomerase	Muscle: skeletal, heart Liver	Glucose-6-P → Fructose-6-P	Cirrhosis Obstructive jaundice Viral hepatitis Malignancy of liver, heart muscle, breast, and prostate gland
Phosphatase (acid)	Prostate Smaller amounts in Bone Liver Kidney RBC	Organic-P-ester + H_2O → Organic alcohol + H_3PO_4	Prostatic carcinoma Multiple myeloma Gaucher's disease Occasionally, leukemia
Phosphatase (alkaline)	Bone Liver Kidney Intestine Placenta	Organic-P-ester + H_2O → Organic alcohol + H_3PO_4	Obstructive and hepato-cellular liver disease Obstructive jaundice Biliary cirrhosis Cholangiolitic hepatitis Occlusion of hepatic duct Viral hepatitis Cirrhosis Infectious mononucleosis Osteoblastic bone disease Hyperparathyroidism Rickets Osteomalacia Neoplastic bone disease Ossification Paget's disease Pregnancy

INTERPRETATION OF LABORATORY TESTS

Young discussed some of the difficulties associated with the interpretation of clinical laboratory data.[10] Because of biological variability it is difficult to establish normal values for tests. The ideal situation would be to compare the individual's test values when he is ill to those obtained when he was healthy.

The major factors that influence laboratory data are defined as genetic, long-term physiological, short-term physiological, specimen collection and processing, and analytical procedures.[10] The major genetic influences are sex, race, and blood group.

The major sex difference can be attributed to the greater muscle mass of the male and the metabolic influence of the female sex hormones.

There are many long-term physiological influences, but age has the greatest effect. Some body constituents change dramatically with age. Body composition is important since obese persons have elevated levels of many blood constituents. An individual's dietary intake affects primarily the nitrogen and lipid components in the body. Other long-term influences on laboratory values are female sex hormones, pregnancy, physical fitness, smoking, and altitude.

An important short-term physiological effect from the standpoint of nutrition is the influence of meals. Some components can only be measured on fasting blood samples, otherwise the time of postprandial sampling would affect the value. Even the time of sampling has an effect because some constituents fluctuate normally throughout the day. In some instances blood values are affected by whether the individual is sitting or lying down. Physical activity and stress can also exert a short-term physiological influence on laboratory tests.

Samples must be carefully collected and processed. Some components are very unstable, and preservatives or freezing, or both, must be employed. Yet this procedure may inactivate enzymes if it is repeated. Certain substances, for example, drugs, may interfere with the analytical test procedure.

In some instances small changes from the normal blood ranges are not treated, yet they may be of significance. Test data may not be used to the greatest advantage. With the advent of a larger number of tests and wider usage the physician in the future may be assisted by computer technology.[10,11] Programs are now available that print out the values for the normal and abnormal test results of the patient. The diagnostic possibilities associated with each of the abnormal values are indicated. This should not only prove useful as a diagnostic aid but serve to inform the physician of the latest interpretation of clinical data.

REFERENCES

1. Normal laboratory values, N. Engl. J. Med. **302:**37, 1980.
2. Faulkner, W. R., and King, J. W.: Manual of clinical laboratory procedures, Cleveland, 1970, Chemical Rubber Co.
3. Holvey, D. N., and Talbott, J. H., editors: Merck manual of diagnosis and therapy, ed. 12, Rahway, N. J., 1972, Merck, Sharp & Dohme Research Laboratories.
4. Krupp, M. A., and Chatton, M. J.: Current diagnosis and treatment, Los Altos, Calif., 1973, Lange Medical Publications.
5. Wallach, J.: Interpretation of diagnostic tests, ed. 2, Boston, 1974, Little, Brown and Co.
6. Tilkian, S. M., and Conover, M. H.: Clinical implications of laboratory tests, ed. 2, St. Louis, 1979, The C. V. Mosby Co.
7. Blume, P., and Freier, E. F., editors: Enzymology in the practice of laboratory medicine, New York, 1974, Academic Press, Inc.
8. Wolf, P. L., Williams, D., and Vander-Muehill, E.: Practical clinical enzymology: techniques and interpretations and biochemical profiling, New York, 1973, John Wiley & Sons, Inc.
9. Manual of clinical enzyme measurements, Freehold, N. J., 1972, Worthington Biochemical Corp.
10. Young, D. S.: Interpretation of clinical laboratory data, Fed. Proc. **34:**2162, 1975.
11. Hobbie, R. K., and Reece, R. L.: Computer interpretation of laboratory test results, Fed. Proc. **34:**2152, 1975.

3 Obesity

The world now faces two extremes of malnutrition—deficiency and excess. The developing countries have the major problem of securing adequate food to combat energy, protein, vitamin, and mineral deficiencies. However, at the opposite extreme, the developed nations have an overabundance of food, and efforts are directed toward reducing dietary intakes. The labor-saving devices of modern technology have contributed to a more sedentary existence. Thus overabundance of food and decreased physical activity subject individuals to nutritional diseases resulting from excessive rather than deficient intakes. The direct effects are manifested as obesity, which predisposes the individual to other diseases such as diabetes mellitus and atherosclerosis.

OBESITY VS OVERWEIGHT

The terms "obesity" and "overweight" have been used interchangeably. This is incorrect. Overweight refers to a condition of overheaviness, and obesity is a result of an excessive amount of fat. Body weight is the sum total of a number of different body components. The most variation is seen in the amounts of fat, muscle, and bone. An individual may be overweight because of an excessive amount of bone, muscle, or even water. An athlete with a high degree of musculature would be considered overweight and not obese. On the other hand a person of average weight might be obese if his bone structure or musculature were small. An individual is considered obese only if there is an excess of adipose tissue.

Weight tables are most often used as a measure of obesity. There are two types of standards employed based either on average or desirable weight. However, these tables do not give any measure of the degree of fatness. The average weight tables are based on life insurance statistics of the general population. The general trend to an increase in weight with age is undesirable; therefore tables of desired weight were developed. The Metropolitan Life Insurance Company used the data from a build and blood pressure study.[1] The lightest and heaviest weights of 5% of men and women between the ages of 25 and 30 were omitted. The remaining weights were then divided into three categories: small, medium, and heavy frame, with ranges. No criteria were given to determine what frame the individual should be put into. Some researchers using these standards consider persons who are 10% above the desirable weight as obese. According to the U.S. Public Health Service 25% to 45% of Americans over 30 years of age are more than 20% above their desirable weight.[2]

METHODS OF ASSESSMENT

Joliffe suggested four practical methods to assess the degree of body fat.[3] The simplest way is to look at oneself nude in the mirror. The pinch test consists of picking up a fold of skin and subcutaneous fat. If the fold is greater than an inch the individual is obese. In the ruler test a ruler should lie flat between the pubic bone and the rib cage of a nonobese person who is lying down. In the girth test, which is used for males, the circumference at the waist should be equal to or less than the circumference of the chest at the nipple level in nonobese men.

More scientific methods have been devised for the measurement of body fat. The only direct method involves the measurement of the fat content of a cadaver. The percentage of fat is about 14% for males. Values above 25% of body weight for males and 30% for females are considered to be an indication of obesity.[4]

More indirect methods have been used. Densitometry measures the body weight in and out of water. Fat is the least dense and most variable component of the body. As the fat increases, the density decreases. The volume of the body can be determined by measurement under water with a correction for the gas in the body. Various isotope dilution techniques using tritiated water, ^{40}K, and ^{42}K can be employed to measure body water and cellular mass. From this information the amount of body fat can be calculated. A chemical method that utilizes cyclopropane has also been developed to measure body fat.

Subcutaneous fat can be measured by the use of x-ray film or anthropometric measurements. Muscle, bone, and adipose tissue show different densities on x-ray film. Soft tissue x-rays are used to measure fat pads. The most widely employed methods are anthropometric measurements of height, weight, and skinfold thickness. Half the body fat is found under the skin, and standardized calipers are available to measure this subcutaneous fat. The triceps and subscapular skinfolds are most frequently measured. The latter is more useful in women.

There are no good statistics as to the incidence of obesity in the United States. However, general observation would indicate that overnutrition is becoming an ever increasing problem. Excessive weight gain is associated with certain ages or physiological conditions. In women weight gain commonly occurs after growth at age 20, during pregnancy, and after menopause. Men tend to gain weight between the ages of 25 and 40 years, after which weight gain is accelerated.

COMPLICATIONS

Obesity not only shortens the life span but also increases the risk of developing other complications. Extremely obese individuals develop respiratory difficulties or, as it is commonly called, the Pickwickian syndrome. Such persons experience periods of somnolence and of turning blue. The fat deposited in the abdominal cavity pushes the diaphragm up, and breathing is inadequate, resulting in insufficient amounts of oxygen and an inability to get rid of excess carbon dioxide. The increased carbon dioxide content of the blood makes the individual sleepy. The insufficient supply of oxygen increases the production of erythrocytes, leading to polycythemia, manifested in a ruddy complexion. Thromboses and blood-clotting problems may also develop.

The excessive weight also increases the stress on the cardiovascular system. Difficulties have been encountered in measuring blood pressure in obese individuals.[5] Generally as weight increases, the blood pressure increases. Hypertension is found frequently in the obese. This presents a greater risk for developing coronary artery disease. Blood pressure is lowered by weight reduction. In some instances cardiac enlargement and congestive heart failure are the result of obesity.

Endocrine disorders also appear with obesity. Cortisol, growth hormone, and insulin are affected.[4] The urinary excretion of 17-hydroxycorticoids is increased and there is an increased production of cortisol by the adrenal glands in obese individuals. Excessive secretion of cortisol is also seen in Cushing's syndrome; however, this is caused by a tumor in the adrenal or pituitary gland, and obesity is seen only in the trunk with the extremities remaining thin. In obesity, growth hormone secretion is decreased. Maturity onset diabetes mellitus appears most often in obese individuals. Glucose tolerance is impaired even though the levels of insulin are high and respond to glucose. Insulin antagonism disappears after weight reduction. It has been shown that the changes in production of cortisol, growth hormone, and insulin are the result of the increase in weight, and thus these hormonal changes do not cause obesity but are the result of obesity.[4]

Pregnancy is also complicated by obesity. Toxemia occurs more frequently when weight gain is excessive.[6] Further difficulties arise during the delivery of the baby. Stillbirths are more frequent in obese women.

Surgery in the obese individual presents even a greater risk. If the surgery is elective, extreme weight reduction methods such as fasting are used prior to the operation. The surgical procedure takes longer when layers of fat must be dissected first, and anesthesia must be maintained for a longer of period of time. If cardiac arrest occurs, it is more difficult to massage the heart through the layers of fat. After surgery it is difficult to find a blood vessel either to start intravenous solutions or to remove a blood sample for a diagnostic procedure.

Psychological disturbances generally are the result of obesity rather than the cause. This must be taken into account when weight reduction is initiated. Thus in times of severe emotional stress, weight reduction is contraindicated. Mayer stated that obese children in psychological testing react as if they were members of a minority group undergoing persecution.[7] One study showed that obese girls have one third the chance of gaining admission to college that nonobese girls do.

Many other disease states are improved by the loss of weight. Obesity compounds the problems of arthritis, particularly in the weight-bearing joints. Hiatal hernia is also improved by a decrease in weight. The incidence of gallbladder disease is much higher in obese individuals, although there is no evidence that obesity is an etiologic factor.

ETIOLOGY

Despite all the research on obesity, the etiology is not completely understood. Since there are a variety of disturbances, the term "obesities" is used. Van Itallie and Campbell proposed three tentative groupings based on a mechanistic approach: regulatory, metabolic, and constitutional.[8] There is no metabolic defect in regulatory obesity. Overeating is the result of a psychological or physiological effect. Metabolic obesity can result from a loss of enzymatic, hormonal, or neurological control. Constitutional obesity is caused by an increased number of fat cells (hyperplasia).

Genetic factors

The role of genetic factors in obesity has been investigated. Most wild animals are not obese but some strains of mice have been found to have hereditary obesity. In humans many studies have shown that heredity plays a role in obesity. In families where both parents are of normal weight, less than 10% of their offspring will be obese. Yet if one parent is obese, 40% of their offspring will be obese, and this increases to 80% if both parents are obese.[9] Furthermore, the weight of adopted children bears little relationship to that of their adopted parents.[10] Identical twins who have been separated and raised in different homes have been found to have similar weights.[11]

Adipocytes

Fat can be stored in the body by increasing the number of fat cells (hyperplasia) or by increasing the size of the cells (hypertrophy). It has been shown that obese individuals have fat cells that are larger, and those who have been excessively obese since childhood have a larger number of fat cells.[4,12,13] Hirsch measured the amount of fat per adipocyte and found that it was 20% higher in obese persons.[7] In addition, individuals of normal weight had approximately 300 billion fat cells, whereas obese individuals had twice that amount. When the obese individual loses weight, the cell number is almost constant but the cells shrink in size. Obesity that appears early in life is primarily hyperplastic, whereas that which appears in adulthood is hypertrophic. The crucial periods of life that determine whether an individual will become obese are the last trimester of pregnancy, the first 3 years of life, and adolescence.

Traumatic factors

Obesity can be created in animals by traumatic factors. In animals physiological traumas resulting from hormonal imbalances result in obesity. Psychic trauma can be caused by punishing the animal. The result is overeating, leading to obesity. People also tend to overeat in times of trauma.

Environmental factors

Environmental factors play an important role in the etiology of obesity. The amount of physical activity has diminished greatly in our present society. Modern technology has turned us into largely a sedentary population. The most popular sports tend to be of the spectator type. Even some golfers ride across the course so as not to get too much exercise! In some locations the automobile reigns supreme, and there are no sidewalks to walk, only highways to ride.

Motion pictures of obese girls showed that they participated in physical activity but to a lesser degree.[14] If they were playing volleyball, they tended to stand around more than the nonobese girls, and if swimming, they spent more time floating. The theory that exercise increases the appetite and thus promotes weight gain has been disproved.

Dietary factors

Much research has centered on the mechanisms that regulate food intake. Animals and humans eat in response to hunger, a complex of unpleasant sensations that appears after deprivation. Appetite consists of more pleasant sensations that are associated with the desire for food. When hunger and appetite are satisfied the individual is satiated and stops eating. Anorexia is the absence of hunger.

The glucostatic theory for short-term regulation of daily food intake was proposed by Mayer.[15] Glucose-sensitive receptors are found in the ventromedial nucleus (satiety center) of the hypothalamus. When the glucose levels are high, the lateral nucleus (feeding center) is shut off; it is activated again when glucose levels are low. Insulin is needed for glucose utilization by the receptor cells. Therefore in diabetes mellitus, hyperglycemia does not affect the receptor cells. When gold thioglucose is injected into animals, the glucoreceptors are destroyed and the animals overeat and become obese.

The regulation of food intake in higher animals and humans is complex. Lepkovsky reviewed some of the newer concepts, for example, the set point in adipose tissues.[16] It has been suggested that the ventromedial nucleus of the hypothalamus controls the amount of adipose tissue by regulating the amount of ingested food. If a lesion develops in the ventromedial area, the control system of the adipose tissue is given a new set point. Since more fat is allowed in the depots, more food is ingested. It has also been suggested that there is feedback from the adipose tissue to the hypothalamus and this in turn regulates the absorption of food from the gastrointestinal tract. Hormonal control is also involved. In lower animals the hypothalamus regulates the intake of food to meet the physiological needs of the animal, but in man higher centers interfere. Habits, customs, prejudices, social pressures, and advertising override the basic hypothalamic response. Humans do not select food wisely and often reject nutritionally adequate diets. Sensory stimuli are important and contribute to the pleasure of eating. Other environmental cues are involved in eating, and obese individuals often react in the opposite manner to people of normal weight. Behavior modification theory attempts to alter the response to some of these cues.

Meal frequency. Leveille and Romsos have concluded that obesity is not caused by faulty metabolism but rather by the human behavior of eating three meals a day.[17] Wild animals are not beset by obesity, and it is only man and his pets who are committed to meal eating rather than nibbling. In one experiment rats were allowed access to food for only 2 hours a day. The control group received the same amount of food, but they were allowed to eat all day long. The rats who received one meal a day ate 15% less than the controls, but they gained as much as the controls. This has often been the contention of obese people that they do not overeat. Humans who eat frequently show less tendency to store calories.[18]

The size of the stomach and intestines increased in meal-fed rats.[17] Measurement of the respiratory quotient indicated that carbohydrate was being converted to fat during the absorptive stage and used as a metabolic energy source only in the postabsorptive state. Of the 70% of absorbed ingested energy in the rat, 20% is converted to glycogen and 50% to fat that is stored in adipose tissue. Further experiments with the meal-fed rats indicated that their adipose tissue was able to convert more radioactive glucose to fatty acids than did the nibblers. The activity of several enzymes involved in lipogenesis was increased in the former group.

It was further shown that when the nibblers are meal fed it takes 9 days to reach maximum fatty acid synthesis. When the animals went back to nibbling, it took 6 weeks to attain normal levels of lipogenesis. Fig. 3-1 shows the enzyme adaptations

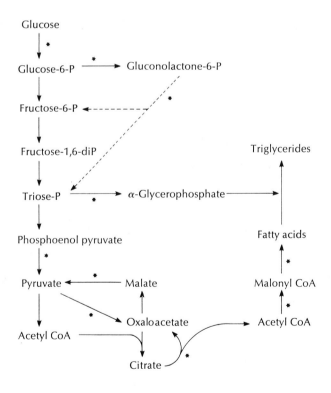

* Meal eating increases the activity of these enzymes.

Fig. 3-1. Enzyme adaptations in adipose tissue of meal-eating rats. (Adapted from Leveille, G. A., and Romsos, D. R.: Meal eating and obesity, Nutr. Today 9(6):8, 1974.)

in adipose tissue of meal-eating rats. The activity of all the enzymes except phospho-fructokinase and malate dehydrogenase is increased.

This situation may also explain why weight reduction programs are unsuccessful. Some individuals on a reducing diet restrict their intake at breakfast and lunch. They eat essentially one meal a day in the evening. This increases the activity of the enzymes needed for lipogenesis. As caloric intake is reduced, weight loss follows, but when normal eating is resumed, there is increased synthesis of fat and weight is rapidly regained. Leveille and Romsos refer to this as the "yo-yo syndrome" of weight reduction.

Sassoon suggested that calorifers (energy carriers) from fat and some starches do not readily promote fat synthesis.[18] On the other hand, sugars are rapidly digested, absorbed, and converted to fat. Enzyme adaptation promotes lipogenesis and not lipolysis. This is further reinforced by increasing the time between meals. Thus both the consumption of sugars and the increased time between the intake of food promotes lipogenesis and then obesity. Therefore the optimal diet would contain restricted protein and sugar, with fats and some starch providing the main source of calories. This diet should be initiated immediately after weaning to prevent obesity.

TREATMENT

Bray and co-workers stated that obesity is treated as if it were a disease when in fact it is a symptom of an underlying disorder.[4] For the most part medical and diet therapy has met with failure. Recently behavior modification methods have met with more success. More emphasis is needed on preventive measures such as proper diet and adequate exercise. These programs must be initiated early in life before bad habits are firmly established.

Drugs

Many drugs have been used to promote anorexia, or a loss of appetite, as an aid to people on reduction diets. These central nervous system stimulants act on the satiety center of the brain and lessen the desire to eat while producing a euphoric state. There are three types of anorectic agents based on their chemical structure: phenyl-ethyl amines (for example, amphetamines), morpholine, and imidazoline.[19] The use of these drugs has been questioned since the anorectic effect is short-term and often is only manifested after a large dose. Various side effects have been noted such as addiction, insomnia, hypertension, cardiac arrhythmias, dry mouth, constipation, impotence, blood disorders, and allergic reactions.

In July 1971 federal regulations issued by the Food and Drug Administration stated that orally used amphetamines or dextroamphetamines should be used for a short time only with weight reduction diets for patients in whom obesity was refractory to other measures.[20] A survey of U.S. physicians showed varying attitudes toward the use of appetite suppressants.[21] About one third of the doctors did not prescribe these drugs. The others prescribed mainly the nonamphetamine types for short periods of time. The most commonly prescribed drug was Tenuate (diethylpro-pion). The amphetamines have given better results but are associated with more side effects. When asked to class the efficacy of these drugs, 7% of the physicians claimed the results were excellent, 24% good, 42% fair, and 27% poor. The physicians did not consider that the use of drugs for weight reduction contributed to drug abuse. Most doctors did not want to ban the use of these drugs even though their usefulness has not been proved.

The drug fenfluramine, which has been used in Europe as an appetite suppres-sant, has been tested in the United States.[22] Patients were given either fenfluramine, dexamphetamine, or a placebo. They were also given instructions on eating, but no diet was prescribed. After 7 weeks of treatment the group on fenfluramine lost 1.9 kg (4.2 lb) and those on dexamphetamine 1.8 kg (4.0 lb). The control group only lost 0.32 kg (0.7 lb). However, drowsiness and gastrointestinal symptoms were reported by 89% of the users of fenfluramine. Side effects appeared in 37% of the placebo group and 44% of the dexamphetamine users. Fenfluramine also exhibited hypoglycemic activity.

Lee and Lichton reported the presence of a fat-mobilizing substance (FMS/A) in the urine of rats,[23,24] This substance, when injected into rats, caused a decrease in food intake and body weight. An injection of 12 mg per rat decreased food consump-tion by 30% in 1 day. Purification of the substance increased the anorexigenic activ-ity. Further analysis was carried on with ultrafiltration, anion exchange chromatog-raphy, and gel filtration. The latter method resulted in a material that when injected in high concentrations caused the death of the animals. It is not known whether this substance plays a role in the regulation of food intake in the rat or if a similar substance exists in humans.

Cellulose and methyl, methylethyl, hydroxymethyl, and sodium carboxymethyl derivatives are used as bulk producers or anorectic agents.[25] These carbohydrates are indigestible and therefore are used to reduce the caloric content of food. In addition, they absorb water and swell, producing the feeling of satiety. A microcrystalline cellulose (Avicel) is a fine powder produced by hydrolysis of cellulose. It is added to ice cream, salad dressings, and syrups. Carrageenin from seaweed and sodium al-ginates from algae are used as thickeners, binders, and emulsifying agents in low-calorie foods.

Hormones (progesterone, human growth, thyroid, and human chorionic gonado-tropin) have been used to treat obese patients.[26] Progesterone has been administered for the pulmonary complications of obesity, in particular, the hypoventilation of the Pickwickian syndrome, although the mechanism of action is not understood. Human growth hormone promotes the breakdown of fat, increases the expenditure of en-ergy, and does not increase nitrogen breakdown. It should be useful in promoting weight reduction in obese patients; however, not enough of the hormone is currently available for testing.

Thyroxine (T4) and triiodothyronine (T3) have been used in obese patients even though many do not have hypothyroidism. There is a loss of weight, but when therapy is discontinued many tend to regain the weight. The hormone can be toxic with either cardiovascular complications or losses of calcium and nitrogen. Rivlin suggested that the thyroid hormones be prescribed only for obese patients with hypothyroidism.[26]

Much controversy has surrounded the use of human chorionic gonadotropin (HCG). This placental hormone is isolated from the urine of pregnant women. HCG was originally used by Simeons to treat obese patients.[27,28] Injections of 125 IU of HCG were given 6 days a week in 40 treatments. The individuals consumed 500 kcal per day in two meals. The weight loss was not attributed to either the hormone or diet therapy. A double-blind study was conducted by Asher and Harper to assess the effect of HCG on weight loss, hunger, and feeling of well-being.[29] Twenty female patients received injections 6 days a week for 6 weeks or until they reached the desired weight. Another group of women received placebo injections. Both groups were instructed to consume between 500 to 550 kcal per day. The mean weight loss in those receiving HCG was 9 kg (20 lb) while the other group lost 5 kg (11 lb). In addition, 87% of those in the HCG group reported that they felt good to excellent, while 70% of those in the placebo group responded in the same way. Hirsch and Van Itallie challenged the study on the basis that the HCG patients received more injections than the placebo group.[30] They suggested that the group receiving more injections might have better adherence to the diet. The difference would then be due to caloric intake rather than to what was injected. The rebuttal of Asher and Harper concluded that the HCG injection made it easier for the patient to follow the low-calorie diet.[31] Maudlin felt that the success of HCG might be due to diet, group therapy, and psychological support.[32]

Stein et al. repeated the experimental protocol of Asher and Harper with 51 obese women.[33] Twenty-five subjects received the human chorionic gonadotropin, and the other 26 received a placebo. Both groups were advised to consume 500 kcal per day. At the end of 32 days of treatment there were no significant differences in weight loss, percent of weight loss, hip and waist circumference, weight loss per injection, or in hunger ratings between the two groups. In a similar double-blind random crossover study with 202 patients, no significant differences were found between those receiving the hormone or the placebo during any part of the experiment.[34]

Fasting

Fasting has been used to treat obese patients who must lose weight rapidly, for example, prior to undergoing surgery. In total fasting only water, vitamins, and minerals are allowed. Semistarvation diets provide 300 to 600 kcal per day. Weight loss is rapid. Men lose more rapidly than women.[4] Some have lost 5 kg (11 lb) per day at the beginning of the fast. Over a 2-month period the average daily weight loss is about 0.45 kg (1 lb).

A lack of carbohydrate in the diet causes the excretion of water, sodium, potassium, calcium, magnesium, and phosphate. Up to 30% of the volume of plasma and extracellular fluid can be lost. This results in postural hypotension. The decrease in circulatory blood volume decreases the blood pressure. If the individual stands up, he may faint. The decrease in fluid loss can be alleviated by giving 1 g of bicarbonate of soda daily. Potassium supplements are given to replace the lost potassium. The decreased blood volume also diminishes the ability of the kidney to clear the blood of wastes. The function of the liver is impaired. Hypertensive agents should not be administered during fasting since the blood pressure generally is lowered.

During fasting approximately 90% of the kilocalories (1800 to 2400) are supplied from the breakdown of fat. Therefore, only 200 to 250 g of fat would be lost per day. Fats are hydrolyzed into fatty acids. When the breakdown is excessive, the fatty acids are converted to the ketone bodies, acetoacetic acid, β-hydroxybutyric acid, and acetone. The levels in blood and urine are elevated. The presence of ketone bodies in the urine confirms the fact that the person is not ingesting food. The serum ketone bodies cause an unpleasant taste sensation, and this helps to decrease the appetite. The keto acids compete with uric acid for excretion in the kidney tubules, and as a result the individual becomes hyperuricemic. Gout and urate stones can develop in patients who are not treated with either allopurinol or probenecid.

The glycogen stores of the liver are depleted and blood glucose levels fall gradually to 40 mg/dl. Since the change is not rapid, no symptoms of hypoglycemia have been observed.

Metabolism continues during the fasting state, and vitamins are needed to form coenzymes. They are excreted, and thus vitamin supplements must be provided daily to avoid deficiency states.

Approximately 1.25 kg of protein, equivalent to 6 kg of muscle, are lost after 3 to 4 weeks of fasting.[35] Protein synthesis is slightly impaired. Sometimes anemia develops. Plasma protein levels are not changed.

A group of 207 morbidly obese patients underwent prolonged fasting.[36] Fifty percent fasted for almost 2 months with an average weight loss of 28.2 kg (62 lb), and 25% fasted for over 2 months and lost on the average 41.4 kg (91.1 lb). Those who had been obese as children had the most difficulty in trying to reach their normal weight. After 1 to 1½ years the majority of 121 follow-up patients were able to maintain their weight, whereas within 2 to 3 years 50% had reverted to their original admission weight. Only seven patients maintained their reduced weights for 7.3 years. Thus fasting of morbidly obese subjects does not result in long-term weight reduction.

Genuth, Castro, and Vertes treated 75 obese outpatients with a semistarvation diet.[37] No food was allowed. Five supplements were taken daily every 4 hours. Alternate feedings of glucose (15 g) and casein calcium (15 g) provided a total daily intake of 300 kcal. The first 45 patients received 45 g of glucose and 30 g of casein calcium while the next 30 patients received 30 g of glucose and 45 g of casein calcium. The amino acid content of the casein calcium (Casec) met the minimum daily adult requirement for essential amino acids. A multivitamin tablet was administered daily and 5 mg of folic acid weekly. Therapy was discontinued when a reasonable weight was attained. The subjects' weights ranged from 80 to 245 kg (176 to 540 lb). Of the 47 patients who successfully reduced their weight, the average weight loss was 41 kg (91 lb) in men and 33 kg (72 lb) in women. Ketone bodies in the patients' blood were lower than those found in fasting patients. No hematologic disorders were found. Liver and kidney function tests were normal. The men excreted more urea and ammonia nitrogen than did the women; thus they most likely had been in negative nitrogen balance although this was not determined. The patients were able to follow the regimen from a minimum of 2 months to a maximum of 1 year. This was accomplished with a minimum disruption of normal routine. Many found it easier to abstain from food completely rather than to consume small amounts.

After fasting or semistarvation diets, patients must be carefully refed. Tea with sugar has been given for 2 to 3 days at the end of a fast.[4] This is followed by small amounts of food providing 500 kcal. Fluid retention results in a rapid weight gain. Since the basal metabolic rate drops during fasting, food intake should be carefully monitored to prevent weight regain. Genuth and his co-workers hospitalized their patients for 3 days at the end of semistarvation and fed a 500 kcal, 250 mg sodium diet.[37]

A supplemented fasting program was adapted for use as a large-scale outpatient regimen.[38] Initially the patients were hospitalized during the first week of fasting; this was later eliminated. After medical examinations a weight reduction goal was set. The patient was fed a protein-glucose supplement five times a day that supplied a daily total of 45 g of protein and 30 g of glucose. A multivitamin tablet and a potassium supplement were also administered. After discharge the patients were instructed to return once a week for a clinic visit. A total of 519 patients participated in the study of which 78% lost a minimum of 18.2 kg (40 lb) in approximately 29.8 weeks of fasting. The average weight loss for females was 1.3 kg (3 lb) per week and for males 2.1 kg (4.6 lb) per week. Most of the patients were able to carry out their normal daily activities with few side effects.

Bistrian et al. have used the protein-sparing modified fast to reduce obese individuals.[39-41] This regimen includes 1 to 1.5 g of meat protein per kilogram of ideal body weight, vitamins, minerals, and fluids. About 400 to 600 kcal are ingested daily. The protein in the diet spares tissue protein and maintains positive nitrogen balance. Body fat is broken down for energy. The ketosis helps to suppress appetite. Approximately 225 g are lost per day without complications. This method has been used primarily with hospitalized patients.

Surgery[42]

Surgery is performed on patients with massive obesity (two to three times ideal weight, or 45 kg [100 lb] overweight) that is accompanied by life-threatening complications.[43] These individuals have been unable to reduce by dietary means. Three types of jejunoileal bypass surgery have been performed.[44] The first operation involves an anastomosis of a short piece of the jejunum directly to the colon. This has been discontinued, since severe diarrhea, electrolyte depletion, and liver failure develop. Now the cut end of the jejunum can be connected to the side of the distal ileum (end to side) or the cut end of the jejunum is joined to the cut end of the ileum (end to end) to allow the bypassed segment to drain into the transverse colon (see Fig. 3-2). This leaves 25 to 35 cm (10 to 14 in) of jejunum, 30 cm (12 in) of ileum, and 480 to 660 cm (16 to 22 ft) of the small intestine in a blind loop. In this way if serious complications develop, the anastomosis can be taken down.

After surgery liquids are administered as soon as peristalsis is initiated.[45] After 3 days solid foods are introduced in small amounts. Large volumes of food and in particular milk and citrus fruits worsen the diarrhea. Since some food reaches the colon without being absorbed it serves as an irritant and results in diarrhea. After 3 to 6 months intestinal absorption increases and the diarrhea lessens. The administration of calcium carbonate has proved helpful.

The average rate of weight loss is 2.3 to 4.5 kg (5 to 10 lb) per month or approximately 34 to 45 kg (75 to 100 lb) during the first year. Weight stabilizes after 18 months. Studies have shown that individuals ingest up to 3000 kcal less per day as a result of the diarrhea. In addition to the decreased caloric intake there is a change in

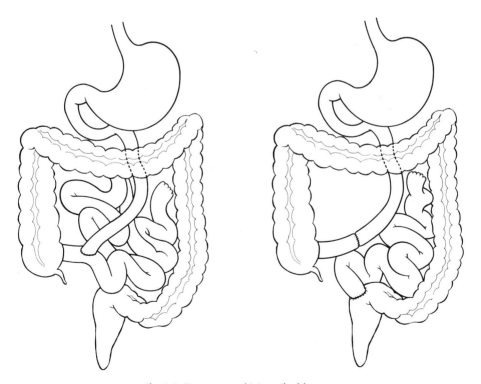

Fig. 3-2. Two types of jejunoileal bypass.

taste preferences.[46] With time there is an increase in the length of the small bowel and an increase in the number of villi. As absorption increases, the diarrhea diminishes, and thus the weight loss decreases.

The following complications have been described in patients after an ileal bypass: feelings of coldness and weakness, anorexia, liver failure, gallstones, bypass enteritis, arthritis, kidney stone formation, and deficiencies of vitamins and minerals.[45,47,48] In cases of severe complications the bypass has been reversed.

Severe liver damage leading to death in some cases has been reported in both the jejunocolic and jejunoileal bypass operations.[49-51] Holzbach and his co-workers reported that 23 massively obese patients 5 to 24 months after a jejunoileal bypass had an increase both in liver total lipids and triglycerides.[52] The values were at least three times the level found in the liver biopsy done during surgery. These liver changes are similar to those found in the protein deficiency disease kwashiorkor.[53] After surgery patients are encouraged to eat at least 60 g of protein per day and to abstain from alcohol in order to avoid liver damage.[45] The treatment for liver damage involves the intravenous administration of amino acids, vitamins, calcium, and magnesium. Neomycin is given to decrease the formation of ammonia and thus prevent hepatic coma.

The relationship of bile acid metabolism to hepatic disease in small-bowel bypass has been studied.[54] Four months after surgery five patients exhibited impaired liver function. In three patients there was an increase in the ratio of glycine to taurine bile acid conjugates, while four patients had elevated levels of serum bile acids, namely cholic and chenodeoxycholic acid. Patients who excrete large amounts of fat synthesize more of the primary bile acids, whereas those who excrete moderate amounts produce more of the secondary bile acids.[45] Higher levels of cholic acid and lower levels of chenodeoxycholic acid are found in bypass patients. The latter bile acid is nonlithogenic, and thus the higher levels of cholic acid predispose the patient to gallstones. Serum cholesterol levels are elevated 3 to 6 weeks postoperatively. Gallstones have developed 5 weeks after a bypass operation.[55] A liver biopsy performed at the time of cholecystectomy showed severe fatty infiltration. However, several months after bypass surgery, serum cholesterol and triglyceride levels have been found to decrease.[56]

Bypass enteritis or colonic pseudo-obstruction is another complication that can appear 1½ to 3 years after surgery.[45,48,57] The symptoms are bloating, distension, cramps, diarrhea, and in some instances chills and fever. It is thought that bacterial overgrowth in the bypassed bowel or colon causes these symptoms. Treatment involves the administration of antibiotics. With some patients there has been only distension of the bowel and no obstruction when surgery was performed.

The intestinal bacterial overgrowth may also be responsible for a form of arthritis that develops in some patients.[45,47,48] The bacteria produce cryoprotein complexes that may be involved in the pathogenesis of the arthritis.[58] Antibiotic administration results in a dramatic improvement of symptoms.

Kidney stone (calcium oxalate) formation also occurs in some patients following an ileal bypass.[45] Prior to surgery the oxalate is bound by calcium and excreted in the feces. Postoperatively fat absorption is decreased, and as a result the fatty acids bind calcium to form soaps. The oxalate is not bound; thus more is absorbed and excreted via the urine. To avoid stone formation the dietary oxalate and fat intake is decreased, while calcium intake is increased. Cholestyramine, which binds bile acids, has been used to decrease oxalate absorption.

Serum electrolyte levels need to be monitored to avoid deficiency states. Decreased intakes of potassium and magnesium may lead to tetany. Vitamin deficiencies may also occur due to decreased absorption. Low levels of 25-hydroxy-vitamin D have been reported in bypass patients.[59] Patients must be observed for skeletal abnormalities since decreases in serum calcium, magnesium, albumin, and alkaline phosphatase have been noted. However, as time passes and the rate of absorption increases, levels approach normal.

Solow and co-workers were interested in the effect of intestinal bypass surgery on personality traits, self-esteem, and level of interpersonal and vocational effectiveness.[60] All 23 patients showed an improvement in all measured indexes of psychosocial functioning. Both physical and social activity increased. The individuals also became more responsive to internal cues in the regulation of eating behavior. The authors felt the most important change was the loss of a sense of entrapment, helplessness, and failure that is associated with morbid obesity.

In another study 18 patients were interviewed 30 months after surgery.[61] They were found to be more stable and productive. Only 28% were satisfied with their weight loss, and only four had attained their ideal weight. A majority of the individuals had experienced medical complications, but many of these individuals recommended the operation to others.

Because of the many complications associated with intestinal bypass, gastric bypass has been used by surgeons for the treatment of morbid obesity.[62] About 80% to 90% of the stomach is bypassed. The distal segment of the stomach is closed off and the proximal stomach is partially closed and anastomosed to the jejunum. After surgery patients are advised to eat three soft meals a day and nothing between meals. It is important that adequate protein and vitamins are ingested. Recovery from this type of surgery is much more rapid than with intestinal bypass. Preoperative and postoperative dietary intakes have shown that postoperatively the patients consume fewer calories due to the small size of the stomach. Anastomotic peptic ulceration has been seen in only a small percentage of gastric bypass patients.

Diets

Millions of dollars are spent annually by the American public on pills, books, and various gimmicks to lose weight quickly. Yet not much success has been attained, and the public continues to search for a magical diet food or pill that will melt away the pounds instantly while eating as if calories don't count.

Dietary treatment has not been very successful. Tullis stated that in the future diet therapy may play a minor role in treating obesity, and behavior modification may become more important.[63] In cases of grand obesity (two to three times ideal weight), there is no rational diet, and other therapeutic measures such as fasting or surgery should be employed.

In order to achieve weight loss, negative caloric balance is necessary; that is, energy output is greater than energy input. This may be accomplished by either a decrease in the amount of calories consumed or an increase in physical activity, or both. Weight loss is often slow and irregular. Plateaus are reached and retention of water tends to make the dieter discouraged. Persistent hunger makes it difficult to adhere to the diet. Even if weight reduction is successful, the maintenance of normal weight is more difficult. Many individuals go through cycles of adding weight and then dieting to lose it. This produces physiological stress on the body.

The diet must be based on the individual's food habits so that it is acceptable. Nutrition education is important because the person must be convinced that he must eat this way for the rest of his life. It is important to achieve satiety on the diet since hunger will result in nonadherence. Although there are many proponents for various proportions of carbohydrate, protein, and fat, no evidence available proves that these regimens are successful for long-term weight reduction. Therefore a balanced diet containing approximately 14% protein, 30% fat, and 56% carbohydrate is recommended. Reasonable short-term goals should be set. It is much easier to set goals for the number of pounds to be lost in a short period of time rather than the total number of pounds that must be lost. The excess weight was gained over a long period of time, and it cannot be lost rapidly by caloric restriction.

Psychological support is also necessary. Weight reduction is contraindicated during periods of emotional stress and certain illnesses.

Various types of liquid formula diets have been developed, at first for hospital use. Many are now available commercially. The advantage to their use is that a measured amount of calories are provided, and decisions do not have to be made about what food and how much to eat. Since these are liquid diets, the individual may miss the experience of chewing. No bulk is ingested and gastrointestinal symptoms may develop. But the main disadvantage in using these formulas is that the individual's dietary habits are not changed by this type of regimen. Resumption of normal eating patterns will only lead to the weight being regained.

Physicians recommend a weight loss of only 0.45 to 0.9 kg (1 to 2 lb) a week. It has been assumed that 0.45 kg (1 lb) of body fat is equivalent to 3500 kcal. Therefore to lose 0.45 kg of fat per week the caloric deficit each day must be 500 kcal, or 1000 kcal to lose 0.9 kg (2 lb) a week.

Water, fat, protein, and glycogen are lost during dieting on a short-term basis, and minerals are lost over a longer period of time.[64] Early in weight reduction, water is lost. It is possible that later in a diet, while fat and protein are being lost, water is retained, resulting in weight gain. There are no easy methods available that can be used to determine the composition of a patient's weight loss. Early in weight loss the calories are not being provided entirely by depot fat; therefore a weight loss of 0.45 kg (1 lb) is not equivalent to an energy deficit of 3500 kcal.

Obese subjects on a 1200 kcal mixed diet lost 0.45 kg (1 lb) per day for the first 5 days, but 66% of that loss was water. When an 800 kcal diet containing 90 g of carbohydrate was fed, the weight loss at the end of a 10-day period was 0.32 kg (0.7 lb) per day. On the other hand, when the diet was ketogenic (800 kcal and 10 g of carbohydrate), the weight loss was 0.41 kg (0.9 lb). The difference between the two diets was caused by the higher rate of water loss on the ketogenic diet. After 10 days of starvation the composition of the weight loss was similar to that obtained on the 800 kcal ketogenic diet. Other experiments have shown that on a long-term caloric restriction, obese subjects are better able to adapt and oxidize a greater proportion of fat and less protein than do nonobese subjects.

According to Bray one of the reasons that obese people do not lose weight is that they become more efficient utilizers of energy on a reduction diet.[13] He calculated that an obese person with a surface area of 3 m² would need 3300 kcal to maintain his weight; however, on a reducing diet he would need only 900 kcal/m², or a total of 2700 kcal. If the individual was placed on a 2300 kcal diet, he would have a daily deficit of 400 kcal (2700 to 2300) or 2800 kcal per week, or the equivalent of 0.36 kg (0.8 lb). When this is calculated on the basis of the maintenance diet, there is a deficit of 1000 kcal (3300 to 2300) for a total loss of 7000 kcal per week, or 0.9 kg (2 lb). Therefore the individual expected to lose 0.9 kg per week, when in actuality he lost only 0.36 kg from the decrease in calories needed to maintain weight when on calorie restriction. In addition, obese individuals have a larger number of adipose cells than do normal weight individuals. During weight reduction the number of cells does not change; the cells merely reduce in size.

Six obese women were maintained for 15 days on a liquid diet containing 12 g nitrogen per day and enough calories to keep their weight constant.[65] For the first 12-day experimental period, 25% of calories needed for weight maintenance and a protein-free liquid diet were fed. For the second experimental period of 12 days the diet contained 3 g of nitrogen. There was no significant difference in the daily weight loss between these two treatments. However, the nitrogen balance was less negative when nitrogen was included in the diet. This meant that there was less breakdown of endogenous protein, and approximately 95% of the endogenous calories came from fat. Potassium balance was more negative in the diet without protein. However, sodium and potassium balance studies were not as useful in predicting changes in body composition.

In a later study eight obese women were fed liquid diets that differed in calorie and nitrogen content.[66] A 15-day stabilization period on a liquid diet containing 12 g of nitrogen per day and calories to maintain weight was followed by four metabolic periods of 12-days' duration. The diet periods included (1) 100% kcal, no nitrogen; (2) 50% kcal, 12 g nitrogen; (3) 25% kcal, no nitrogen; and (4) 25% kcal, 3 g nitrogen. For four subjects who completed the study the most negative nitrogen balance appeared when no nitrogen was fed (periods 1 and 3). Even though the caloric intake was different, the nitrogen balance was the same. Nitrogen balance was positive when 12 g of nitrogen and 50% of calories were fed, but negative nitrogen balance resulted on 3.5 g nitrogen and 25% of calories. The data indicated that obese individuals are able to conserve body protein when faced with caloric restriction. Obese individuals on low intakes of calories and proteins are able to stay in nitrogen balance when persons of normal weight could not.

Kasper, Thiel, and Ehl studied the effect of low-carbohydrate and high-fat diets.[67] Nonobese subjects were fed a diet containing 168 g of carbohydrate supplemented with up to 600 g of corn or olive oil daily. When the fat intake was 300 to 400 g the subjects felt very hot. Despite the high caloric intake of up to 6800 kcal per day, there was only a slight weight gain. The same effect was observed in obese subjects. With a diet containing 50 to 60 g of carbohydrate and 150 g of fat, the average daily weight reduction was 0.3 kg. The authors suggested that on a high-fat, low-carbohydrate diet the increased energy output is dissipated as heat.

The Kempner rice diet has been used for the treatment of renal insufficiency, hypertension, and diabetes mellitus, and it is now being used for obesity by reducing the caloric intake.[68] The diet provides 400 to 800 kcal (90% to 95% carbohyrate) per day from rice and fruit. Since the intake of sodium is less than 60 mg per day, the intake of fluid is restricted. After 1 month vegetables are added to the diet, and then later lean meats and poultry are allowed. The caloric intake is kept at less than 1000 kcal per day, and the sodium intake is maintained at less than 100 mg per day.

The patients on the Kempner diet reported daily to a satellite facility ("rice house") of Duke University for meals and weight and blood pressure measurements. Twice weekly, urine samples were collected and measured for sodium or chloride content to ascertain the degree of adherence to the diet. Motivational techniques, peer pressure, and exercise were used as adjuncts to diet therapy.

Of 106 patients who were studied, all had lost at least 45 kg (99 lb), and 43 patients had reached their normal weight. The average daily weight loss was 0.24 ± 0.09 kg (0.53 ± 0.2 lb) per day; the length of the treatment ranged from approximately 6 months to over a year for 26 patients. There were also significant decreases in systolic and diastolic blood pressure, fasting and 2-hour postprandial blood glucose levels, heart size, serum triglycerides, and serum uric acid levels. Serum cholesterol levels varied; patients whose levels were initially normal showed increased levels, whereas decreased blood cholesterol levels were observed in those patients whose initial levels were elevated. The authors concluded that massively obese subjects can lose weight as outpatients without resorting to the more drastic methods of intervention.

Fad diets. The American public is being continually assaulted with one fad diet after another. Since they are ineffective, one diet fades away and another one with a slightly new gimmick takes its place. Fineberg described some of the popular fad diets: Calories Don't Count, All-the-Meat-You-Want, Doctor's Quick Weight Loss

Diet, The Drinking Man's Diet, the Mayo Clinic Diet, Air Force Diet, Dr. Atkins' Diet Revolution, the Rockefeller Diet, Grapefruit Diet, Skimmed Milk and Banana Diet, and the Doctor's Quick Inches Off Diet.[69]

Many of these fad diets are based on a severe restriction of carbohydrate with unlimited amounts of fat and protein. The Calories Don't Count diet calls for unlimited consumption of proteins and fats in the form of safflower oil.[70] The Doctor's Quick Weight Loss Diet allows the individual to eat all he wants of foods that are high in protein and fat.[71] One can consume lean meat, poultry, lean fish, other seafood, eggs, and cheese. Eight glasses of water must be consumed daily. These diets purport to allow unrestricted eating, but in fact they are very restrictive, and most individuals soon abandon the regimen.

Rickman and his co-workers studied the effect of the Stillman diet on serum lipid levels.[72] Twelve volunteers followed the diet for a period of 3 to 17 days. The average daily intake was 1400 to 1500 kcal. Fats and proteins each provided about 50% of the total caloric intake. The average cholesterol intake was 1.215 g, or twice that of the normal intake. It was difficult to get the subjects to adhere to the diet for more than a week. The average weight loss at the beginning was 1.4 to 2.3 kg (3 to 5 lb), but after a week this dropped to 0.9 to 1.4 kg (2 to 3 lb). However, a week after the end of the experiment, eight subjects experienced a weight gain of 0.9 to 3.6 kg (2 to 8 lb). There was a significant increase in serum cholesterol from 215 mg/dl to 248 mg/dl while on the Stillman diet. Serum triglyceride levels increased in six of the subjects and decreased in the other 10. The authors concluded that the elevated serum cholesterol levels observed during the diet may present a potential risk to persons prone to coronary artery disease. They had little reason to recommend this diet.

In a similar study 10 women were placed on the Stillman diet and 10 on a balanced low-calorie diet for 14 days.[73] The high-protein, low-carbohydrate diet contained 142.7 g protein and 58.3 g of fat, while the control diet had 61.2 g protein and 62.3 g of fat. After the initial week the average weight loss was 3.7 kg (8.2 lb) on the experimental diet and 2.5 kg (5.6 lb) for the control group. A higher weight loss of 5.4 kg (12 lb) was observed at the end of the second week of the high-protein, low-carbohydrate diet compared with 3.9 kg (8.7 lb) on the balanced low-calorie diet; however, the weight losses during this week were similar for both groups. No significant changes in blood urea nitrogen, serum uric acid, and 2-hour postprandial blood sugar levels were noted between the two groups.[74] However, ketonemia was more pronounced in the high-protein, low-carbohydrate group. The degree of ketosis did not contribute to anorexia since most of the individuals experienced hunger and had difficulty adhering to the diet.

The Council on Foods and Nutrition of the American Medical Association reviewed the low-carbohydrate ketogenic weight reduction regimens.[75] On these diets only carbohydrate is restricted but not calories. This produces ketonuria, and it has been suggested by some that this accounts for the weight loss. It has been shown that this would produce a loss of only 100 kcal a day. The carbohydrate restriction increases sodium and water losses, and thus this results initially in a rapid weight loss that could lead to dehydration. The average diet contains 45% carbohydrate. On the restricted diet the calories must be supplied by protein and fat. This is difficult for Americans to adjust to, so as a result the diet becomes low in calories and thus the weight loss ensues. The ingestion of large amounts of fat may, lead to hypercholesterolemia and hypertriglyceridemia and eventually to coronary artery disease. Hyperuricemia, gout, and postural hypotension have also been reported on these low-carbohydrate diets.

Atkins stated in his book that carbohydrates are responsible for obesity.[76] In the body they stimulate the synthesis of fat. He suggested that a fat-mobilizing hormone (FMH) is produced on a carbohydrate-restricted diet and that FMH converts the stored fat into carbohydrates, which are released into the blood. FMH has never been isolated from humans, nor can fat be converted into carbohydrate in the body. Sugar is said to have antinutrient properties. Atkins stated that most obese people are hypoglycemic when in actuality they are most often resistant to their own insulin. The American Medical Association Council concluded that the rationale for the diet was unscientific.[75] The diet is not new since it is just another variation on a low-carbohydrate diet that has been promoted for years. It is not practical for long-term weight reduction or for maintenance of weight, and the high intake of fats would increase the risk of coronary artery disease. The council advised physicians to warn patients of the harmful effects of the ketogenic diet.

In 1976 a protein-sparing fast program, or the so-called Last Chance Diet, was introduced by Linn.[77] The regimen consists of the daily ingestion of a predigested protein product—112 to 140 g (4 to 5 oz) for women and 196 to 224 g (7 to 8 oz) for men (15 g protein per 30 ml). In addition, vitamin and mineral supplements including 2 to 4 g (0.07 to 0.14 oz) of potassium and higher than normal amounts of folic acid are prescribed. The dieter must consume 1.4 to 1.9 L (1½ to 2 qt) of fluid such as water, coffee, tea, or sugarless soda. In some instances medication may be necesary to lower serum uric acid levels. The Last Chance Diet is not advocated for pregnant women or for those who have liver, kidney, or heart disease.

When the dieters reach their goal, a refeeding period is instituted for 3 to 4 weeks. Breakfast consists of tea or coffee. For lunch and dinner 112 g (4 oz) of meat and 0.12 to 0.16 l (½ to ⅔ c) of vegetables and gelatin are allowed. Before and after the evening meal, 14 g (½ oz) of the predigested protein product is consumed. This is followed by the maintenance diet where breakfast consists of juice and coffee or tea, and for lunch and dinner one selection is made from each of four groups of food, namely, meat, vegetables, bread, and fruit.

Since the introduction of this diet many liquid, partially digested protein hydrolysates and whole protein products have been manufactured. The low biological quality proteins collagen and gelatin that are obtained from cowhides and connective tissue are used in these preparations. Some are supplemented with essential amino acids, vitamins, and minerals, but none have been found to be nutritionally complete.[78]

Some of these dietary products have a low protein-efficiency ratio and are deficient in trace elements.[79]

Several side effects have been observed with the use of these products such as fatigue, dehydration, hair loss, skin dryness, cold intolerance, amenorrhea, nausea, vomiting, diarrhea, muscle cramps, postural hypotension and faintness, cardiac arrhythmias, dysphoria, constipation, blackout episodes, peroneal palsy, and gout.[78,79] In 1977, 10 deaths of women who had been on the liquid protein, modified fast diet were investigated by the Center for Disease Control.[80] These women had been dieting for 2 to 8 months and had lost from 18 to 62 kg (40 to 136 lb) under a physician's care. All had taken vitamin and mineral supplements, and nine had received additional potassium. Eight women died in the hospital of arrhythmia. The autopsies revealed cardiac pathological states in five of the women.

Several other case studies of individuals on protein-sparing modified fasting who died suddenly have been reported.[81-83] An examination of the heart, skeletal muscle, and liver of a woman who had followed the diet for 8 months showed evidence of starvation.[81] Since many more deaths have been reported, the Food and Drug Administration has proposed the following label for the protein supplements used for weight reduction: "Warning: Very low-calorie protein diets may cause serious illness or death. Do not use for weight reduction without medical supervision. Do not use for any purpose without medical advice if you are taking medication. Not for use by infants, children, or pregnant or nursing women."[84] This diet regimen is not recommended for those who want to lose less than 9 to 11.3 kg (20 to 25 lb) or those who are morbidly obese. Refeeding programs must be carefully monitored to avoid fluid and electrolyte imbalance.

These diets are not recommended by the American Dietetic Association because of the many dangers associated with their use.[85] The long-term effects of this regimen are not known. A balanced diet that is low in kilocalories in addition to exercise is the weight reduction method advocated by this association.

Group therapy

More success has been observed in weight reduction by means of group therapy. The group TOPs (Take Off Pounds Sensibly) was founded in 1948. There are an estimated 300,000 members in the United States. Weekly meetings are held, and each member is weighed in. Recognition is given to those who have lost weight, and a penalty is administered to those who have gained. These tactics are successful, for an average weight loss of 6.8 kg (15 lb) or more that persisted for 16 months or longer has been reported.[6]

Weight Watchers is a commercial organization that also utilizes group therapy. The program consists of a weight-reducing plan to reach a weight goal and a leveling plan to provide an incentive when a person is 4.5 kg (10 lb) away from an ideal weight. Then the person goes onto a maintenance plan to stay at the desired weight. A fee must be paid to attend the weekly weigh-in meetings. Dietary advice is available from the leader of the group. Special foods are manufactured by Weight Watchers. This organization was recently purchased by the Pillsbury Company.

Behavior modification

For the past several years the principles of behavior modification have been applied to obese patients. This method has been unusually successful. In one study it was reported that 25% of the patients lost 9 kg (20 lb), and 5% lost 18 kg (40 lb).[86] In another study 53% lost more than 9 kg, 13% more than 18 kg, while others reported that 80% lost more than 9 kg and 30% more than 18 kg.[86]

Levitz summarized the basic techniques used in treating obesity by means of behavior therapy.[87] The process starts with the assessment of the individual's eating habits. It is of importance to determine the habit patterns and frequencies, the cues that signal these habits, and the situations that maintain them. A food record is kept of all foods consumed for several days. With this information the therapist can then decide how best to alter eating behavior. Some suggestions that have been made are to chew food thoroughly, leave food on the plate, eat in only one location, and during mealtimes not to engage in any other activity. Since various emotional states trigger eating habits, individuals are taught how to program incompatible behavior. When patients have the desire to eat they are told to engage in another activity. Positive reinforcement is also employed. If a certain objective is achieved, such as a reduction in food intake for the day, the individual is rewarded with, for example, money or participation in a pleasurable activity. Although the program is aimed at reducing food intake it is also possible to set up a plan to increase the energy expenditure of the individual by increasing his physical activity. It is also advantageous to involve family members in the behavior modification program. Such techniques are described in detail in a program devised by Ferguson entitled Learning to Eat, Behavior Modification for Weight Control.[88] A leader's and student's manual are available for those who are interested in starting a weight control group.

Since both group therapy and behavior modification have been successful, a pilot study combining these two methods was run.[89] A business executive was the leader of a group of 13 people. During the first 12 weeks when only social pressure was applied to the group, the average weight loss was 1.4 kg (3 lb). Then the leader was instructed in behavior modification techniques. In the next 12 weeks of this therapy the average weight loss was 4.5 kg (10 lb), and at the end of the second 12 weeks it was only 1.4 kg (3 lb). During the latter period the leader was away for several sessions. The initial success indicated that it might be possible to train lay leaders for behavior modification programs, since this type of therapy involves a great deal of time.

Musante suggested that patients should weigh in and receive a menu of 21 predesigned meals each week.[86] He felt that it was too difficult for obese patients to plan their own menus from food group lists. The term "unstructured eating" (USE) is used rather than "cheating" to indicate the number of times a day the plan is not followed. A diary of food intake and activity is kept along with the reason for USE. This information is then employed to determine what behaviors to alter. The final part of the program involves a discussion of the misconceptions about obesity. Patients receive valuable information from each other, making group meetings important.

Behavior modification techniques were tried with a mixed racial group.[90] Of eight women in this group, three were white, four black, and one Puerto Rican. Two other untreated control groups received the regular clinical procedure either as individuals or as a group. The untreated control group was interviewed by a nutritionist and given a diet. For 3 weeks they met individually with the nutritionist. The other untreated control group followed the same procedure except that they met as a group with the nutritionist. The behavior modification group met weekly for 16 weeks with the nutritionist and a psychologist. At the meeting they weighed in and discussed their difficulties. They agreed to keep a food diary, make a list of the positive and negative results of weight loss with reasons for losing weight, not keep favorite foods at home, slow their rate of eating, and set up a point system to reward themselves when weight was lost. However, many of the women did not follow the recommendations. Analysis showed that the behavior modification was less effective than the other two standard methods, or not significantly different. However, differences were found within the racial groups. For blacks, behavior modification was the least successful method. On the other hand, individual treatment was the least effective method for whites and Puerto Ricans. It may be that the lack of success was due primarily to the mixed racial group. The authors recommended that perhaps a fee should be collected and used as a reinforcer, and when the person achieved a certain behavior, part of this money would be returned.

At the University of Kentucky a weight reduction program for students utilized a combination of behavior and diet therapy.[91] The program was directed by graduate students in nutrition who had previously completed a course given by a psychiatrist on behavioral techniques. Nine subjects out of 15 completed the 12-week program; the mean weight loss was 0.3 kg (⅔ lb) a week. Three of the subjects reached their weight reduction goals.

In another university clinic, senior dietetic students were used as group leaders for an 11-week behavior modification program.[92] The 10 subjects in the behavioral modification group lost an average of 6.9 kg (15.2 lb), whereas the 12 control subjects lost an average of 4.5 kg (9.9 lb). However, 1 year after treatment both the control and behavioral subjects had regained part of the weight loss. Thus behavior modification has been more successful on the short-term rather than on the long-term basis.

Similar results were found by Currey et al. with a group of older individuals.[93] Of 165 patients who were enrolled in a behavior modification program, 144 completed 10 weeks of treatment. Of these individuals, 81% had been in previous weight reduction programs. In a 12-month period, 56 patients who had completed the program were contacted for evaluation. It was found that 70% had either regained their pretreatment weights or were heavier, 10% had maintained their weight, and 20% had continued to lose weight during the ensuing year. The authors concluded that behavioral techniques have not been as successful with older obese individuals who have other health problems.

Dahms et al. studied the effectiveness of behavior modification, two anorectic drugs (mazindol and diethylpropion), and a placebo.[94] Originally 144 subjects were screened, but only 120 actually participated. After 8 to 10 weeks, 50% were still enrolled, but only 33 completed the 14-week program. There was no significant difference in weight loss between those receiving behavioral therapy, drugs, or a placebo. However, the weight loss of the individuals in the treatment groups was greater than that of the control group subjects who were not treated. Behavioral therapy produced weight loss without the cost or potential side effects that were observed with the use of drugs. More efficient use of professional time resulted from the behavioral therapy also; since it was done with a group of patients at one time rather than with separate individuals, it proved to be less costly.

Since in some behavior modification programs the emphasis is primarily on changing eating habits rather than on dietary instruction, a study was initiated to determine whether a change in nutrient intake occurs.[95] Prior to a 20-session behavioral weight control program 15 subjects were found to have met two thirds of the recommended daily dietary allowances. During the fifteenth week of the study, self-recorded, 7-day food records indicated that two thirds of the RDA for iron, thiamine, and calcium were not met. The nutrient density for fiber, phosphorus, iron, vitamin A, thiamine, ascorbic acid, niacin, riboflavin, and cholesterol increased, while it decreased for calcium, carbohydrate, and fat. The percentage of calories from protein increased, while the percentage of fat and carbohydrate decreased. There was a decreased intake of fruits other than citrus, milk, cheese other than cottage, ice cream, meat, eggs, nuts, legumes, bread, cereal, and soft drinks.

Health education campaigns to get people to change certain aspects of their life-style such as diet, physical activity, cigarette smoking, and consumption of alcohol have not been very successful. Behavior modification has met with success in treating obesity, and similar techniques have been used in the treatment of smokers and alcoholics. When such a method was used to treat individuals who were at high risk for cardiovascular disease, it produced the greatest change. Pomerleau and his co-workers suggested that behavior modification would be an appropriate procedure to use in preventive medicine since this method has resulted in the greatest alteration in health habits.[96]

The National Heart, Lung, and Blood Institute has initiated programs for the prevention and control of heart, lung, and blood disorders.[97] The principles of behavioral science have been utilized in these programs in an attempt to change health behavior. In the Multiple Risk Fitness Intervention Trial, nutritionists and behaviorists are working together to try to change dietary practices in order to prevent cardiovascular disease. Thus it is useful for behavioral scientists to have some knowledge of nutrition and for dietitians to be aware of two areas of behavioral science—social psychology and behavior modification—so that nutritional counseling can be more effective.

Since altering human health behavior patterns is not accomplished by simply supplying information, Mahoney and Caggiula have summarized some of the most effective techniques that can be used to accomplish a change.[98] Human behavior is determined by three environments: physical (nonhuman factor), social (other persons), and private (basic physiological systems). These environments are complex and overlap in controlling human behavior. Most bad health practices results in short-term pleasurable sensations, and it is the long-term effect that is deleterious to health. Yet man is more strongly influenced by the short-term rather than the long-term consequences.

To have an impact in nutritional counseling, Mahoney and Caggiula suggest the following: patients must take responsibility for their own behavioral changes, short-term and long-term goals must be established, and an adequate assessment of the patients' environments is necessary.[98] For example, if an obese individual has difficulty avoiding evening snacks, the counselors would suggest changes in the physical, social, and private environment to deter the patient from this negative behavior. It is helpful to develop a contract for a specific goal. If the goal is attained, then the patient is rewarded. The authors recommend that the counseling stress changes in eating patterns rather than in weight loss. It is important to emphasize the positive changes that have been accomplished rather than punishing the individual for negative behavior.

Evans and Hall have suggested the formation of a "therapeutic alliance" between the health professional and the patient.[99] In the past a medical model was used in which the patient was dependent upon the health professional. In the new alliance the patient must be an active participant and decide to follow the treatment and to reinforce his own behavior. In this way a long-term change can be brought about that becomes an automatic part of the patient's life-style. These researchers also stress the development of precise goals in which the patient is involved. It is also important for the health professional to understand the patient and obtain information about his past experiences. Then the health professional practices his area of expertise in a behavior modification program. A positive approach may be a more successful motivator than fear in changing negative health behavior. This may also apply to the process of altering eating behavior.

Thus behavior modification programs stress the importance of subjects' being responsible for changing their own life-styles. It is necessary to gather information and then instruct the individual to set precise goals. The health professional can then use the obtained knowledge to assist the patient in changing his behavior to more healthful practices for the remainder of his life. As newer techniques of behavior modification are put into practice and behavioral scientists and dietitians collaborate, more long-term successes in changing eating behavior will be realized.

REFERENCES

1. Society of Actuaries: Build and blood pressure study, vols. 1 and 2, Chicago, 1959, Society of Actuaries.
2. U.S. Public Health Service, Division of Chronic Diseases: Obesity and health: a source book of current information for professional health personnel, Public Health Service Publication 1485, Washington, D.C., 1966, U.S. Government Printing Office.
3. Joliffe, N.: Reduce and stay reduced, ed. 3, New York, 1963, Simon & Schuster, Inc.
4. Bray, G. A., Davidson, M. B., and Drenick, E. J.: Obesity: a serious symptom, Ann. Intern. Med. 77:797, 1972.
5. Mann, G. V.: The influence of obesity on health (Part 1), N. Engl. J. Med. 291:178, 1974.
6. Mann, G. V.: The influence of obesity on health (Part 2), N. Engl. J. Med. 291:226, 1974.
7. Winick, M.: Childhood obesity, Nutr. Today 9(3):6, 1974.
8. Van Itallie, T. B., and Campbell, R. G.: Multi-disciplinary approach to the problem of obesity, J. Am. Diet. Assoc. 61:385, 1972.
9. Johnson, M. L., Burke, B. S., and Mayer, J.: Relative importance of inactivity and overeating in the energy balance of obese high school girls, Am. J. Clin. Nutr. 4:37, 1956.
10. Withers, R. F. J.: Problems in the genetics of human obesity, Eugenics Reviews 56(2):81, 1964.
11. Newman, H. H., Freeman, F. N., and Holzinger, J. J.: Twins, a study of heredity and environment, Chicago, 1937, University of Chicago Press.
12. Hirsch, J., and Knittle, J. L.: Cellularity of obese and nonobese human adipose tissue, Fed. Proc. 29:1516, 1970.
13. Bray, G. A.: The myth of diet in the management of obesity, Am. J. Clin. Nutr. 23:1141, 1970.
14. Bullen, B. A., Monello, L. F., Cohen, H., and Mayer, J.: Attitudes toward physical activity, food and family in obese and nonobese adolescent girls, Am. J. Clin. Nutr. 12:1, 1963.
15. Mayer, J.: Why people get hungry, Nutr. Today 1(2):2, 1966.
16. Lepkovsky, S.: Newer concepts in the regulation of food intake, Am. J. Clin. Nutr. 26:271, 1973.
17. Leveille, G. A., and Romsos, D. R.: Meal eating and obesity, Nutr. Today 9(6):4, 1974.

18. Sassoon, H. F.: Time factors in obesity, Am. J. Clin. Nutr. 26:776, 1973.
19. Calesnick, B.: Anorectics, Am. Fam. Physician 10(3):193, 1974.
20. Anderson, B. J.: Do federal regulations permit physicians to prescribe amphetamines for obesity? J.A.M.A. 230:900, 1974.
21. Lasagna, L.: Attitudes toward appetite suppressants. A survey of U.S. physicians, J.A.M.A. 225:44, 1973.
22. Fenfluramine helps obese patients lose weight, J.A.M.A. 224:975, 1973.
23. Lee, Y., and Lichton, I. J.: Partial purification of rat urinary anorexigenic substance, J. Nutr. 103:1616, 1973.
24. Anorexigenic substances in rat urine, Nutr. Rev. 32:123, 1974.
25. Fletcher, D. C.: Artificial "bulk producers" as anorectic agents, J.A.M.A. 230:901, 1974.
26. Rivlin, R. S.: Drug therapy: therapy of obesity with hormones, N. Engl. J. Med. 292:26, 1975.
27. Simeons, A. T. W.: The action of chorionic gonadotrophin in the obese, Lancet 2:946, 1954.
28. Simeons, A. T. W.: Chorionic gonadotropin in geriatrics, J. Am. Geriat. Soc. 4:36, 1956.
29. Asher, W. L., and Harper, H. W.: Effect of human chorionic gonadotrophin on weight loss, hunger and feeling of well-being, Am. J. Clin. Nutr. 26:211, 1973.
30. Hirsch, J., and Van Itallie, T. B.: The treatment of obesity. Letters to the editor, Am. J. Clin. Nutr. 26:1039, 1973.
31. Asher, W. L., and Harper, H. W.: Human chorionic gonadotrophin treatment for obesity: a rebuttal. Letters to the editor, Am. J. Clin. Nutr. 27:450, 1974.
32. Maudlin, R. K.: Gonadotropins in obesity, Am. Fam. Physician 8:202, 1973.
33. Stein, M. R., et al.: Ineffectiveness of human chorionic gonadotropin in weight reduction: a double-blind study, Am. J. Clin. Nutr. 29:940, 1976.
34. Young, R. L., Fuchs, R. S., and Woltjen, M. J.: Chorionic gonadotropin in weight control. A double-blind crossover study, J.A.M.A. 236:2495, 1976.
35. Flatt, J. P., and Blackburn, G. L.: The metabolic fuel regulatory system: implications for protein-sparing therapies during caloric deprivation and disease, Am. J. Clin. Nutr. 27:175, 1974.

36. Johnson, D., and Drenick, E. J.: Therapeutic fasting in morbid obesity, Arch. Intern. Med. 137:1381, 1977.

37. Genuth, S. M., Castro, J. H., and Vertes, V.: Weight reduction in obesity by outpatient starvation, J.A.M.A. 230:987, 1974.

38. Vertes, V., Genuth, S. M., and Hazelton, I. M.: Supplemented fasting as a large-scale outpatient program, J.A.M.A. 238:2151, 1977.

39. Bistrian, B. R., et al.: Nitrogen metabolism and insulin requirements in obese diabetic adults on a protein-sparing modified fast, Diabetes 25:494, 1976.

40. Bistrian, B. R., Winterer, J., and Blackburn, G. L.: Effect of a protein-sparing diet and brief fast on nitrogen metabolism in mildly obese subjects, J. Lab. Clin. Med. 89:1030, 1977.

41. Bistrian, B. R., Blackburn, G. L., and Stanbury, J. B.: Metabolic aspects of a protein-sparing modified fast in the dietary management of Prader-Willi obesity, N. Engl. J. Med. 296:774, 1977.

42. Faloon, W. W.: Symposium on jejunoileostomy for obesity, Am. J. Clin. Nutr. 30:1, (Jan) 1977.

43. Payne, J. H., et al.: Is the intestinal bypass operation an accepted method of treatment for obesity? J.A.M.A. 223:1281, 1973.

44. Current status of jejuno-ileal bypass for obesity, Nutr. Rev. 32:333, 1974.

45. Faloon, W. W.: Ileal bypass for obesity: postoperative perspective, Hosp. Pract. 12(1):73, 1977.

46. Bray, G. A.: Intestinal bypass surgery for obesity decreases food intake and taste preferences, Am. J. Clin. Nutr. 29:779, 1976.

47. Pi-Sunyer, F. X.: Jejunoileal bypass surgery for obesity, Am. J. Clin. Nutr. 29:409, 1976.

48. Bray, G. A., et al.: Surgical treatment of obesity: current status, Am. Fam. Physician 15(3):111, 1977.

49. Obesity, jejuno-ileal bypass and death, Nutr. Rev. 33:38, 1975.

50. Intestinal bypass surgery for obesity, Nutr. Rev. 33:78, 1975.

51. Moxley, R. T., Pozefsky, T., and Lockwood, D. H.: Protein nutrition and liver disease after small bowel bypass for obesity, Clin. Res. 21:520, 1970.

52. Holzbach, R. T., et al.: Hepatic lipid in morbid obesity, N. Engl. J. Med. 290:296, 1974.

53. Moxley, R. T., Pozefsky, T., and Lockwood, D. H.: Protein nutrition and liver disease after jejunoileal bypass for morbid obesity, N. Engl. J. Med. 290:921, 1974.

54. Sherr, H. P., et al.: Bile acid metabolism and hepatic disease following small bowel bypass for obesity, Am. J. Clin. Nutr. 27:1369, 1974.

55. Neshat, A. A., and Flye, M. W.: Early formation of gallstones following jejunoileal bypass for treatment of morbid obesity, Am. Surg. 41:486, 1975.

56. Bendezu, R., et al.: Certain metabolic consequences of jejunoileal bypass, Am. J. Clin. Nutr. 29:366, 1976.

57. Barry, R. E., et al.: Colonic pseudo-obstruction: a new complication of jejunoileal bypass, Gut 16:903, 1975.

58. Wands, J. R., et al.: Arthritis associated with intestinal-bypass procedure for morbid obesity, N. Engl. J. Med. 294:121, 1976.

59. Teitelbaum, S. L., et al.: Abnormalities of circulating 25-OH vitamin D after jejunal-ileal bypass for obesity, Ann. Intern. Med. 86:289, 1977.

60. Solow, C., Silberfarb, P. M., and Swift, K.: Psychosocial effects of intestinal bypass surgery for severe obesity, N. Engl. J. Med. 290:300, 1974.

61. Rigden, S. R., and Hagen, D. Q.: Psychiatric aspects of intestinal bypass surgery for obesity, Am. Fam. Physician 13(5):68, 1976.

62. Sorrell, V. F., and Burcher, S. K.: Gastric bypass for morbid obesity, N. Z. Med. J. 84:96, 1976.

63. Tullis, I. F.: Rational diet construction for mild and grand obesity, J.A.M.A. 226:70, 1973.

64. Van Itallie, T. B., and Yang, M.: Current concepts in nutrition. Diet and weight loss, N. Engl. J. Med. 297:1158, 1977.

65. Jourdan, M. H., and Bradfield, R. B.: Body composition changes during weight loss estimated from energy, nitrogen, sodium, and potassium balance, Am. J. Clin. Nutr. 26:144, 1973.

66. Jourdan, M., Margen, S., and Bradfield, R. B.: Protein-sparing effect in obese women fed low-calorie diets, Am. J. Clin. Nutr. 27:3, 1974.

67. Kasper, H., Thiel, H., and Ehl, M.: Response of body weight to a low carbohydrate, high fat diet in normal and obese subjects, Am. J. Clin. Nutr. 26:197, 1973.

68. Kempner, W., et al.: Treatment of massive

obesity with rice reduction diet program, Arch. Intern. Med. **135**:1575, 1975.

69. Fineberg, S. K.: The realities of obesity and fad diets, Nutr. Today **7**(4):23, 1972.

70. Taller, H.: Calories don't count, New York, 1961, Simon & Schuster, Inc.

71. Stillman, I. M., and Baker, S. S.: The doctor's quick weight loss diet, Englewood Cliffs, N. J., 1967, Prentice-Hall, Inc.

72. Rickman, F., Mitchell, N., Dingman, J., and Dalen, J. E.: Changes in serum cholesterol during the Stillman Diet, J.A.M.A. **228**:54, 1974.

73. Worthington, B. S., and Taylor, L. E.: Balanced low-calorie vs high-protein-low-carbohydrate reducing diets. I. Weight loss, nutrient intake and subjective evaluation, J. Am. Diet. Assoc. **64**:47, 1974.

74. Worthington, B. S., and Taylor, L. E.: Balanced low-calorie vs high-protein-low-carbohydrate reducing diets. II. Biochemical changes, J. Am. Diet. Assoc. **64**:52, 1974.

75. A critique of low-carbohydrate ketogenic weight reduction regimens. A review of Dr. Atkins' diet revolution, J.A.M.A. **224**:1415, 1973.

76. Atkins, R. C.: Dr. Atkins' diet revolution, the high calorie way to stay thin forever, New York, 1972, David McKay Co., Inc.

77. Linn, R., and Stuart, S. L.: The Last Chance Diet, Secaucus, N.J., 1976, Lyle Stuart (New York, Bantam Books, Inc. 1977).

78. Gunby, P.: FDA asks for warning labels on weight control liquid protein, J.A.M.A. **238**:2243, 1977.

79. Van Itallie, T. B.: Liquid protein mayhem, J.A.M.A. **240**:144, 1978.

80. Details released on deaths of ten on liquid protein diets, J.A.M.A. **238**:2680, 1977.

81. Michiel, R. R., et al.: Sudden death in a patient on a liquid protein diet, N. Engl. J. Med. **298**:1005, 1978.

82. Singh, B. N., et al.: Liquid protein diets and torsade de pointes, J.A.M.A. **240**:115, 1978.

83. Brown, J. M., et al.: Cardiac complications of protein-sparing modified fasting, J.A.M.A. **240**:120, 1978.

84. Warning labels proposed for diet protein, FDA Consumer **12**:24, Feb., 1978.

85. Statement by the American Dietetic Association on diet protein products, J. Am. Diet. Assoc. **73**:547, 1978.

86. Musante, J.: Obesity: a behavioral treatment program, Am. Fam. Physician **10**(6):95, 1974.

87. Levitz, L. S.: Behavior therapy in treating obesity, J. Am. Diet. Assoc. **63**:22, 1973.

88. Ferguson, J.: Learning to Eat. Behavior modification for weight control, Palo Alto, Calif., 1975, Bull Publishing Co.

89. Jordan, H. A., and Levitz, L. S., Behavior modification in a self-help group. A pilot study, J. Am. Diet. Assoc. **63**:27, 1973.

90. Weisenberg, M., and Fray, E.: What's missing in the treatment of obesity by behavior modification? J. Am. Diet. Assoc. **65**:410, 1974.

91. Sloan, C. L., et al.: A weight control program for students using diet and behavior therapy, J. Am. Diet. Assoc. **68**:466, 1976.

92. Cormier, A., and Préfontaine, M.: Does behavior modification work for obese young adults? J. Nutr. Educ. **9**(1):31, 1977.

93. Currey, H., et al.: Behavioral treatment of obesity. Limitations and results with the chronically obese, J.A.M.A. **237**:2829, 1977.

94. Dahms, W. T., et al.: Treatment of obesity: Cost-benefit assessment of behavioral therapy, placebo, and two anorectic drugs, Am. J. Clin. Nutr. **31**:774, 1978.

95. Ritt, R. S., Jordan, H. A., and Levitz, L. S.: Changes in nutrient intake during a behavioral weight control program, J. Am. Diet. Assoc. **74**:325, 1979.

96. Pomerleau, O., Bass, F., and Crown, V.: Role of behavior modification in preventive medicine, N. Engl. J. Med. **292**:1277, 1975.

97. Barlow, D. H., and Tillotson, J. L.: Behavioral science and nutrition: a new perspective, J. Am. Diet. Assoc. **72**:368, 1978.

98. Mahoney, M. J., and Caggiula, A. W.: Applying behavioral methods to nutrition counseling, J. Am. Diet. Assoc. **72**:372, 1978.

99. Evans, R. J., and Hall, Y.: Social-psychologic perspective in motivating changes in eating behavior, J. Am. Diet. Assoc. **72**:378, 1978.

4 Gastrointestinal disorders

DIGESTION

Food must be hydrolyzed into smaller compounds before it can be absorbed by the body. Carbohydrates are converted to monosaccharides, proteins to amino acids, and fats to fatty acids and glycerol. These changes are brought about by enzymes at various sites in the digestive tract.

The major parts of the digestive tract are mouth, esophagus, stomach, the small intestine (duodenum, jejunum, ileum), and the large intestine (cecum, ascending, transverse, descending, sigmoid colon, rectum), which terminates at the anus (Fig. 4-1).

A limited amount of digestion begins in the mouth. Approximately 1 to 1½ L of saliva are secreted by the salivary glands daily. Saliva consists of 99.5% water. The remaining 0.5% contains salivary amylase, proteins, ammonia, amino acids, urea, uric acid, cholesterol, and the ions—calcium, sodium, potassium, magnesium, phosphate, chloride, and bicarbonate. The pH of saliva is 6.8.

Salivary amylase, formerly called ptyalin, is the only digestive enzyme secreted in the mouth. It acts on starch and hydrolyzes the $\alpha1,4$ glucosidic linkages to dextrins. If the action proceeds for a long period of time, maltose can be formed. Chloride ions activate the enzyme, whose optimum pH is 6.6. This digestive action proceeds in the stomach until the acidity destroys the enzyme.

Salivary amylase activity can be measured by determining the achromic point. This is the point at which starch after having been acted on by amylase gives no color with iodine. As starch is broken down by amylase, the color with iodine proceeds from blue to purple to red and finally to colorless.

The other important component in saliva is mucin, which is a glycoprotein. It is responsible for the ropy consistency of saliva. Its function is to lubricate the food and allow it to move more easily from the esophagus into the stomach.

The surface of the stomach is covered with a single layer of epithelium made up of columnar cells. These cells secrete mucus, a mixture of proteins and carbohydrates. This adheres to the surface of the stomach and protects it from endogenous and exogenous substances that might irritate it.

Between the epithelial cells are the pits or openings of the gastric glands. Parietal, chief, mucus, and argentaffin cells make up the gastric gland. They are situated around a central canal into which their secretions are released.

It has been estimated that there are approximately 1 to 1.5 billion parietal cells.[1]

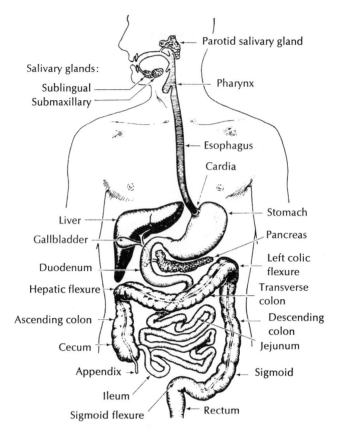

Fig. 4-1. Alimentary canal and associated structures in man. (From Schottelius, B. A., and Schottelius, D. D.: Textbook of physiology, ed. 18, St. Louis, 1978, The C. V. Mosby Co.)

These cells secrete hydrochloric acid. The acid content of the stomach is 100 millimoles per liter for a pH of approximately 1. The parietal cells also produce the intrinsic factor (IF). This glycoprotein is needed for the absorption of vitamin B_{12} in the ileum.

The chief cells secrete the enzyme pepsinogen. This is the inactive form of the enzyme pepsin. Since this enzyme digests protein, it is secreted in the inactive form to prevent the self-digestion of the stomach.

The argentaffin cells are so named because they take up a silver stain. These cells secrete the compound serotonin into the blood. Serotonin has many physiological functions.

Thoughts of food and the taste of it cause the vagus nerve to stimulate the stomach to release gastric juice. When food reaches the stomach, the hormone gastrin is released, and it also initiates the secretion of gastric juice. When the contents of the stomach become acid, gastrin release ceases. Histamine, solutions of amino acids, alcohol, and caffeine stimulate gastric secretion. Another hormone, gastric inhibitory peptide (GIP), inhibits the release of gastric acid.

Approximately 2 to 3 L of gastric juice are secreted into the stomach per day. It is composed of 99% water and 0.5% hydrochloric acid. The remaining 0.5% contains mucin, pepsin, rennin, lipase, and the electrolytes sodium, potassium, chloride, and phosphate. Gastric juice mixes with the extracellular fluid of the stomach that contains, in addition, the electrolytes calcium, magnesium, and bicarbonate.

Most of the digestion in the stomach is concerned with breaking down protein. However, the action of salivary amylase continues in the stomach until it is deactivated by the acid pH. The proenzyme pepsinogen in the presence of hydrochloric acid is converted to pepsin by the removal of a blocking peptide. Pepsin can also activate pepsinogen. This enzyme acts on the aromatic amino acids (phenylalanine, tyrosine) in the protein. The peptide bond is broken on the amino side. The action is rapid, and the protein may be broken up into peptides containing from 2 to 50 amino acids.

Rennin is an enzyme that is important in infants. It coagulates milk by acting on the protein casein. In the presence of calcium ions, calcium paracaseinate or a milk clot (curd) is formed. This slows the passage of milk through the gastrointestinal tract and thus allows more time for the enzymes to act on the milk.

A gastric lipase is secreted by the gastric mucosa. It hydrolyzes fat containing short-or medium-chain fatty acids.

The stomach contents (chyme) are intermittently introduced into the duodenum through the pyloric valve. The pancreatic and bile ducts open into the duodenum near this valve. The secretions from the pancreas and bile are alkaline and thus neutralize the acid chyme. This shift of pH is necessary because the enzymes in pancreatic and intestinal juice are active at an alkaline pH.

An analysis of gastric juice is used as a diagnostic technique. Achlorhydria (absence of free acid and pepsin) occurs in pernicious anemia and carcinoma of the stomach. Decreased levels of hydrochloric acid (hypochlorhydria) are found in carcinoma of the stomach, constipation, chronic gastritis, and appendicitis. Elevated levels of hydrochloric acid (hyperchlorhydria) are seen in gastric and duodenal ulcers and cholecystitis.

Pancreatic juice and bile are released from their respective organs by hormonal action. The presence of hydrochloric acid, fats, proteins, carbohydrates, and partially digested food stuffs results in the secretion of hormones into the duodenum and upper jejunum. These are absorbed from the small intestine through the blood and are carried either to the pancreas, liver, or gallbladder. The hormone secretin stimulates the pancreas to release bicarbonate ions. Cholecystokinin also exhibits the same action, but in addition, it stimulates the release of pancreatic enzymes and causes the gallbladder to contract. Enterocrinin starts the flow of intestinal juice (succus entericus).

Pancreatic juice is a nonviscous watery fluid whose main constituent is water. It contains protein, organic compounds, and the ions—sodium, potassium, calcium, zinc, chloride, bicarbonate, sulfate, and monohydrogen phosphate. The pH of pancreatic juice is alkaline, approximately 7.5 to 8.0. Many digestive enzymes are found in pancreatic juice. The protein-digesting enzymes are secreted in an inactive form to prevent self-digestion.

Trypsinogen is converted to trypsin by the enzyme enterokinase. It acts on the carboxyl side of the peptide linkages of arginine and lysine.[2] The three forms of the enzyme chymotrypsinogen are activated by trypsin to chymotrypsin. All act on the carboxyl side of the peptide linkage. Chymotrypsin A breaks adjacent to the amino acids phenylalanine, tyrosine, and tryptophan; B splits peptide bonds adjacent to leucine; and C splits the bonds next to methionine and glutamine. Procarboxypeptidase is an exopeptidase that is converted to carboxypeptidase by trypsin. There are two forms, A and B. Carboxypeptidase A acts on protein to split off the terminal amino acid, which has a free carboxyl group but has an aromatic or aliphatic side chain. The B enzyme removes basic amino acids only. Thus proteins are broken down into smaller fragments until all peptide bonds are broken and only amino acids are left.

Pancreatic amylase hydrolyzes starch to dextrins and then to maltose.

For fat digestion to proceed, the fat particles must be emulsified. Bile is secreted into the small intestine. The bile salts (sodium taurocholate and sodium glycocholate) in this secretion lower the surface tension of the fat particle and thus emulsify it. Digestion by pancreatic lipase occurs on the interface of the oil and water. Bile salts render the products of enzyme digestion soluble and thus remove them from the site of enzyme action by forming micelles that consist of a mixture of bile salts, fatty acids, and monoglycerides. These micelles are taken up by the intestinal mucosal cells. Bile salts inhibit the resynthesis of triglycerides from fatty acids and monoglycerides, thus promoting the breakdown of triglycerides into fatty acids and glycerol.[3]

Approximately 3 L of intestinal juice are secreted every day. Aminopeptidase acts on the peptide linkage of the terminal amino acid with a free amine group and splits it off. Other peptidases act on the peptides to yield finally amino acids.

Disaccharides are broken down into monosaccharides. Maltase acts on maltose from starch digestion to produce glucose. Lactose (milk sugar) is converted to glucose and galactose by lactase. Sucrose is hydrolyzed by sucrase to glucose and fructose.

Food is moved through the intestines by peristalsis. These rhythmic contractions mix the digestive enzymes with the food and move it along. Monosaccharides, dipeptides, amino acids, glycerol, and fatty acids are absorbed in the small intestine. Water is absorbed from the undigested food and wastes in the large intestine.

ABSORPTION

The small intestine is approximately 300 cm (10 ft) long but has an absorbing area larger than half a basketball court.[4] This is a result of an invagination of the inner surface of the small intestine to form fingerlike projections called villi. There are 5 ×

10^6 villi in the intestine of man with about 30 per square millimeters of mucosa.[5] These range in size from 0.5 to 1.5 mm long.[4] The surface area of each of these villi contain bristles or microvilli 1 μm long and 0.1 μm wide. These are referred to as the brush border.

The lining of the intestinal lumen consists of one layer of epithelial cells, beneath which is the lamina propria. This is made up of capillaries and lacteals embedded in connective tissue. Substances must pass from the lumen through the lipoprotein membrane of the intestinal cell into the lamina propria. Pores also appear along the epithelial membrane. The small molecules are able to pass through these small holes.

The end products of digestion are for the most part too large to pass through the pores. Passive diffusion occurs because of the difference in concentration gradients but ceases when the concentration on both sides of the membrane is equal. It is postulated that carriers transport water-soluble substances across the lipoprotein membrane but do not enter the intestinal epithelial cell. Sodium ions move from the lumen into the lamina propria even though the solutions on both sides of the membrane are isotonic. This sets up a positive charge and causes the movement of ions from the lumen into the mucosa. This process requires energy in that adenosine triphosphate (ATP) is needed to remove sodium from the cell.

The brush border of the villi in the jejunum contains most of the disaccharidases that hydrolyze the disaccharides into monosaccharides. Of the monosaccharides, glucose and galactose are thought to be actively and passively absorbed. Both compete for the same carrier. Fructose undergoes diffusion into the mucosal cell, where it is metabolized to glucose and lactic acid.

Dipeptides and amino acids are also absorbed by diffusion and active transport. Pyridoxal phosphate is needed for active transport.

Another substance that needs a carrier for absorption is vitamin B_{12}. The intrinsic factor, a glycoprotein, is elaborated in the stomach. It brings vitamin B_{12} to the receptor sites in the ileum, where it is absorbed.

The monosaccharides, amino acids, and fatty acids of 10-carbon atoms or less are absorbed directly into the capillaries. The capillaries empty into the portal vein, which brings the nutrients directly to the liver. The longer chain fatty acids and monoglycerides in the mucosal cell are resynthesized into triglycerides. Cholesterol and a lipoprotein coat are added to these particles, called chylomicrons. These are absorbed into the lacteals of the lymphatic system. At the juncture of the thoracic duct and the subclavian vein the chylomicrons enter the circulation.

DISORDERS OF THE ESOPHAGUS
Achalasia

In achalasia a neural disturbance dilates the esophagus. The lower end gradually narrows in diameter. Peristalsis is absent, and the lower esophageal sphincter does not open.[6] The individual experiences difficulty in swallowing (dysphagia).

Prior to treatment only soft or liquid foods at moderate temperatures are allowed.

The muscles in the lower esophageal sphincter are either dilated or slit by means of surgery to allow food to be swallowed more easily.

Esophagitis

The inflammation of the esophagus is a result of the reflux of gastric juice. It may be caused by a short esophagus, excessive vomiting, hiatus hernia, or the inability to empty the stomach. The initial symptoms are dysphagia, substernal pain, and hypochromic anemia. Later there is hemorrhaging and stricture.

Normally the lower esophageal sphincter (LES) maintains a higher pressure on the esophagus than is found in the stomach. This prevents the reflux of the acid gastric contents into the esophagus. If the pressure is low, regurgitation can occur.

Hormones and various foods affect this pressure.[7] Gastrin increases the LES pressure, while secretin and cholecystokinin have the opposite effect. Protein, which stimulates the release of gastrin, also increases the LES pressure. Other foods that cause heartburn such as citrus juices and spicy foods do not lower the LES pressure. It is suggested that the effect may be due to a direct irritation rather than a lowering of the pressure.

Treatment involves antacids to decrease gastric acidity and a diet similar to that for ulcer patients, namely, bland and fiber restricted. Small frequent feedings are necessary.

Hiatus hernia

In this condition the stomach passes through the esophageal hiatus of the diaphragm into the thoracic cavity. Coughing, lifting, bending, or eating precipitate pain behind the sternum. Reflux of the stomach contents may lead to heartburn, dysphagia, or gastrointestinal bleeding. Pulmonary and cardiac symptoms may also appear.

Antacids such as aluminum hydroxide and magnesium oxide are given between and after meals. The effects of gastric acidity can also be reduced by avoiding alcohol, coffee, and tobacco.[8] Liquids should be consumed between meals. Bland fiber-restricted diets with between-meal feedings are prescribed. Foods with a high-fat content should be restricted, since they stimulate the release of secretin, a hormone that increases gastroesophageal reflux.[9] Large amounts of food should not be consumed at any one time. If the individual is obese, a reduction diet is necessary. In some instances surgical repair may be required to alleviate the symptoms.

DISORDERS OF THE STOMACH
Gastritis

Gastritis is an inflammation of the mucosa of the stomach. It may be acute or chronic. Acute gastritis is caused by bacterial infections or toxins, viral infections, chemical irritants, or allergy. The only symptom may be anorexia. No food or liquids are allowed until pain and nausea have ceased. During this time parenteral feeding is needed. A clear liquid diet is followed by a soft bland diet as tolerated.

The cause of chronic gastritis is unknown. It is often found in conjunction with gastric carcinoma, pernicious anemia, excessive ingestion of aspirin, diabetes mellitus, thyroid disease, and pituitary and adrenal insufficiency. Recurrent inflammation leads to an atrophy of the gastric glands with a decrease in the secretion of hydrochloric acid and enzymes.

The patient may be asymptomatic or have mild nausea, pain, or discomfort on eating. No specific treatment is prescribed. Foods that produce symptoms and alcohol, caffeine, and aspirin should be avoided. A bland diet may be helpful to some. Antacids are prescribed to neutralize gastric acidity.

Gastric carcinoma

Cancer of the stomach is the second most common form found in the digestive tract. It appears mainly in men over 40 years of age. In the early stages there are no symptoms. Individuals with gastritis, gastric ulcer, or achlorhydria may develop gastric carcinoma. If it is detected early, a surgical resection can be performed. The dumping syndrome may develop after surgery (see postgastrectomy syndrome). When the carcinoma is inoperable, small frequent feedings low in fiber should be used. It is important to provide foods that are appetizing to the patient.

Peptic ulcer

A peptic ulcer is an erosion of a portion of the mucosal lining of the digestive tract that has been in contact with gastric juice. Those that occur in the stomach are called gastric ulcers. These are found predominantly in males over the age of 40. Most of the duodenal ulcers appear in the first 2 cm of the duodenum. The average age at onset is 33 years. Again men are more susceptible than women. In general these individuals experience epigastric distress about 1 hour after eating or at night. The pain is relieved by food, antacids, or vomiting. X-ray films are used to confirm the presence of an ulcer.

The etiology of peptic ulcer is not completely understood. One of the factors that has been implicated is the overproduction of gastric acid. Hypersecretion may be caused by an increase in parietal cell mass. Normal individuals have about 1 billion parietal cells, whereas ulcer patients have two to four times that number.[10] Overstimulation of the vagus nerve causes the parietal cells to release more acid. The hormone gastrin, which is released by the mechanical stimulation of food in the antrum of the stomach, also promotes acid secretion. Although fasting levels of gastrin are the same in normal and ulcer patients, levels in ulcer patients are elevated after they have eaten.[11] Histamine increases the blood flow through the gastric mucosa, and thus it promotes parietal cell secretions. Alcohol and caffeine act as stimulants on parietal cells.

There are two immunochemically distinct pepsinogens: pepsinogen I and pepsinogen II. Elevated levels of pepsinogen I have been found in some patients with duodenal ulcer. Rotter and his co-workers measured pepsinogen I by radioimmuno-assay in two families with a history of duodenal ulcer.[12] The results suggested that elevated levels of this enzyme are inherited as an autosomal dominant trait, and this is a marker for the genetic predisposition to duodenal ulcer. It is hypothesized that hyperpepsinogenemia is a result of an increased mass of chief cells, which in turn is associated with an increase in parietal cells that produce acid.[12,13] The increased levels of acid and pepsin in conjunction with a decrease in mucosal resistance predispose the individual to the development of an ulcer.

Ulcers have been found in individuals with diseases that result in gastric hypersecretion, namely, hyperparathyroid disease, chronic pulmonary disease, diabetes mellitus, central nervous system disease, and collagen vascular disease.[10]

Decreased tissue resistance may arise from a decrease in mucus production. The mucosal protective barrier of the stomach can no longer function. The administration of "ulcerogenic drugs" such as salicylates, phenylbutazone, cinchophen, corticosteroids, and reserpine interferes with the production of mucus.[10]

Psychological aspects are also important since emotional stress and pressure may predispose the individual to hypersecretion of acid. Ulcers tend to appear in tense, competitive individuals.

Alcohol and caffeine increase the secretion of gastric acid and thus may make an individual susceptible to peptic ulcer. The role of cigarette smoking is not completely understood. Friedman and his co-workers reported a greater incidence of peptic ulcers both in men and women cigarette smokers.[14] Both alcohol and coffee consumption correlated with smoking, but the consumption of either beverage was not related to the incidence of ulcers. Since coffee or alcohol may precipitate ulcer symptoms, it is possible that individuals restrict their own intake and thus no correlation was observed.

Men who were either smokers or coffee drinkers while in college showed a greater risk of developing ulcers in later life.[15] Those who smoked and also drank coffee showed an even greater risk. However, coffee consumption was found to be a better predictor than smoking of the risk of developing an ulcer.

Medical treatment. During the acute phase both physical and mental rest are prescribed. Alcohol, aspirin, and smoking should be avoided. Sedation may be necessary for extremely tense individuals.

Since the buffering of gastric contents lasts for only 1 to 2 hours after a meal, antacids are prescribed. The drugs are taken hourly during the day for 2 weeks and then four doses daily for an additional 2 to 4 weeks.[16] Duodenal ulcers may heal within 6 weeks. Several different types of antacids are used: sodium bicarbonate, calcium carbonate, aluminum hydroxide, magnesium hydroxide, and magnesium-aluminum mixtures; however, side effects will occur if any of these are used in excess.[16,17] Sodium bicarbonate is effective in neutralizing the hydrochloric acid of gastric juice for only a short time. An excess can cause alkalosis. In addition, it should not be taken by patients with heart and kidney disease who must restrict their sodium intake. Although calcium carbonate functions as an effective antacid, it can cause hypercalcemia, impaired renal function, and constipation. It was also shown to increase gastrin and gastric juice secretion.[18] Aluminum hydroxide gels bind phosphates and create a phosphate deficiency. Bone resorption, increased calcium absorption, hypercalciuria, renal stone formation, and constipation have been noted after administration of large doses. Magnesium hydroxide causes diarrhea and can be toxic to patients in renal failure. Hendrix suggested that mixtures of magnesium and aluminum hydroxide would be best for the treatment of peptic ulcers.[19] However, this has not been proved clinically.

Anticholingeric drugs are administered hourly to block the vagal stimulation of parietal cells and thus diminish the secretion of gastric juice.[10] Gastric emptying is delayed, and this allows the antacid to remain in the stomach for a longer period of time. Other drugs under study are 16,16-methylated prostaglandin E_2 and the histamine H_2-receptor antagonist metiamide.[20] Metiamide inhibits gastric acid and pepsin secretion and has given ulcer patients relief from their symptoms.[21,22]

Cimetidine (Tagamet), another histamine H_2-receptor antagonist, is currently being used to treat peptic ulcers, as it causes less serious side effects than the anticholinergics and prostaglandins.

Diet therapy. Diet therapy has been the subject of much controversy. In 1915 Sippy prescribed hourly feedings of 84 ml (3 oz) of equal parts of milk and cream for bleeding ulcers.[23] After 2 to 3 days soft eggs and strained cereals were added. Then bland and easily digested foods such as custards, cream soups, and vegetable purees replaced or were added to the milk-cream mixture. No one feeding contained more than 168 ml (6 oz). Meulengracht in 1935 prescribed a more liberal diet.[24] It consisted of milk, eggs, custard, ice cream, gelatin, pudding, crackers, bread, butter, pureed fruits, and vegetables. After 48 hours ground meats and fish were included. Spices, pickles, nuts, pastries, coffee, tea, soft drinks, and alcohol were not permitted. The Andresen diet consisted of a mixture of meat, cream, gelatin, and glucose (168 g [6 oz]) given every 2 hours.[25] On the fifth or sixth day an egg or 84 g (3 oz) of cereal, custard, gelatin, or ice cream were added to three or four of the daily feedings. This was followed by a bland diet.

For many years ulcer dietotherapy followed a conservative approach. The patient progressed through a series of bland diets, in some cases as many as four. Foods that were chemically, mechanically, and thermally irritating were to be avoided. This provided physiological rest for the stomach. Thus the patient started with a bland I diet, or the Sippy diet, which consisted of hourly feedings of milk. The patient progressed to a bland II diet, which was comprised of small frequent feedings primarily of milk and dairy products throughout the day. Meat, fish, poultry, fried foods, fruits, fruit juices, and certain vegetables were not allowed. The bland III diet was a more liberal diet in that more foods were allowed, but foods strongly flavored, spicy, fried, or fibrous, fruit juices, raw fruits, and vegetables were not permitted. The bland IV diet contained even fewer restrictions, and patients were advised to avoid spicy and fibrous foods such as whole grains. None of the diets permitted coffee.

Such diets were not understood by some patients who followed a more restrictive diet than was prescribed.[26] Ulcer patients (152) and some of their wives (30) were asked to categorize a list of 43 foods as good or bad for an ulcer. More than 90% rated milk, soft-boiled eggs, toast, baked potatoes, oatmeal, butter, baby food, custard and cottage cheese as good. Less than 10% classed pop, sausage, onions, fried potatoes, salami, and chili as good for ulcers. Fat or fried, seasoned or spicy, rough or scratchy, and acid or gassy foods were classed as bad for ulcers. Some patients based the harmfulness of a food on the symptoms it caused upon ingestion. Others eliminated foods they thought kept the stomach from being scratched or irritated. Many patients did not understand that the aim of diet therapy was to decrease the secretion of acid. As a result they followed diets that were very strict. Fats were omitted from the diet since they were felt to be difficult to digest when, in fact, fats are prescribed to decrease gastric motility and acid secretion.

In a later study ulcer patients (92), their wives (30), dietitians (42), physicians (41), college students (27), and nonulcer patients (30) were asked to check a list of 43 foods as to whether each was good or bad for an ulcer diet.[27] Most of the ulcer patients agreed on their designation of foods as good or bad. The following nine foods were checked as good by about 90% of the ulcer patients: milk, soft-boiled eggs, toast, baked potatoes, oatmeal, butter, strained baby food, custard, and cottage cheese. Eleven foods were considered bad by over 90%: salami, fried potatoes, gassy foods, fatty foods, onions, sausage, pop-cola, cabbage, fried eggs, chili, and acid foods. These findings were similar to the earlier study. The selections of foods by the other groups surveyed were similar to those of the ulcer patients. Patients still held to a restricted diet even though current diet therapy had been liberalized.

The previous rationale for the restrictive diets for ulcer patients has had little scientific basis. Many of the practices have been attributed to folklore.[28] In addition, bland diets differ from one hospital to another. A bland food is interpreted as one that has a particular color, consistency, and taste.[28] However, the appearance of a food prior to ingestion has nothing to do with its effect on the gastrointestinal tract.

The American Medical Association and the American Dietetic Association proposed that foods with a pH of 4 or less and those that are irritating should be restricted in inflammatory or ulcerative states of the esophagus or stomach.[29] Protein and moderate amounts of fat are recommended for chronic peptic disorders resulting from excessive gastric acidity. All other restrictions are unnecessary.

The 1971 position paper of the American Dietetic Association on the bland diet for the treatment of chronic ulcer disease discusses some of the controversies.[30] Many spices, condiments, and highly seasoned foods have been found nonirritating to the gastric mucosa. Therefore, only black pepper, chili powder, caffeine, coffee, tea, cocoa, alcohol, and certain drugs that are irritating should be restricted for the ulcer patient. Milk has been the basis for many ulcer diets. It has been prescribed to reduce and neutralize the acid stomach contents. Proteins do function as buffers for a period of time, but they also stimulate the secretion of acid. The amino acid histidine is decarboxylated to histamine, which is a potent stimulator of gastric juice.

Ippoliti et al. found that whole, low-fat, and nonfat milk increased gastric acid secretion in normal and duodenal ulcer patients.[31] Low-calcium milk increased acid secretion in the ulcer patients but not in the normal individuals. It is known that both protein and calcium stimulate gastric acid secretion. In addition, the combination of milk and the antacid calcium carbonate may lead to the development of the milk-alkali syndrome. Therefore the authors questioned the frequent use of milk in patients with peptic ulcer.

Caffeine is known to be a potent stimulator of gastric acid secretion and therefore is not permitted in peptic ulcer diets. Decaffeinated coffee, on the other hand, has been allowed in some diets. However, it has been found that both coffee and decaffeinated coffee are more potent stimulators of acid secretion than caffeine.[32] In addition, coffee and decaffeinated coffee increase the lower esophageal sphincter pressure, whereas the effect of caffeine is minimal. In another study caffeine was found to decrease the pressure.[7] However, other substances in regular or decaffeinated coffee may be potent stimulators of gastric acid secretion. Therefore both regular and decaffeinated coffee should be banned from peptic ulcer diets.

There is no evidence that foods high in roughage such as fruit skins, celery, lettuce, and nuts should be omitted from a peptic ulcer diet. However, if the individual is not able to chew well, then these foods must be well ground.

Fats should be included in the diet since they inhibit gastric secretion. Gastric motility is decreased and food remains in the stomach for a longer time. This allows, for more neutralization of gastric acid. There is no evidence that cream is more effective than other fats or fried foods. All fats have the same effect.

It has been suggested that gas-producing foods should be avoided. There is little data available as to the amount of gas that is generated by foods in the gastrointestinal tract. A more reasonable approach is to allow the individual a free choice of foods. Those that produce discomfort are quickly removed from the diet. When this approach is followed, the ulcers heal more rapidly.

Currently the Sippy diet is used to treat the acute phase of an active ulcer. Alternate feedings of milk and antacids are prescribed. There is evidence of an increased tendency to coronary thrombosis in ulcer patients.[33] This has resulted in the substitution of skim milk for the milk and cream. Polyunsaturated oils can be added to the milk. Since the diet is nutritionally inadequate, the patient proceeds to a bland diet with between-meal feedings to provide maximum neutralization of acid secretion. Generally the patient is the best judge of which foods he can tolerate. A severely restricted diet that the patient cannot follow only leads to stress, and this aggravates his condition. Sapp suggested that the content of meals is not as important as the regularity, and antacids are the important part of the treatment.[10] Tumen stated that bad habits, such as spacing of meals and eating too much and too fast, contribute to gastrointestinal dysfunction. Teaching a patient how to eat is more important than what he eats.[34]

In 1975 Welsh surveyed 326 hospital dietitians as to the diets prescribed for peptic ulcer patients.[35] The following were listed in the diet manuals: 5% specific peptic ulcer diet, 45% modified Sippy diet, and 72% some gradations of a bland diet, of which 73% has three or four gradations. Eighty-two of the later diets were selected for analysis. Bland I diets in sixty-four manuals were comprised only of milk feedings. The bland II, III, IV diets were compared as to whether 14 food items were or were not permitted. Bland II was the most restrictive diet, and in the majority of manuals the 14 food items (meat, poultry, fish, fruit, fruit juices, chocolate, cocoa, decaffeinated coffee, fried foods, lunch meats, nuts, tea, coffee, and carbonated drinks) were not allowed. The majority of hospitals did not permit the last six food items on a bland IV diet.

The survey revealed many differences in ulcer dietotherapy. Welsh commented that bland diets are routinely prescribed, yet there is no evidence that these diets are more effective in healing peptic ulcers. In most diets, milk, decaffeinated coffee, and frequent feedings were advocated, yet all of these tend to increase secretion of gastric acid. This information must be made available to all those who are treating ulcer patients. It was also found that lactose malabsorption was rarely considered when diets were issued for patients with peptic ulcer. [36] Further research is needed to determine what dietary restrictions are necessary for the ulcer patient.

Complications. Perforation of a duodenal ulcer occurs more frequently than with gastric ulcers. Immediate surgery is necessary.

Obstruction may be caused by spasm, edema, or scar tissue. Only the scar tissue must be treated by surgery.

When the ulcer hemorrhages, a nasogastric tube is passed into the stomach for suctioning. If the bleeding is excessive, a larger tube is inserted and the stomach is washed out with iced saline or water. When the bleeding stops, milk with an antacid is administered hourly.[10] Blood transfusions are given as needed. Surgery is initiated after 48 hours if the hemorrhaging has not stopped. It may also be recommended for persons with repeated episodes of severe bleeding.

Surgery. Several surgical procedures have been devised for gastric carcinoma and peptic ulcer. There is no general consensus as to which operation is the best.[37] Generally a vagotomy is also performed when a duodenal ulcer is present. The severing of the vagus nerve disrupts the stimulation of parietal cells and thus decreases the amount of gastric juice that is released.

Four general types of gastric surgery have been employed.[38,39] A total gastrectomy is performed in patients with proximal gastric cancer and those with the Zollinger-Ellison syndrome (peptic ulceration in conjuction with a tumor of the pancreas). The esophagus is connected to the jejunum. A subtotal gastrectomy (Billroth II) is used in cases of distal gastric carcinoma and proximal gastric ulcers. This involves a 75% gastric resection and gastrojejunostomy. Antrectomy (Billroth I) involves the removal of 50% to 60% of the stomach. The remaining part is anastomosed to the duodenum. This procedure has been used for duodenal and distal gastric ulcers. The safest operation is vagotomy and pyloroplasty. By this method gastric juice production is diminished and drainage is established.

Postgastrectomy syndrome. After gastric surgery some patients may experience the dumping syndrome, reactive hypoglycemia, and diarrhea. This is referred to as the postgastrectomy syndrome.[38] The stomach is not large enough to hold the food, and thus it is passed into the duodenum 10 to 15 minutes after ingestion. The individual experiences nausea, dizziness, sweating, pallor, tachycardia, abdominal cramps, and weakness. The presence of hyperosmolar chyme in the jejunum causes a flow of fluid from the surrounding plasma and extracellular tissues. As a result, blood volume and pressure drop. Carbohydrates are rapidly digested and absorbed. The pancreas releases additional insulin, and within 2 to 3 hours hypoglycemia occurs.

Factors other than rapid glucose absorption might be responsible for the hypoglycemia seen in individuals who have had gastric surgery.[40] More insulin was released when glucose was administered orally or intraintestinally rather than intravenously in subjects who had undergone gastric surgery. Those individuals who were hypoglycemic after oral glucose loads were shown to have higher serum insulin levels. It is known that gastric inhibitory peptide and glucagon stimulate insulin secretion. The authors suggested that these hormones were secreted in excessive amounts in postgastrectomy patients and thus were responsible for the hypoglycemia. Glucose tolerance tests may not be useful in diagnosing chemical diabetes mellitus in such patients.

The syndrome can be alleviated by dietary means. Small frequent feedings that are high in protein, moderate in fat, and low in carbohydrate should be given. Concentrated sweets should be avoided. Liquids should be consumed between meals.

INTESTINAL DISORDERS
Regional enteritis (Crohn's disease, terminal ileitis)

Regional enteritis is a disease of unknown etiology that appears most frequently in young adults. The ileum becomes chronically inflamed and filled with granulomas. Occasionally the colon and duodenum become involved. The individual experiences cramps, diarrhea, fever, anorexia, and weight loss. The symptoms may be aggravated by the ingestion of milk, milk products, and foods that are chemically and mechanically irritating.

The initial dietary treatment consists of a high-calorie, high-protein diet low in residue. Raw fruits and vegetables should be excluded. Vitamin supplements are administered.

Eight patients with Crohn's disease were fed by total parenteral nutrition for 1 month.[41] The solution provided daily 3000 to 3500 kcal, 150 to 175 g of protein, electrolytes, and vitamins. Iron, vitamin K, folic acid, and vitamin B_{12} were not included in the preparation but instead were administered as needed. Every 10 days two eggs were given to stimulate the gallbladder. The patients experienced relief of pain, improvement of their diarrhea, and an average weight gain of 10.4 kg (23 lb). Calcium malabsorption has been found infrequently in individuals with Crohn's disease.[42]

Irritable colon syndrome (spastic syndrome)

The irritable colon syndrome is characterized by abdominal pain, constipation, and diarrhea. It appears in tense individuals who tend to eat irregular meals, overuse laxatives, and get inadequate rest. The normal peristaltic action of the colon is replaced by irregular contractions that do not move the intestinal contents along. Constipation is caused by spasms, increased water absorption, and decreased motility. On the other hand, diarrhea results when there is a decrease in absorption of water and increased contractions. Abdominal pain is caused by the accumulation of gas, spasms, and the increase in contractions.

An important part of therapy is the establishment of regular habits. It may be necessary to restrict the intake of alcohol and smoking. Mild sedation or tranquilizers may be prescribed.

The dietary treatment varies from individual to individual. Milk and milk products may be irritating to some patients with diarrhea. To alleviate constipation, bulk should be provided in the diet. However, large amounts of raw fruits and vegetables promote peristalsis, and this should be avoided. Piepmeyer administered 40 to 50 ml (8 to 10 rounded tsp) of unprocessed bran to 30 patients with irritable bowel syndrome for 4 months.[43] Twenty-three of them showed improvement in that their bowel habits became more regular, and there was a decrease in abdominal distention and cramps. Texter and Butler also advocate a high-fiber diet that contains a large amount of unprocessed bran.[44]

Diverticular disease

Diverticula are small sacs that protrude through weak spots in the muscle of the colon. A high intraluminal pressure forces these pouches through the wall. This syndrome is called spastic colon diverticulosis and is thought to precede irritable bowel syndrome.[45]

In diverticulitis the sacs become filled with food residues, and bacterial action leads to inflammation. Perforation or abscess formation can occur. The symptoms include lower abdominal pain, abdominal distention, spasm, fever, and constipation. Diverticular disease was unknown before the twentieth century but has now become common in Western civilizations.[46] The incidence is related to the economic development in the country, and thus is rare in developing countries. The economic improvement has paralleled a change from a high- to a low-residue diet; therefore, Painter and Burkitt concluded that diverticular disease was due to a deficiency of fiber.[46] For 50 years the treatment has been a low-residue diet. Yet in many patients with diverticular disease, bran relieved abdominal aching, pain, and distention.

High-fiber diets have been prescribed for diverticulosis. When diverticulitis develops, a low-residue diet and antibiotics are prescribed. If the individual does not respond to these measures, then surgery may be necessary.

Diets low in residue tend to contract the colon more tightly and so compound the problem by increasing intraluminal pressures. On the other hand, high-residue diets distend the wall of the colon and relieve the pressure. Bulk agents have been used in the past to relieve the symptoms. Goldstein suggested that large quantities of raw fruits and vegetables should be avoided because of their laxative effect.[45] He also suggested that the low-residue diets are responsible for the increase in noninfective bowel disease in the developed nations. This is probably a result of the increased intraluminal pressures caused by such diets.

Connell suggested that there are two distinct forms of diverticular disease: one in which there is a thickening of the muscle and narrowing of the colon with a resulting high intracolonic pressure, and the second in which the muscle is not thickened and intracolonic pressure is not elevated.[47] Fiber has been found to decrease intracolonic pressure after eating; others have reported a decreased pressure in the resting state. Different fibers may have different effects on pressure and influence other factors such as transit time. Fiber may act primarily through increasing the bulk of the stool, influencing gastric emptying and excretion of bile acids, and stimulating enzymes and hormones of the small intestine.

Plumley and Francis treated 48 patients suffering from spastic colon diverticulosis with a high-fiber crispbread made from 52% wheat gluten, 7% wheat flour, and 41% wheat bran.[48] The patients consumed six slices daily of the crispbread, which contained 16% total unavailable carbohydrate. On this regimen 71% reported that their symptoms (pain, alteration in bowel habit, and mucus) were controlled satisfactorily. When they consumed a standard crispbread with a 0.5% total unavailable carbohydrate, the symptoms reappeared.

For 1 month patients with symptomatic diverticular disease received either a high-roughage diet with bran supplements, a bulk laxative with an antispasmodic, or 18 g of bran as tablets that were taken throughout the day.[49] The treatments were crossed over; those on bran tablets received a high-roughage diet or a bulk laxative, and the others received bran. The bran tablets were the most effective treatment, resulting in an increased daily stool weight, decreased intestinal time, and improvement of symptoms.

The crude fiber intake of 40 patients with diverticular disease was significantly lower (2.6 g per day) than that of a control group (5.2 g per day).[50] For 6 months patients with diverticular disease were treated with 24 g of wheat bran daily. Those with an uncomplicated form of the disease reported fewer symptoms and improved colonic function, namely an increase in stool weight, change in transit time, and a reduced intraluminal pressure.

In another study lasting 3 months, patients eating 6.7 g of fiber per day from bran crispbread reported fewer symptoms than those consuming 0.6 g of fiber from a wheat crispbread.[51]

However, other researchers have found that fiber has no effect on irritable bowel syndrome. After an initial 3-week control period, patients consumed either a placebo or muffins containing 12 g of bran daily for two 6-week periods.[52] Subjective improvement was noted during the initial control period and in those patients with intermediate transit times when they received bran.

In a double-blind study, patients with irritable bowel or mild diverticular disease were divided into two groups.[53] One group received wheat biscuits with a small amount of bran, and the others received biscuits with a total of 30 g of bran daily. After 6 weeks there was no difference in symptoms between the two groups.

Ulcerative colitis

In this disease abscesses, hyperemia, edema, and hemorrhages appear in the mucosa of the colon. The etiology of the disease, which is found primarily in young adults, is unknown. The symptoms are bloody diarrhea, anemia, weight loss, and abdominal pain. Some individuals cannot tolerate milk products. This suggests that the disease may be caused by food allergies. Others have noted that it is more common in tense individuals.

Adrenocorticoid hormones and sulfonamides are prescribed along with mild sedatives. A bland, high-protein, high-calorie diet is prescribed initially. During the acute phase when diarrhea is present, dairy products and wheat should be eliminated from the diet.

FIBER

Recent interest has been focused on the nondigestible portion of the dietary fiber. Epidemiological evidence seems to suggest that a lack of fiber may play a role in the increased incidence of diverticular disease, appendicitis, hiatal hernia, bowel cancer, gallstones, constipation, hemorrhoids, varicose veins, atherosclerosis, diabetes mellitus, obesity, and dental caries.[54] In addition to these, ulcerative colitis, Crohn's disease, ischemic heart disease, deep vein thrombosis, cholecystitis, peridontal disease, and duodenal ulcer have been classed as fiber deficiency diseases.[55]

Definition

Dietary fiber is a complex mixture of a variety of substances that are difficult to measure. It cannot be defined precisely, and as a result many definitions have been proposed. The first term used was "crude fiber," the residue that remains after plant material is extracted with a series of chemicals. Crude fiber consists of cellulose, hemicellulose A, hemicellulose B, pectic substances, and the noncarbohydrate lignin.[56] Hemicellulose A is a polymer consisting of xylose, galactose, glucose, mannose, and arabinose units. Hemicellulose B contains these sugars plus the uronic acid derivatives. Lignin in the plant cell is made up of phenylpropane units. As the plant cell ages, the lignin content increases. Unavailable carbohydrate refers to the plant polysaccharides that are not hydrolyzed in the digestive tract, therefore excluding lignin.

The term "dietary fiber" refers to plant residues and plant cell walls that are resistant to animal digestive enzymes.[57] Others consider that dietary fiber also includes the residues that remain after digestion of animal foods. For the most part, the mixture found in dietary fiber consists of the structural components of the plant cell wall (noncellulosic polysaccharides, cellulose, lignin) and nonstructural polysaccharides (gums, mucilages, algal polysaccharides, modified celluloses, and other substances such as protein, lipids, waxes, cutins, etc.).[58]

Trowell has proposed that the term "dietary fiber complex" be used to include the components of dietary fiber (structural polymers, cellulose, matrix polysaccharides, and lignin) plus all the other chemical substances associated with and around the structural polymers (phytates, nitrogen-containing material, complex unavailable lipids, minerals, and trace elements).[59]

The undigested plant materials form a matrix in the digestive system of humans. The action of colonic bacteria on this matrix results in many physiological effects. The term "plantix" has been suggested as a combination of the words plant and matrix.[60] Plantix consists of cellulose, hemicellulose, mucilages, pectins, gums, and lignin. The plantix content has been approximated by measuring pectin and neutral detergent fiber (cellulose + hemicellulose + lignin).

Measurement of fiber

Crude fiber is the residue of plant material that remains after treatment with sulfuric acid, sodium hydroxide, water, alcohol, and ether. It consists primarily of cellulose and lignin. By this method 50% to 90% of lignin, 85% of hemicellulose, and 0% to 50% of cellulose are lost.[61] There is little relationship between crude and dietary fiber. Food composition tables contain crude fiber values; therefore, it is very difficult to calculate true dietary fiber intakes from this data.

Three basic methods are used to estimate the dietary fiber content of foods.[62] Biochemical analysis involves separating the fiber components and hydrolyzing the carbohydrates into hexoses, pentoses, and uronic acids. These are then analyzed separately and the values totaled. This procedure is time consuming and costly. In the second method the food is treated with digestive enzymes, and the remaining indigestible residue is dietary fiber. The third method uses chemicals to separate the fiber components. The acid-detergent method developed by Van Soest primarily measures lignin and cellulose.[63] Neutral-detergent fiber essentially is composed of lignin, cellulose, and hemicellulose. The approximate hemicellulose content is obtained by subtracting the amount of acid-detergent fiber from that of neutral-detergent fiber. Pectin is removed by these extractions and must be analyzed separately.

Consumption

The crude fiber intake in the United States is about 8 to 11 g per day, whereas in Great Britain it is about 4 to 8 g per day. It may be as high as 12 to 24 g per day in vegetarians.[56] The major source of dietary fiber is whole grain. Wheat grain is composed of the outer coat or bran, 25%; endosperm, 72%; and the germ or embryo, 3%. Bran consists of 6% cellulose, 24% hemicellulose, and 4% lignin. Milling operations remove most of the fiber in the endosperm. Whole wheat bread contains 1.6% crude fiber, while white bread has 0.2%, and bran has 9%. Fruits and vegetables contain about 0.5% to 1% crude fiber. This amount is further reduced by processing.

Food consumption patterns in the twentieth century have changed. There has been a decrease in the consumption of whole wheat flour from 72 kg (160 lb) per capita in 1900 to 45 kg (100 lb) in 1970.[64] The use of processed fruits and vegetables has increased from 29.5 kg (65 lb) in 1940 to 50 kg (110 lb) per capita in 1970, while there has been a decline in the use of fresh fruits and vegetables in this same period (114 kg [250 lb] per capita to 81 kg [180 lb]). Scala has estimated that the dietary fiber intake has dropped by about five to one in this century.[45] The greatest change has been in the consumption of cereal fiber.

However, Heller and Hackler calculated the crude fiber intake from food consumption data and found that in 1909, 6.8 g per day was ingested, and presently 4.9 g per day are being consumed.[65] The greatest decline has been in the use of potatoes, fruits, cereals, dry peas, and beans. The consumption of vegetables decreased slightly, but the amount of nuts ingested increased.

Digestion

It has been found that various fractions of dietary fiber can be digested in different segments of the gastrointestinal tract. Polysaccharides are fermented by the microbial flora.[66] The breakdown products are the volatile fatty acids—acetic, propionic, and butyric—hydrogen, methane, and carbon dioxide. Approximately 50% of the fiber can be digested, but there is great individual variation.

The digestion of cellulose, hemicellulose, and lignin was studied in normal subjects and in those who had ileostomies.[67] Fiber components were extracted from the feces for analysis. It was found that 84.5% of cellulose digestion occurred mainly in the large bowel, whereas 96% of hemicellulose digestion took place in the small bowel.

Physiological function

The addition of fiber to the diet modifies gut motility. Generally there is an increase in fecal output with an increasing excretion of fecal energy from fat and nitrogen sources. A decrease in transit time has also been observed.[54] Yet in some instances transit time has increased or has not been affected. In addition, bran inhibits the action of bacteria on bile salts and thus may prevent the formation of

Table 4-1. Classification of dietary fiber by structure and human physiological function*

Fiber class	Chemical structure of main chain	Human function†
I. Noncellulosic polysaccharides		
A. Gums (secretions)	Galacturonic acid, mannose	1. May slow gastric emptying
	Galacturonic acid, rhamnose	2. Provides fermentable substrate for colonic bacteria with produc-
B. Mucilages (secretions, plant seeds)	Galactose, mannose	tion of gas and volatile fatty acids
	Galacturonic acid, rhamnose	
	Arabinose, xylose	3. Binds bile acids variably
C. Algar polysaccharides (from algae and seaweeds)	Mannose, xylose, glucuronic acid, glucose	
D. Pectin substances (intercellular cement)	Galacturonic acid	
E. Hemicelluloses (from the cell wall of many plants)	Xylose, mannose, galactose, glucose (branching chains)	1. Holds water, increases stool bulk
		2. May reduce elevated colonic intraluminal pressure
		3. Binds bile acids variably
II. Cellulose (principal cell wall constituent)	Polyglycan, unbranched glucose polymer	1. Depending on particle size, holds water
		2. May reduce elevated colonic intraluminal pressure
		3. May bind zinc
III. Lignin (woody part of plants)	Polymeric phenylpropane, noncarbohydrate	1. Serves as antioxidant
		2. May bind metals

*From Mendeloff, A. I.: Fiber Part 1. Dietary fiber and health: an introduction in nutrition in disease, Columbus, Ohio, 1978, Ross Laboratories.
†Incompletely understood

carcinogens. All these factors may be implicated in colon cancer (see Chapter 11). The increase in fecal bulk and the decrease in transit time may be the result of the increased production of the volatile fatty acids (acetic, butyric, and propionic) by bacterial action on dietary fiber.[56] These fatty acids may act as cathartics. Fiber may absorb water and function as a bulking agent, promoting peristalsis, and thus decreasing transit time.

Negative balances of calcium, magnesium, zinc, and phosphorus resulted from the feeding of high-fiber diets to two persons for 20 days.[68] This was due to an increased excretion of these minerals. Sanstead et al. found that 26 g of standard, soft white wheat bran decreased the retention of zinc but improved copper balance.[69] Corn bran did not affect zinc and copper balance. There was no influence on iron balance by either type of bran.

Table 4-1 summarizes the human physiological function of the various components of fiber.

Relationship to disease

Appendicitis is thought to result from the blockage of the lumen of the appendix. This could be brought about by the formation of fecaliths or by muscular contraction, which produce an increase in intraluminal pressure.[70] Some diverticular disease is also brought about by an increase in intraluminal pressure that blows out the diverticula.

Straining at stool and increased abdominal pressure could result in varicose veins, hemorrhoids, and hiatal hernia.[54] When the fiber content of the diet is low, the amount of available carbohydrate is increased. Carbohydrate overconsumption and rapid absorption could lead to dental caries, obesity, diabetes mellitus, and coronary heart disease. Trowell proposed the hypothesis that dietary fiber protects against ischemic heart disease.[71,72] His study of 1154 age-matched Irish brothers in Ireland and Boston suggested that the higher intake of crude fiber of the brothers in Ireland caused their lower serum cholesterol levels.

Many plant polysaccharides have been found to lower blood cholesterol levels in animals. However, this has not been proved, and many conflicting reports exist as to the effect of fiber on serum cholesterol.[56] Groen reported a decrease in serum cholesterol when bread replaced the saturated fat of the diet.[73] The fiber content of the bread was low, and its effect was probably negligible. Story and Kritchevsky have suggested that the interactions between bile salts, fiber, and intestinal flora result in an increased excretion of bile salts in the feces.[74] Fiber seems to have an effect on bile and blood cholesterol levels.

Trowell also proposed the hypothesis that the ingestion of starch low in fiber can lead to diabetes mellitus in susceptible genotypes.[72] The diabetic mortality rate for women in England and Wales started to decrease in 1941. Between 1955 and 1959 it remained stable, but after that it began to increase. During the war, milling procedures were changed because of a shortage of wheat. As a result, from 1941 to 1954 the fiber content of the flour was increased. This is the period when the mortality rates were lower.

The rise of blood glucose and insulin after a carbohydrate meal was decreased in normal and diabetic subjects who had consumed pectin or guar gum.[75] It has been suggested that these compounds form gels that affect the absorption of glucose and the secretion of gastrointestinal hormones and pancreatic hormones.[75,76] In another study, insulin-requiring diabetics who consumed diets containing 20 g of crude fiber had significantly lower plasma glucose levels than those eating 3 g of crude fiber.[77] More hypoglycemic reactions were reported on the high-fiber diet. Diabetics consuming high-fiber, high-carbohydrate (75% kcal) diets had improved glucose tolerance, possibly due to an increased sensitivity to insulin.[78,79]

Several hospitals are using high-fiber diets for the treatment of diverticulosis, irritable bowel syndrome, and constipation.[80] The diets include whole grain breads and cereals (especially bran), fresh and cooked vegetables, and fruits. At Shands Teaching Hospital and Clinic in Gainesville, Florida, bran and raw fruit plus 240 ml (8 oz) of water are prescribed for between-meal feedings. Eight to ten glasses of fluid per day are also recommended. The Mayo Clinic in Minnesota is studying the effect of a high-fiber (20 to 25 g [0.7 to 0.9 oz]), low-cholesterol, and low-animal-fat diet on patients with type IIa hyperlipoproteinemia. The fiber comes mainly from a special bread (2 g per slice) and the remainder from fruits and vegetables.

Although much research has been conducted, many conflicting opinions exist as to the role of dietary fiber and its relationship to disease. The initial interest in fiber arose from epidemiological evidence that low-fiber intakes are associated with a high incidence of a large number of diseases—the so-called fiber deficiency diseases of Western civilization. Experiments to prove this relationship have not been forthcoming for many reasons. Fiber is not a single entity but a complex, made up of a variety of substances. Early definitions alluded to an indigestible residue, yet it has been shown that microorganisms in the colon can digest some components of fiber. At present there are no simple analytical techniques for measuring the various fiber components. Further experimentation has been hampered by a lack of a standard for fiber components, since their physiological effects vary, and divergent experimental results have been obtained.

Confusion has also been created by the use of a variety of animals with differing gastrointestinal tracts; the laboratory results are not always applicable to humans. On the basis of anatomical structure the pig and the baboon are the most appropriate experimental animal models. Recently it has been found that different animal species have distinct bacterial species, and therefore no animal model is appropriate for fiber studies. However, it is sometimes useful to use animals prior to human experimentation.

In the past, fiber experiments with humans have not been subjected to rigid controls. Often fiber intake is increased, but the type of fiber is not defined. No attempt is made to assess the amount of fiber from the diet that is being consumed.

The experiments generally are of short duration, and the long-term effects of fiber ingestion may be different. The previous fiber intake and perhaps the amounts of other nutrients in the diet may influence the experimental results. The health of the subjects in the study may also have a bearing on the experimental outcome. Thus there is a need for more rigorously controlled studies on the nutritional significance of fiber.

The Life Sciences Research Office Report for the Food and Drug Administration concluded that an increased intake of dietary fiber is beneficial for diverticular disease, atonic constipation, and some hemorrhoidal conditions, but the relationship to other diseases needs to be confirmed.[81] A high-fiber intake supplies bulk, gentle laxation, and ease of defecation. Since there was little experimental evidence available, the report concluded that there was no reason to increase the dietary intake of fiber except for individual cases where it was considered medically beneficial.

Several bibliographies on fiber have been compiled.[82-84]

REFERENCES

1. Ingelfinger, F. J.: Gastric function, Nutr. Today 6(5):2, 1971.
2. Beck, I. T.: The role of pancreatic enzymes in digestion, Am. J. Clin. Nutr. 26:311, 1973.
3. Holt, P. R.: Fats and bile salts. I. Physiologic considerations, J. Am. Diet. Assoc. 60:491, 1972.
4. Ingelfinger, F. J.: Gastrointestinal absorption, Nutr. Today 2(1):2, 1967.
5. Luckey, T. D.: Introduction: the villus in chemostat man, Am. J. Clin. Nutr. 27:1266, 1974.
6. Ingelfinger, F. J.: How to swallow and belch and cope with heartburn, Nutr. Today 8(1):4, 1973.
7. Castell, D. O.: Diet and the lower esophageal sphincter, Am. J. Clin. Nutr. 28:1296, 1975.
8. Ellis, F. H., Jr.: Esophageal hiatal hernia, N. Engl. J. Med. 287:646, 1972.
9. Katz, D., and Pitchumoni, C. S.: Management of the hiatal hernia–esophagitis complex in the elderly, Geriatrics 28:84, 1973.
10. Sapp, O. L., III: Treatment of duodenal ulcer, Am. Fam. Physician 7(2):129, 1973.
11. McGuigan, J. E., Trudeau, W. L.: Differences in rates of gastrin release in normal persons and patients with duodenal ulcer, N. Engl. J. Med. 288:64, 1973.
12. Rotter, J. I., et al.: Duodenal-ulcer disease associated with elevated serum pepsinogen I: an inherited autosomal dominant disorder, N. Engl. J. Med. 300:63, 1979.
13. Grossman, M. I.: Elevated serum pepsinogen I: a genetic marker for duodenal-ulcer disease, N. Eng. J. Med. 300:89, 1979
14. Friedman, G. D., Siegelaub, A. B., and Selter, C. C.: Cigarettes, alcohol, coffee, and peptic ulcer, N. Engl. J. Med. 290:469, 1974.
15. Paffenburger, R. S., Jr., Wing, A. L., and Hyde, R. T.: Coffee, cigarettes, and peptic ulcer, N. Engl. J. Med. 290:1091, 1974.
16. Morrissey, J. T., and Barreras, R. F.: Drug therapy: antacid therapy, N. Engl. J. Med. 290:550, 1974.
17. Texter, E. C., Jr., Smart, D. F., and Butler, R. C.: Antacids, Am. Fam. Physician 11(4):111, 1975.
18. Levant, J. A., Walsh, J. H., and Isenberg, J. I.: Stimulation of gastric secretion and gastrin release by single oral doses of calcium carbonate in man, N. Engl. J. Med. 289:555, 1973.
19. Hendrix, T. R.: Antacids, Am. Fam. Physician 9(3):184, 1974.
20. Isenberg, J. L.: Peptic ulcer disease, Postgrad. Med. 57:163, 1975.
21. Mainardi, M.: Metiamide, an H_2-receptor blocker as inhibitor of basal and meal stimulated gastric acid secretion in patients with duodenal ulcer, N. Engl. J. Med. 291:393, 1974.
22. Haggie, S. J., et al.: Clinical experience with metiamide, Fed. Proc. 35:1948, 1976.
23. Sippy, B. W.: Gastric and duodenal ulcers: medical cure by an efficient removal of gastric juice erosion, J.A.M.A. 64:1625, 1915.

24. Meulengracht, E.: Treatment of haematemesis and melaena with food, Lancet **2**:1220, 1935.

25. Andresen, A. F. R.: Results of treatment of massive gastric hemorrhage, Am. J. Dig. Dis. **6**:641, 1939.

26. Roth, H. P., and Caron, H. S.: Patients' misconceptions about their peptic ulcer diets: potential obstacles to cooperation, J. Chronic Dis. **20**:5, 1967.

27. Caron, H. S., and Roth, H. P.: Popular beliefs about peptic ulcer diet, J. Am. Diet. Assoc. **60**:306, 1972.

28. Donaldson, R. M., Jr.: The muddle of diets for gastrointestinal disorders, J.A.M.A. **225**:1243, 1973.

29. Diet as related to gastrointestinal function, J. Am. Diet. Assoc. **38**:425, 1961.

30. Position paper on bland diet in the treatment of chronic duodenal ulcer disease, J. Am. Diet. Assoc. **59**:244, 1971.

31. Ippoliti, A. F., Maxwell, V., and Isenberg, J. I.: The effect of various forms of milk on gastric-acid secretion. Studies in patients with duodenal ulcer and normal subjects, Ann. Intern. Med. **84**:286, 1976.

32. Cohen, S., and Booth, G. H., Jr.: Gastric acid secretion and lower-esophageal–sphincter pressure in response to coffee and caffeine, N. Engl. J. Med. **293**:897, 1975.

33. Hartroft, W. S.: The incidence of coronary artery disease in patients treated with the Sippy diet, Am. J. Clin. Nutr. **15**:205, 1964.

34. Tumen, H. J.: Diets for gastrointestinal disorders, J. A. M. A. **226**:1231, 1973.

35. Welsh, J. D.: Diet therapy of peptic ulcer disease, Gastroenterology **72**:740, 1977.

36. Welsh, J. D.: Diet therapy in adult lactose malabsorption practices, Am. J. Clin. Nutr. **31**:592, 1978.

37. Jordan, P. H., Jr.: Elective operations for duodenal ulcer, N. Engl. J. Med. **287**:1329, 1972.

38. Moore, F. D.: Operative treatment of duodenal ulcer. Transatlantic data and opinion, N. Engl. J. Med. **290**:906, 1974.

39. Behn, V., Murchie, G., and King, D. R.: Nutritional care of the patient following gastric surgery, Dietetic Currents **1**(2):1, 1974.

40. Leichter, S. B., Arnold, A. C., and Lewis, S. B.: Glucose tolerance, insulin secretion, and glucose utilization in subjects after gastric surgery, Am. J. Clin. Nutr. **30**:2053, 1977.

41. Total parenteral nutrition and Crohn's disease, Nutr. Rev. **32**:72, 1974.

42. Drawitt, E. L., Beeken, W. L., and Janney, C. D.: Calcium absorption in Crohn's disease, Gastroenterology **71**:251, 1976.

43. Piepmeyer, J. L.: Use of unprocessed bran in treatment of irritable bowel syndrome, Am. J. Clin. Nutr. **27**:106, 1974.

44. Texter, E. C., Jr., and Butler, R. C.: The irritable bowel syndrome, Am. Fam. Physician **11**(3):167, 1975.

45. Goldstein, F.: Diet and colonic disease, J. Am. Diet. Assoc. **60**:499, 1972.

46. Painter, N. S., and Burkitt, D. P.: Diverticular disease of the colon: a deficiency disease of Western civilization, Br. Med. J. **2**:450, 1971.

47. Connell, A. M.: The effects of dietary fiber on gastrointestinal motor function, Am. J. Clin. Nutr. **31**:S-152, 1978.

48. Plumley, P. F., and Francis, B.: Dietary treatment of diverticular disease, J. Am. Diet. Assoc. **63**:527, 1973.

49. Taylor, I., and Duthie, H. L.: Bran tablets and diverticular disease, Br. Med. J. **1**:988, 1976.

50. Brodribb, A. J. M., and Humphreys, D. M.: Diverticular disease: three studies, Br. Med. J. **1**:424, 1976.

51. Brodribb, A. J. M.: Treatment of symptomatic diverticular disease with a high-fibre diet, Lancet **1**:664, 1977.

52. Lyford, C. J., et al.: Controlled clinical trial of bran on irritable bowel syndrome, Clin. Res. **23**:253A, 1975.

53. Soltoft, J., et al.: A double-blind trial of the effect of wheat bran on symptoms of irritable bowel syndrome, Lancet **1**:270, (Feb.), 1976.

54. Burkitt, D. P., Walker, A. R. P., and Painter, N. S.: Dietary fiber and disease, J.A.M.A. **229**:1068, 1974.

55. Burkitt, D. P., and Trowell, H. C., editors: Refined carbohydrate foods and disease. Some implications of dietary fibre, London, 1975, Academic Press.

56. Cummings, J. H.: Dietary fiber, Gut **14**:69, 1973.

57. Van Soest, P. J.: Workshop I. Component analysis of fiber in foods. Summary and recommendations, Am. J. Clin. Nutr. **31**:S-75, 1978.

58. Southgate, D. A. T.: Dietary fiber: analysis and food sources, Am. J. Clin. Nutr. **31**:S-107, 1978.

59. Trowell, J.: Definition of dietary fiber and hypothesis that it is a protective factor in certain diseases, Am. J. Clin. Nutr. **29**:417, 1976.

60. Spiller, G. A. Fassett-Cornelius, G., and Briggs, G.: A new term for plant fibers in nutrition, Am. J. Clin. Nutr. **29**:934, 1976.

61. Van Soest, P. J.: Dietary fibers: their definition and nutritional properties, Am. J. Clin. Nutr. **31:**S-12, 1978.
62. Schaller, D.: Fiber content and structure in foods, Am. J. Clin. Nutr. **31:**S-99, 1978.
63. Van Soest, P. J., and Robertson, J. B.: What is fibre and fibre in food? Nutr. Rev. **35:**12, 1977.
64. Scala, J.: Fiber—the forgotten nutrient, Food Tech. **28:**34, 1974.
65. Heller, S. N., and Hackler, L. R.: Changes in the crude fiber content of the American diet, Am. J. Clin. Nutr. **31:**1510, 1978.
66. Cummings, J. H.: Nutritional implications of dietary fiber, Am. J. Clin. Nutr. **31:**S-21, 1978.
67. Holloway, W. D., Tasman-Jones, C., and Lee, S. P.: Digestion of certain fractions of dietary fiber in humans, Am. J. Clin. Nutr. **31:**927, 1978.
68. Reinhold, J. G., et al.: Decreased absorption of calcium, magnesium, zinc, and phosphorus by humans due to increased fiber and phosphorus consumption as wheat bread, J. Nutr. **106:**493, 1976.
69. Sandstead, H. H., et al.: Influence of dietary fiber on trace element balance, Am. J. Clin. Nutr. **31:**S-180, 1978.
70. Burkitt, D. P.: Epidemiology of large bowel disease: the role of fiber, Proc. Nutr. Soc. **33:**145, 1973.
71. Trowell, H.: Ischemic heart disease and dietary fiber, Am. J. Clin. Nutr. **25:**926, 1972.
72. Trowell, H.: Dietary fiber, ischemic heart disease and diabetes mellitus, Proc. Nutr. Soc. **33:**151, 1973.
73. Groen, J. J.: Why bread in the diet lowers serum cholesterol, Proc. Nutr. Soc. **33:**159, 1973.
74. Story, J. A., and Kritchevsky, D.: Bile acid metabolism and fiber, Am. J. Clin. Nutr. **31:**S-199, 1978.
75. Jenkins, D. J. A., et al.: Decrease in postprandial insulin and glucose concentrations by guar and pectin, Ann. Intern. Med. **86:**20, 1977.
76. Jenkins, D. J. A., et al.: Carbohydrate tolerance in man after six weeks of pectin administration, Proc. Nutr. Soc. **36:**624, 1977.
77. Miranda, P. M., and Horwitz, D. L.: High fiber diets in the treatment of diabetes mellitus, Ann. Intern. Med. **88:**482, 1978.
78. Kiehm, T. G., Anderson, J. W., and Ward, K.: Beneficial effects of a high carbohydrate high fiber diet on hyperglycemic men, Am. J. Clin. Nutr. **29:**895, 1976.
79. Anderson, J. W.: High polysaccharide diet studies on patients with diabetes and vascular disease, Cereal Foods World **22:**12, 1977.
80. Idea exchange: fiber in the diet, J. Am. Diet. Assoc. **66:**50, 1975.
81. FASEB: The nutritional significance of dietary fiber, Bethesda, Md., 1977, Life Sciences Research Office, Federation of American Societies for Experimental Biology.
82. Selected bibliography on dietary fiber, Am. J. Clin. Nutr. **31:**S-285, 1978.
83. Trowell, H.: Dietary fibre bibliography. In New developments in the importance of dietary fibre in health, Manchester, England, 1978, Kelloggs.
84. Kelsay, J. L.: A review of research on effects of fiber intake in man, Am. J. Clin. Nutr. **31:**142, 1978.

5 Liver and gallbladder disease

LIVER FUNCTION

The liver is the largest gland in the body. It is also the most diverse organ in that it has been estimated that each liver parenchymal cell can perform from 60 to 100 functions. These can be divided into four basic categories: circulation, metabolism, (carbohydrate, amino acid, lipid, vitamin, and mineral), production of bile, and detoxification. The liver regulates and integrates the activities of the human body as does no other organ.

Circulation

The two major vessels that bring substances to the liver are the hepatic artery and the portal vein. Oxygen is brought in via the hepatic artery. The digested nutrients (carbohydrates, amino acids, short-chain fatty acids, water-soluble vitamins, and minerals) are absorbed into the capillaries of the villi, which are located in the small intestine. The capillaries then empty into the portal vein, which goes to the liver. Therefore, after digestion the nutrients that are absorbed into the blood are brought directly to the liver for metabolism or redistribution to other tissues.

In addition, if there is too much blood in the body, it can be stored in the liver; when the blood volume is low, blood is then released from the liver.

Metabolism

Carbohydrates. Fifty percent of the calories that we ingest daily are obtained from carbohydrates. Lactose (milk sugar) and sucrose (table sugar) are the main disaccharides, and starch is the major polysaccharide found in the diet. Salivary and intestinal enzymes break down starch to glucose, lactose to glucose and galactose, and sucrose to glucose and fructose. These simple sugars, or monosaccharides (glucose, galactose, and fructose), enter the portal vein and are carried to the liver.

Glucose is the sugar most commonly utilized for energy purposes by the cells in our body. To obtain energy from glucose, it must be broken down stepwise in a series of reactions that can proceed either with or without oxygen. The process that does not require oxygen is called anaerobic metabolism, or glycolysis (Fig. 5-1). Glucose is broken down to pyruvic acid by glycolysis. In the absence of oxygen this pyruvic acid can be converted to lactic acid. Thus some energy can be produced for muscular activity even though enough oxygen is not available to oxidize glucose completely to carbon dioxide and water.

The next sequence of reactions in the metabolism of carbohydrates requires

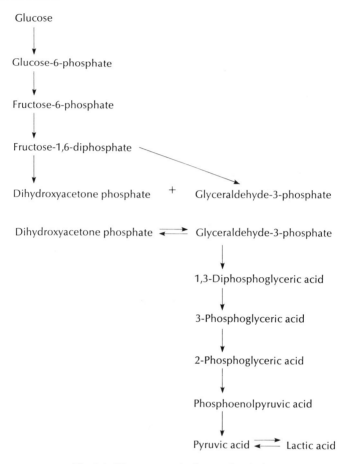

Fig. 5-1. Glucose metabolism—glycolysis.

oxygen (aerobic metabolism). Pyruvic acid is metabolized to acetyl coenzyme A (CoA) and is then broken down to carbon dioxide and water through the reactions of the citric acid cycle (Fig. 5-2). During both glycolysis and the citric acid cycle some of the energy released is used to make adenosine triphosphate (ATP). This is the compound that provides the energy for metabolic reactions in the cell.

Liver cells are able to synthesize glucose from deaminated amino acids. This process is called gluconeogenesis. The monosaccharide galactose is also converted to glucose by a series of reactions (Fig. 5-3). Fructose is converted to metabolites that appear in the glycolytic pathway (Fig. 5-4).

The liver also plays a part in regulating the amount of glucose in the blood. The normal concentration of blood glucose is 70 to 100 mg/dl of blood. The circulation affords a means of transporting glucose to other cells of the body. For example, glucose is the major source of energy for the central nervous system; however, when blood glucose levels are high, the excess glucose is converted to glycogen. This

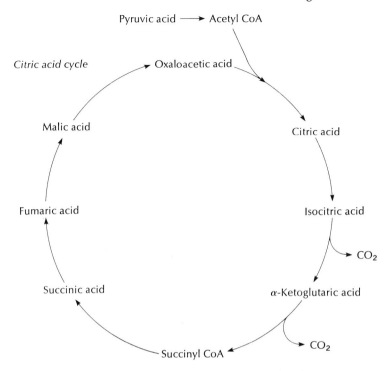

Fig. 5-2. Glucose metabolism—citric acid cycle.

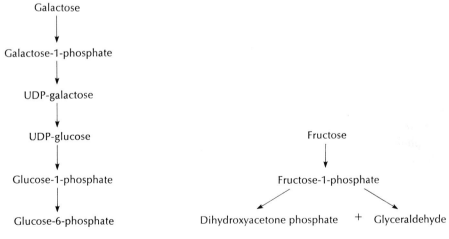

Fig. 5-3. Metabolism of galactose.   **Fig. 5-4.** Metabolism of fructose.

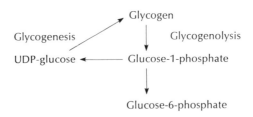

Fig. 5-5. Metabolism of glycogen.

process is glycogenesis (Fig. 5-5). On the other hand, when blood glucose levels drop, liver glycogen is hydrolyzed to give glucose (glycogenolysis, Fig. 5-5). During the time when food is not being ingested, glycogenolysis can help maintain blood glucose levels. Muscle cells also have the ability to synthesize glycogen, thus providing a ready source of energy that enables them to begin activity immediately.

Lipids. Another source of energy available to cells is the triglycerides, or neutral fats. These are digested into fatty acids and glycerol. The short-chain fatty acids (10 carbons or less) are transported to the liver by means of the portal vein, but the longer chain fatty acids must be resynthesized into triglycerides. In addition, cholesterol and protein are added to these triglycerides to form chylomicrons, which are absorbed into the lacteals of the villi and eventually enter the blood system. They then reach the liver via a different route.

In the liver the fatty acids may be metabolized for energy. Initially, the acetyl CoA that is formed can enter the citric acid cycle to be metabolized to carbon dioxide and water. Acetyl CoA can also be converted to ketone bodies (acetoacetic acid, β-hydroxybutyric acid, and acetone). Other tissues may then metabolize acetoacetic acid to acetyl CoA, but the enzyme for the conversion is not present in the liver. When the oxidation of fats becomes excessive, such as in starvation, uncontrolled diabetes mellitus, or in low carbohydrate intake, the production of ketone bodies increases. This increase may lead to acidosis.

Triglycerides may be synthesized in the liver from glycerol and fatty acids. In addition to the synthesis of these simple lipids, liver cells have the ability to manufacture compound lipids. Lipoproteins of the alpha, beta, and pre-beta varieties are made that serve as transport forms of lipids in the blood. Conversion to these soluble forms also prevents the deposition of fats in the liver. Other compound lipids synthesized by liver cells that contain both nitrogen bases and phosphates include the phospholipids. Examples of phospholipids are lecithin, cephalin, plasmalogen, and sphingomyelin. Cholesterol is another lipid synthesized from the two-carbon precursor acetyl CoA. Cholesterol belongs to a class of compounds called sterols. It is the precursor for bile acids and steroid hormones. Cholesterol contains a hydroxyl group that can be esterified with a fatty acid. The esterification provides another method of transporting fatty acids.

The metabolism of lipids is summarized in Fig. 5-6.

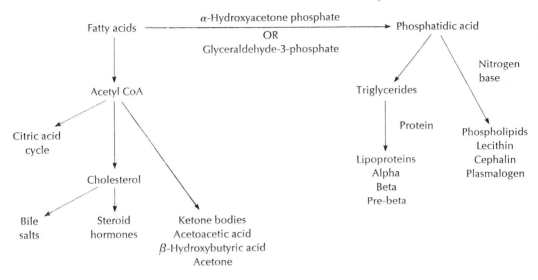

Fig. 5-6. Metabolism of lipids.

Amino acids. The amino acids reach the liver via the portal vein. They may be used to make protein for the liver cell. Plasma proteins are also synthesized in this organ. Examples of these are albumin, globulin, fibrinogen, and prothrombin. The latter two proteins are two of the factors involved in the complex process of blood clotting.

The nonessential amino acids may be synthesized from other amino acids by a reaction called transamination. This reaction involves the transfer of an amino group from one amino acid to a keto acid. Thus a second amino acid is synthesized. An example of this is:

Glutamic acid + Oxaloacetic acid → α-Ketoglutaric acid + Aspartic acid

Each of the 20 amino acids found in structural protein can be metabolized by its own pathway; however, in general, all amino acids can be catabolized by two reactions—decarboxylation and deamination. Decarboxylation involves the removal of a carboxyl group as carbon dioxide. The remaining compound is called an amine. For example:

Alanine → Ethylamine + Carbon dioxide

Many of these amines have a physiological function such as histamine, dopamine, serotonin, and γ-aminobutyric acid.

Deamination involves the removal of an amine group as in ammonia and leaves a carbon skeleton. For example:

Alanine → Pyruvic acid + Ammonia

Minerals. Minerals are utilized as structural components of the body and as cofactors for enzymatic reactions. The liver is an important storage site for minerals: iron is stored in combination with a protein as ferritin, and copper is also stored. Both iron and copper are necessary for the synthesis of the respiratory pigment, hemoglobin. Other minerals such as zinc, manganese, and magnesium are also stored in the liver.

Vitamins. Vitamins are supplied in microquantities from ingested food. Some vitamins are soluble in water, such as ascorbic acid and the B complex (thiamine, riboflavin, pyridoxine, vitamin B_{12}, niacin, folic acid, pantothenic acid, and biotin). The water-soluble vitamins, except for ascorbic acid, are used primarily as coenzymes in enzymatic reactions. The fat-soluble vitamins (A, D, E, and K) are involved in specific physiological functions. High concentrations of the fat-soluble vitamins A, D, and K are found in the liver. The B-complex vitamins and C are also present in substantial amounts in this organ.

Some vitamins are metabolized into an active form in the liver. Most carotene is converted into vitamin A in the intestine, but any unconverted carotene is hydrolyzed in the liver. The fat-soluble vitamin K is necessary for the synthesis of the protein prothrombin by the liver. This is one of the factors involved in blood clotting.

Production of bile

The liver synthesizes the secretion known as bile. It is composed of cholesterol and the primary bile salts, cholate and chenodeoxycholate. These salts can be conjugated to either glycine or taurine. The color of the bile is due to the presence of the bile pigments, bilirubin and biliverdin. When the erythrocyte dies, the hemoglobin is broken into heme and globin in the reticuloendothelial cells. The heme is metabolized to biliverdin, and this is reduced to the principal bile pigment, bilirubin. In the liver, bilirubin is conjugated with glucuronic acid to form bilirubin diglucuronide. The conjugated and unconjugated bilirubin are released into the bile.

Bile is stored and concentrated in the gallbladder. The presence of fat in the small intestine releases the hormone cholecystokinin. This causes the gallbladder to contract, and bile is released into the intestine. The main function of bile is to aid in the digestion and absorption of fats and fat-soluble substances. The bile salts act as emulsifying agents; that is, they assist in solubilizing the insoluble fat particles so that digestion and absorption may proceed.

Secondary bile salts are formed in the small intestine as a result of bacterial action; cholate is converted to deoxycholate, and chenodeoxycholate is metabolized to lithocholate. The bile salts are reabsorbed in the ileum and are returned to the liver by the so-called enterohepatic circulation.

Jaundice or icterus, an excessive accumulation of bile pigments in the body that produces an intense yellow coloration of the skin, may be the result of hemolysis or the inability of the liver to metabolize bilirubin. In hemolytic jaundice the liver is unable to conjugate all the bilirubin produced from the heme, so it then appears in the blood. Hepatocellular jaundice is the result of a defect in the metabolism of bilirubin in the liver. Obstructive jaundice is due to a blockage in the bile duct. As a result, conjugated bilirubin appears in the circulation.

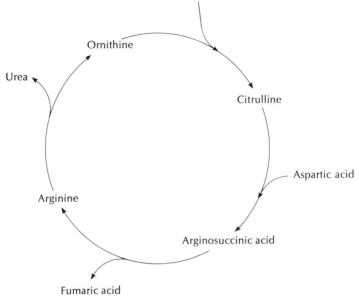

Fig. 5-7. Urea cycle.

Detoxification

A specialized function of the liver is its ability to remove injurious substances such as ingested toxins from food, drugs, metabolites, or toxins produced by bacteria in the body. Ammonia, a by-product of the metabolism of amino acids, is also removed. In the liver, ammonia is combined with carbon dioxide and synthesized into urea (Fig. 5-7), which is then excreted in the urine.

There are several reactions by which toxic substances may be rendered innocuous. These may involve oxidation, reduction, or methylation of the substance. Another method available to the liver is the conjugation of the toxic compound with an amino or organic acid; this substance is then excreted via the kidneys into the urine.

LIVER DISEASE
Tests for diagnosis of liver disease

Many tests can be used to evaluate the function of the liver. The van den Bergh reaction can be used to measure either the free bilirubin (unconjugated) or bilirubin diglucuronide (conjugated). Serum levels are elevated in liver disease and extrahepatic bile duct obstruction. The measurement of urinary bilirubin, urobilirubin, or fecal urobilinogen may prove useful. Serum prothrombin is synthesized in the liver, so in the case of hepatic disease the prothrombin time would be increased; however, a deficiency of vitamin K, which is needed for prothrombin synthesis, could also cause an increase.

Another test involves the intravenous injection of sulfobromophthalein (Bromsulphalein or BSP) and the subsequent measurement of the BSP concentration in the plasma. BSP is conjugated with glutathione and is excreted in a manner similar to that of bilirubin; therefore an increase in the retention of BSP is indicative of liver dysfunction.

Hepatic protein synthesis is altered when disease occurs in the liver. Serum albumin levels are decreased, but in most instances serum globulin levels are elevated because of the immune response. Flocculation tests are performed by adding serum to reagents such as thymol, zinc sulfate, and cephalin-cholesterol. Albumin will retard the precipitation or turbidity when these reagents are added, whereas globulin will tend to cause precipitation. Abnormal values are seen in liver disease, chronic infections, kidney disease, rheumatoid arthritis, collagen disease, and multiple myeloma.

Carbohydrate metabolism is also affected by liver disease. Glucose, galactose, and glucagon tolerance tests are abnormal. However, glucose tolerance test results are variable and thus are of little practical use. In liver dysfunction, glycogen storage is impaired, and the administration of glucagon leads to hypoglycemia. Galactose tolerance tests are abnormal in liver disease, since the ability to convert galactose to glucose is impaired.

Enzyme levels are elevated in liver disease because of the destruction of hepatic cells followed by release of enzymes into the circulation. Lactic dehydrogenase, transaminases (glutamic-oxaloacetic and glutamic-pyruvic), alkaline phosphatase, leucine aminopeptidase, and 5'-nucleotidase are elevated in liver disease. For further details see Chapter 2, Laboratory Diagnosis.

A new test that measures the clearance of bile acids from the plasma shows promise of being useful in diagnosing liver disease at an early stage.[1] Sodium cholylglycinate was injected intravenously, and blood samples were taken periodically. Radioimmunoassay was used to measure the remaining conjugated bile acid. Since cholylglycine is rapidly cleared from the plasma, a sampling time of 10 minutes was selected. A delayed clearance of cholylglycine was seen in 25 patients who had abnormal liver function tests.[2] The same result was seen in 9 patients out of 11 who had normal liver function tests but who had liver disease.

Hepatitis

Hepatitis is an inflammatory condition of the liver characterized by injury to the liver cells. It can be caused by toxic agents such as chloroform, carbon tetrachloride, arsenicals, phosphorus, anesthetics, and antibiotics. Infectious agents such as viruses, spirochetes, protozoa, bacteria, and helminths can also cause hepatitis.

Viral, or infectious, hepatitis can be transmitted through food, sewage, contaminated water, and wastes. Serum hepatitis may develop through the use of nonsterile medical instruments and blood transfusions.

Nausea, loss of appetite, vomiting after meals, headache, fever, abdominal discomfort, and loss of muscle tone are common in hepatitis. Jaundice may develop in a few days or weeks, and the liver becomes enlarged (hepatomegaly). The organ has remarkable regenerative powers; individuals usually recover after 6 to 8 weeks. In the elderly, however, liver damage may be severe and result in fatty infiltration of the liver, followed by hepatic coma.

The dietary treatment of hepatitis is important. In the acute stage when vomiting is severe, it may be necessary to administer an intravenous solution of 10% glucose. If this period is prolonged, parenteral or tube feeding may be instituted. The patient should be encouraged to take liquids and solids by mouth as soon as possible. Small frequent meals may be necessary at first to keep the patient from becoming nauseous.

The daily intake of calories should be 3000 to 4000 kcal. Protein levels of 1.5 to 2 g/kg of body weight (100 to 150 g) provide enough protein for the regeneration of liver cells. The carbohydrate intake should be high (300 to 400 g per day) in order to spare protein and promote the synthesis of liver glycogen as protection against further liver damage. In past years the amount of fat in the diet was restricted to 50 g per day, but today a liberal intake (150 g) is prescribed. More fat not only increases the palatability of the diet, but it also serves to increase the caloric density. Vitamin and mineral supplements are not necessary when adequate food is being consumed.

Acute fulminant hepatitis is a variant of infectious hepatitis that develops rapidly and is often fatal. Exchange transfusions, cross circulation, liver perfusions, and charcoal hemoperfusions have not been very successful. Increased survival rates were reported in patients who were treated with electrolyte solutions, plasma, and blood.[3] Magnesium sulfate was administered to clear the gastrointestinal tract of protein, and neomycin sulfate was given to reduce the bacterial production of nitrogen. The diet was free of protein.

It has been suggested that perhaps diet therapy should consist of the administration of essential amino acids, especially the branched-chain amino acids, and alpha keto acids rather than a protein-free diet.[4]

Fatty liver

Under some conditions large amounts of fat are deposited in the liver, causing it to become enlarged. Fatty liver is characteristic of alcoholism, uncontrolled diabetes mellitus, starvation, nutritional deficiencies (such as kwashiorkor and pellagra), tuberculosis, and inanition due to gastrointestinal abnormalities.

This condition has been produced experimentally in rats fed low-protein diets with high amounts of either carbohydrate or fat.[5] When the low-protein diets were also deficient in lipotropes and vitamins, even more triglycerides accumulated in the liver. The results were similar to those observed in children with kwashiorkor. When lipotropes such as choline, betaine, and methionine are ingested, less fat is deposited in the liver.

Lieber and DeCarli fed rats varying amounts of fat (2%, 5%, 10%, 15%, 25%,

35%, or 43% of total calories) while they were given alcohol.[6] As the caloric content from fat increased from 25% to 43%, the hepatic lipid content also increased. When the caloric value contributed by fat was reduced from 25% to 2%, there was no concomitant decrease in hepatic lipid. The substitution of medium-chain triglycerides reduced the capacity of ethanol to produce lipid deposition in the liver. However, a diet in which 25% of calories was supplied by protein produced no change in the ability of ethanol to produce a fatty liver. Thus the liver cannot be fully protected from alcohol-induced steatosis by dietary modifications.

In the case of alcoholics, it is necessary that they abstain from the consumption of alcohol. The dietary treatment is similar to that for hepatitis. Adequate amounts of calories are provided in the form of fat and carbohydrate. Carbohydrate promotes the deposition of glycogen in the liver and also exerts a protein-sparing effect. The diet should be high in protein, especially from animal sources, to support the synthesis of lipotropic agents. The aim of diet therapy is to promote the synthesis of liver cells.

Cirrhosis

Cirrhosis is a most serious form of liver disease. The liver cells are gradually replaced by fibrous connective tissue, and the liver becomes smaller and loses its function. The disease may result from chronic alcoholism, malnutrition, infectious hepatitis, obstruction or inflammation of the biliary tract, poisons, drugs, metabolic abnormalities (for example, Wilson's disease and hemochromatosis), congestive heart failure, and atherosclerosis.

The cirrhotic patient shows a loss of appetite, nausea, vomiting, pain, and abdominal distension. If the bile tract is involved, jaundice is also present. The impairment of the portal circulation caused by the accumulation of fibrous tissue in the liver results in hypertension. Varicose veins develop in the esophagus (esophageal varices) and abdominal region. These veins rupture easily, and the ensuing hemorrhage may be fatal. Ascites, the accumulation of fluid in the abdominal cavity, and edema may occur in the event of low serum protein levels.

The aim of diet therapy is to provide sufficient protein to promote liver regeneration but not enough to cause hepatic coma. Positive nitrogen balance has been achieved in cirrhotics by feeding 65 to 75 g of protein per day.[7] Larger amounts have not been proved beneficial. Gabuzda and Shear recommended that a patient without hepatic coma be given 50 g per day and 1600 kcal.[7] If no symptoms appear, this is increased weekly by 10 to 15 g until 65 to 85 g per day are reached with a total intake of 2000 to 3000 kcal. This regimen should improve hepatic function and nutritional status. The protein intake is lowered to 25 to 35 g if symptoms of hepatic encephalopathy develop.

Additional studies are needed on the quality of protein to be fed, since some proteins yield more ammonia than do others.[7] Rudman and co-workers fed dosages of 0.063 to 2 g ammonium chloride per 50 kg (110 lb) body weight to normal individuals with no effect on blood ammonia levels.[8] Hyperammonemia was observed in all the cirrhotic patients tested, with three individuals responding to the lowest dose level. Foods were then tested for their ammonia content. Those containing the highest amounts (ammonia nitrogen as percent of total nitrogen) were mayonnaise 23%, margarine 22%, French dressing 14%, and onions, grape wine, catsup, and pickle relish 11% respectively. Three patients with Laennec's cirrhosis were fed three "high ammonia" foods (domestic blue cheese, salami, cheddar cheese) and three "low ammonia" foods (lima beans, egg yolk, bacon) in doses equivalent to the ammonium chloride previously fed. Two to four hours later blood ammonia levels were higher in the individuals ingesting the "high ammonia" foods. Therefore, diets for individuals with liver disease should be composed of foods low in ammonia content. However, the authors suggested that ammonia formed from urea generated by the gastrointestinal tract and from the removal of amine groups from amino acids should also be evaluated.

In a later study Rudman and co-workers fed amino acids to normal and cirrhotic patients and measured blood ammonia levels.[9] The amino acids were classified into three categories of ammonigenic potency: group A (highest)—glycine, serine, threonine, glutamine, histidine, lysine, and asparagine; group B (intermediate)—leucine, alanine, valine, phenylalanine, isoleucine, tyrosine, and proline; and group C (lowest)—arginine, aspartic acid, glutamic acid, and tryptophan. (Because of its possible role as an intermediary in production of NH_3 from amino acids, urea was also tested in this group.) When neomycin was administered to reduce intestinal synthesis of ammonia, no change in ammonigenic potency of the amino acids was observed. Likewise the route of administration, whether oral or intravenous, had no effect. This suggested that the pathways by which these three groups of amino acids are metabolized may be different. Group A amino acids may be preferentially deaminated or deamidated, while group B and group C amino acids may undergo transamination and enter the urea cycle as aspartic acid rather than as ammonia. The authors recommended that patients with cirrhosis should restrict their intake of the group A amino acids, which generate the most ammonia. Since, for the most part, these are nonessential amino acids, the diets should provide sources of the essential amino acids.

Milk has been used successfully as a source of protein. Low-sodium milk may be used for patients who have ascites and edema. It is important to continually monitor cirrhotic patients to maintain them in optimal protein nutriture.

Moderate amounts of fat and a high intake of carbohydrate are needed to provide adequate calories. However, cirrhotic patients may have hepatogenous diabetes,[10] in which no clinical symptoms are seen and insulin therapy is not needed. In cases of hepatic coma, high carbohydrate intakes are necessary even though the cirrhotic is diabetic. Quite often cirrhosis is associated with diabetes mellitus.[11] Hyperglucagonemia has been observed in cirrhotic patients and to a greater degree in those with portacaval shunts.[12] This may be the result of the decreased ability of the liver to deactivate glucagon. It does not explain, however, the abnormal carbohydrate intolerance that is observed. Similar elevations of glucagon were reported by Sherwin and co-workers in patients with Laennec's cirrhosis.[13] They suggested that the elevated levels may be because of an increase in secretion of the hormone rather than a decrease in degradation. These researchers postulated that the hyperglucagonemia may cause a diabetic state by stimulating gluconeogenesis rather than glycogenolysis.

In liver dysfunction, vitamin deficiencies may arise from a number of factors such as malabsorption, decreased liver storage, and diminished conversion into metabolically active forms. Pyridoxine deficiency in chronic liver disease may be due to an increase in the catabolism of pyridoxal phosphate to pyridoxic acid.[14] Leevy and co-workers reported the correction of vitamin depletion in cirrhotic patients by the parenteral administration of vitamins to overcome malabsorption, plus a vitamin-supplemented diet.[15] For complete recovery from deficiency states, all the vitamins must be provided. A survey of 80 individuals with chronic liver disease revealed lowered blood levels of the vitamins A, E, C, B_1, B_2, B_{12}, folate, and iron and decreased urinary excretion of N-methyl-nicotinamide as compared to normal subjects.[16] However, the incidence of deficiency states of the fat-soluble vitamins was higher than that of the water-soluble vitamins.

Additional problems are seen in patients with biliary cirrhosis caused by chronic cholestasis (slowing or cessation of the flow of bile). A lack of bile salts results in the malabsorption of fats, fat-soluble vitamins, and cholesterol. The steatorrhea (fat in the feces) results in the formation of insoluble calcium salts of fatty acids (soap); thus, calcium absorption is decreased. Dietary treatment involves a low neutral fat diet of 30 g supplemented with medium-chain triglycerides (MCT).[10] Vitamins A, D, and K must be injected intravenously since they are poorly absorbed.

The amount of protein in the diet must be carefully regulated. If liver damage is severe, the breakdown of amino acids will yield large amounts of ammonia that cannot be converted to urea. As a result, toxic levels of ammonia appear in the blood and lead to hepatic coma. The protein level of the diet should be reduced to 20 to 60 g per day.[17] During the comatose state, parenteral feedings containing no protein may be used for a few days.

Ammonia may be released as a result of the action of the intestinal bacteria on endogenous and exogenous protein. Neomycin is administered to reduce the production of this bacterial ammonia.

The protein content of the diet is gradually increased to the amount that can be tolerated by the patient without precipitating hepatic coma.

Elevated levels of hepatic, serum, and urinary copper and serum ceruloplasmin have been found in patients with primary biliary cirrhosis. Recently pigmented corneal rings that are characteristic of Wilson's disease have been observed in four patients.[18] Further research is indicated as to whether low-copper diets should be prescribed.

Portacaval shunts are surgical procedures designed to relieve the pressure on the veins of the esophagus and stomach. The portal vein is connected to the vena cava; thus the nutrients absorbed from the small intestine are not carried to the liver but instead enter the general circulation directly. Controversy now exists as to whether this procedure is beneficial.

When there is edema and ascites, diuresis may be initiated on a 10 mEq sodium-restricted diet. However, it is not always safe to prescribe a diuretic.[19] Generally 0.5 to 1 g of sodium is allowed per day.

To avoid hemorrhage of the esophageal varices, roughage should be eliminated from the diet. If there is bleeding, it may be necessary to use tube feeding.

Frequent small feedings and the use of antacids may prove useful.[19]

Hepatic encephalopathy

Ammonia, mercaptans, thiols, short-chain fatty acids, and amines and their precursor amino acids have been thought to produce hepatic encephalopathy.[20] Abnormal amino acid patterns have been found, namely, elevated levels of the aromatic amino acids and decreased levels of the branched-chain amino acids. Patients on parenteral nutrition were able to tolerate a synthetic amino acid solution that provided from 100 to 120 g protein per 24 hours. Plasma amino acid levels were normalized.[21] Intravenous or oral administration of the alpha keto acids of valine, leucine, isoleucine, methionine, and phenylalanine helped to diminish encephalopathy.[22]

Alcoholism

It is estimated that there are currently 10 million alcoholic Americans in the United States.[13] These individuals may develop fatty liver, alcoholic hepatitis, and fibrosis. The latter is characterized by necrosis, ballooned liver cells, alcoholic hyaline (Mallory bodies), polymorphonuclear leukocytic infiltration, fat, and connective tissue in the liver.[14]

Alcoholics generally consume an inadequate diet with the major source of calories being the alcohol. It has been felt that malnutrition associated with a diet of this type contributes to the liver damage. Animals allowed to drink ethanol ad libitum do not consume sufficient quantities and so do not develop liver injury. By feeding a nutritionally adequate, totally liquid diet with ethanol, sufficient quantities are consumed and liver damage results.[25] Rats develop a fatty liver, while primates develop alcoholic hepatitis and cirrhosis.[26] Thus good nutrition offers no protection against the hepatotoxic effects of alcohol.

One liter of alcohol a day can be metabolized by the liver. In general a man can metabolize 10 ml per hour. Therefore it takes 5 or 6 hours to metabolize the ethanol of 120 ml (4 oz) of whiskey or 1.2 L (2½ pt) of beer.[27] Excessive amounts of alcohol must be consumed before there is evidence of liver damage. It is not understood why only a small percentage of alcoholics develop cirrhosis.

Alcohol is rapidly absorbed both from the stomach and small intestine. Food in the stomach, but not in the intestine, will delay its absorption. Approximately 90% of the ingested alcohol is metabolized in the liver. Although ethanol yields 7 kcal per gram, this energy cannot be used for muscular activity. It is mainly used to maintain

1. $C_2H_5OH + NAD^+ \xrightarrow{\text{ADH}} CH_3CHO + NADH + H^+$

2. $C_2H_5OH + NADPH + H^+ + O_2 \xrightarrow{\text{MEOS}} CH_3CHO + NADP^+ + 2H_2O$

3. $NADPH + H^+ + O_2 \xrightarrow[\text{oxidase}]{\text{NADPH}} NADP^+ + H_2O_2$

$+$

$H_2O_2 + C_2H_5OH \xrightarrow{\text{catalase}} CH_3CHO + 2H_2O$

ADH = Alcohol dehydrogenase

MEOS = Microsomal ethanol oxidizing system

Fig. 5-8. Hepatic metabolism of ethanol.

body temperature or is dissipated as heat. Ethanol becomes the preferred fuel for the liver, so less fat is oxidized for energy. Because of the increased proliferation of the smooth endoplasmic reticulum, alcohol and drugs can be metabolized at a faster rate. Three enzyme systems have been postulated for the metabolism of ethanol in the liver (Fig. 5-8). The relative significance of these pathways has not been elucidated.[28-31] Acetaldehyde is metabolized to acetate and released into the blood. This excess NADH is used to synthesize fatty acids. Such synthesis, in conjunction with the decreased oxidation of fatty acids, leads to fat deposition in the liver. Excess lipids are also released into the bloodstream as lipoproteins and ketone bodies.

Lactic acid levels increase and cause the kidney's excretion of uric acid to decrease, resulting in hyperuricemia (elevated serum uric acid). Lactate is also thought to stimulate the synthesis of collagen, a protein contributing to the fibrotic conditions of the liver in cirrhosis.[32]

Ethanol also blocks hepatic gluconeogenesis and thus contributes to hypoglycemia. On the other hand, hyperglycemia also has been observed in alcoholics.

Alcohol depresses the appetite. The gastric mucosa are irritated, resulting in gastritis. The mucosal protective barrier is lost. Gastric juice acts on the stomach wall, and hemorrhaging results. The amount of pancreatic enzymes secreted is decreased. These enzymes are released into the pancreas and begin their action there.[27] The structure of the intestinal mucosa is affected. Alcohol decreases the absorption of sugars, amino acids, fats, fat-soluble vitamins, folic acid, vitamin B_{12}, pyridoxine, and calcium.[33-35] Iron overload has been reported in chronic alcoholics with anemia and other complications; bone marrow smears showed plasma cells containing iron.[36] Iron supplements should not be prescribed for patients with severe liver disease.[37]

Dietary treatment involves an adequate diet with supplemental vitamins. No alcohol is allowed. Low-fat diets decrease the amount of fat deposited in the liver especially if the fat consists of medium-chain triglycerides.[38] However, these diets tend to be unpalatable.

The substitution of medium-chain triglycerides (70 g) for long-chain triglycerides (100 g) in the diet of alcoholics with cirrhosis resulted in a change in liver lipids in that the short-chain fatty acids (myristic and pentadecanoic acid) increased and the long-chain fatty acids (stearic and oleic acid) decreased.[39] The amount of linoleic acid in the liver was not altered by these diets. No significant change in liver fatty acid composition was observed when medium-chain triglycerides were fed to alcoholics who did not have cirrhosis. After 2 weeks of feeding the medium-chain triglycerides to the cirrhotic patients, the serum albumin levels increased. This indicates a recovery of liver function, and thus medium-chain triglycerides are valuable for treatment of cirrhotic patients.

Ketoacidosis is another disorder associated with alcoholism. Metabolic acidosis is due to the accumulation of primary keto acids and lactate. The mechanism is unknown, but low levels of insulin and high levels of growth hormone, epinephrine, glucagon, and cortisol are seen.[35] These hormones stimulate the release and metabolism of fatty acids, and this could lead to elevated levels of the keto acids. Treatment involves the administration of glucose.[40] If serum phosphorus levels are low, phosphorus should be given.

Register and co-workers fed rats the typical foods of a teenage diet.[41] They found that rats consuming coffee and caffeine ingested more alcohol than did the animals fed no caffeine. The authors suggested that dietary factors may affect the metabolic controls of drinking.

GALLBLADDER

The bile that is synthesized in the liver is stored in the gallbladder, which has a capacity of 40 to 70 ml. Here liver bile is concentrated so that it contains primarily bile salts, bilirubin, cholesterol, and fatty acids.

Cholecystitis is an inflammation of the gallbladder. It generally results from the obstruction of the cystic duct by a gallstone. Gallstones (cholelithiasis) are made up of cholesterol, bilirubin, and calcium. A small percentage are calcium bilirubinate pigment stones or crystalline cholesterol stones. Cholesterol precipitates when the bile is so saturated that the bile salts and phospholipids are unable to keep it solubilized.[42]

In the age group 55 through 64 years, approximately 10% of males and 20% of females, or perhaps as many as 15 million Americans, may have gallstones.[43] The symptoms include abdominal discomfort, bloating, belching, and intolerance of fried foods and some vegetables.

Prior to the surgical removal of the gallbladder (cholecystectomy), the daily fat intake should be restricted to 20 to 30 g. For those who can tolerate it, up to 60 g may be allowed. For obese individuals, caloric restriction is necessary. Most of the calories should be provided by carbohydrates. No general food intolerances are exhibited by patients with gallbladder disease; however, foods that cause distress to the individual should be avoided.

After surgical removal of the gallbladder a fat-restricted diet may be followed for a few months. Then a normal diet is resumed. Bile is necessary for the absorption of fat-soluble vitamins; hence care should be taken to provide adequate amounts of these vitamins in the diet after cholecystectomy to avoid malabsorption.

Recent success has been achieved with the dissolution of gallstones by the oral administration of chenodeoxycholic acid.[44-46] It is absorbed and enters the bile acid pool, where it is thought to suppress hepatic cholesterol synthesis.[47] Therefore the secreted bile would be less lithogenic. Chenodeoxycholic acid has been shown to be toxic in monkeys. However, humans have an increased ability to sulfate the hydroxyl groups of the bile acids and thus increase their excretion.

Gallstones are commonly found in obese and diabetic individuals. Gallbladder bile in diabetics undergoing treatment with insulin has been shown to contain more cholesterol.[48] This same effect was observed in women taking oral contraceptives.[49]

Data from the Coronary Drug Project indicated that gallstones are an associated risk when estrogen and clofibrate were prescribed as hypolipidemic drugs.[50] Estrogen was withdrawn during the trial due to an increased mortality rate. Both clofibrate and estrogens have been shown to increase the cholesterol content of bile.

REFERENCES

1. Korman, M. G., et al.: Development of an intravenous bile acid tolerance test. Plasma disappearance of cholylglycine in health, N. Engl. J. Med. **292:**1205, 1975.
2. LaRusso, N. F., et al.: Validity and sensitivity of an intravenous bile acid tolerance test in patients with liver disease, N. Engl. J. Med. **292:**1209, 1975.
3. Auslander, M. O., and Gitnick, G. L.: Vigorous medical management of acute fulminant hepatitis, Arch. Intern. Med. **137:**599, 1977.
4. Role of nutrition in medical management of acute fulminant hepatitis, Nutr. Rev. **35:**167, 1977.
5. Porta, E. A., and Hartroft, W. S.: Protein deficiency and liver injury, Am. J. Clin. Nutr. **23:**447, 1970.
6. Lieber, C. S., and DeCarli, L. M.: Quantitative relationship between amount of dietary fat and severity of alcoholic fatty liver, Am. J. Clin. Nutr. **23:**474, 1970.
7. Gabuzda, G. J., and Shear, L.: Metabolism of dietary protein in hepatic cirrhosis, nutritional and clinical considerations, Am. J. Clin. Nutr. **23:**479, 1970.
8. Rudman, D., et al.: Ammonia content of food, Am. J. Clin. Nutr. **26:**487, 1973.
9. Rudman, D., et al.: Comparison of the effect of various amino acids upon the blood ammonia concentration of patients with liver disease, Am. J. Clin. Nutr. **26:**916, 1973.
10. Sherlock, S.: Nutritional complications of biliary cirrhosis. Chronic cholestasis, Am. J. Clin. Nutr. **23:**640, 1970.
11. Sherlock, S.: Carbohydrate changes in liver disease, Am. J. Clin. Nutr. **23:**463, 1970.
12. Marco, M. L., et al.: Elevated plasma glucagon levels in cirrhosis of the liver, N. Engl. J. Med. **289:**1107, 1973.
13. Sherwin, R., et al.: Hyperglucagonemia in Laennec's cirrhosis. The role of systemic shunting, N. Engl. J. Med. **290:**239, 1974.
14. Labadarios, D., et al.: Vitamin B_6 deficiency in chronic liver disease—evidence for increased degradation of pyridoxal-5¹-phosphate, Gut **18:**23, 1977.

15. Leevy, C. M., Thompson, A., and Baker, H.: Vitamins and liver injury, Am. J. Clin. Nutr. **23:**493, 1970.
16. Morgan, A. G., et al.: Nutrition in cryptogenic cirrhosis and chronic aggressive hepatitis, Gut **17:**113, 1976.
17. Gabuzda, G. J.: Nutrition and liver disease, Med. Clin. North Am. **54:**1455, 1970.
18. Fleming, C. R., et al.: Pigmented corneal rings in non-Wilsonian liver disease, Ann. Intern. Med. **86:**285, 1977.
19. Davidson, C. S.: Dietary treatment of hepatic disease, J. Am. Diet. Assoc. **62:**515, 1973.
20. Fischer, J. E.: Amino acid infusion in hepatic encephalopathy, Dietetic Currents **3(2):**1, 1976.
21. Fischer, J., et al.: The effects of normalization of plasma amino acids on hepatic encephalopathy, Surgery **80:**77, 1976.
22. Maddrey, W., et al.: Effects of keto-analogues of essential amino acids in portal systemic encephalopathy, Gastroenterology **71:**190, 1976.
23. Popper, H.: Alcoholic hepatitis—an experimental approach to a conceptual and clinical problem, N. Engl. J. Med. **290:**159, 1974.
24. Scheig, R.: Effects of ethanol on the liver, Am. J. Clin. Nutr. **23:**467, 1970.
25. Lieber, C. S., and Decarli, L. M.: Animal models of ethanol dependence and liver injury in rats and baboons, Fed. Proc. **35:**1232, 1976.
26. Rubin, E., and Lieber, C. S.: Fatty liver, alcoholic hepatitis and cirrhosis produced by alcohol in primates, N. Engl. J. Med. **290:**128, 1974.
27. Iber, F. L.: In alcoholism, the liver sets the pace, Nutr. Today **6(1):**2, 1971.
28. Lieber, C. S., et al.: Differences in hepatic and metabolic changes after acute and chronic alcohol consumption, Fed. Proc. **34:**2060, 1975.
29. Thurman, R. G., et al.: Significant pathways of hepatic ethanol metabolism, Fed. Proc. **34:**2075, 1975.
30. Pirola, R. C., and Lieber, C. S.: Hypothesis: energy wastage in alcoholism and drug abuse: possible role of hepatic microsomal enzymes, Am. J. Clin. Nutr. **29:**90, 1976.
31. Thurman, R. G.: Hepatic alcohol oxidation and its metabolic liability, Fed. Proc. **36:**1640, 1977.
32. Lieber, C. S.: Liver adaptation and injury in alcoholism, N. Engl. J. Med. **288:**356, 1973.
33. Linscheer, W. G.: Malabsorption in cirrhosis, Am. J. Clin. Nutr. **23:**488, 1970.
34. Baker, H., et al.: Inability of chronic alcoholics with liver disease to use food as a source of folates, thiamin and vitamin B$_6$, Am. J. Clin. Nutr. **28:**1377, 1975.
35. Isselbacher, K. J.: Metabolic and hepatic effects of alcohol, N. Engl. J. Med. **296:**612, 1977.
36. Karcioglu, G. L., and Hardison, J. E.: Iron-containing plasma cells, Arch. Intern. Med. **138:**97, 1978.
37. Shaw, S., and Lieber, C. S.: Nutrition and alcoholic liver disease, Nutr. Dis., March 1978, Ross Laboratories.
38. Lieber, C. S.: Alcohol, nutrition and the liver, Am. J. Clin. Nutr. **26:**1163, 1973.
39. Malagelada, J. R., et al.: Effect of medium-chain triglycerides on liver fatty acid composition in alcoholics with or without cirrhosis, Am. J. Clin. Nutr. **26:**738, 1973.
40. Miller, P. D., Heinig, R. E., and Waterhouse, C.: Treatment of alcoholic acidosis. The role of dextrose and phosphorus, Arch. Intern. Med. **138:**67, 1978.
41. Register, U. D., et al.: Influence of nutrients on intake of alcohol, J. Am. Diet. Assoc. **61:**159, 1972.
42. The metabolic disorder in cholesterol gallstone disease, Nutr. Rev. **36:**45, 1978.
43. Binder, S. C., and Katz, B.: The benefits of surgery for asymptomatic gallstones, Am. Fam. Physician **18(4):**171, 1978.
44. Dissolution of gallstones, Nutr. Rev. **31:**113, 1973.
45. Thistle, J. L., and Hofmann, A. F.: Efficacy and specificity of chenodeoxycholic acid therapy for dissolving gallstones, N. Engl. J. Med. **289:**655, 1973.
46. Thistle, J. L., et al.: Chenotherapy for gallstone dissolution. I. Efficacy and safety, J.A.M.A. **239:**1041, 1978.
47. Chenodeoxycholic acid in the dissolution of gallstones, Nutr. Rev. **34:**20, 1976.
48. Bennion, L. J., and Grundy, S. M.: Effects of diabetes mellitus on cholesterol metabolism in man, N. Engl. J. Med. **296:**1365, 1977.
49. Bennion, L. J., et al.: Effects of oral contraceptives on the gallbladder bile of normal women, N. Engl. J. Med. **294:**189, 1976.
50. Gallbladder disease as a side effect of drugs influencing lipid metabolism. Experience in the coronary drug project, N. Engl. J. Med. **296:**1185, 1977.

6 Renal disease

KIDNEY

The major excretory organ of the body is the kidney. It is capable of excreting all waste materials except carbon dioxide, which is expired through the lungs.

Function

The kidney performs many functions and is second in diversity only to the liver. One of its functions is the removal of wastes from the blood. Metabolic end products such as urea, uric acid, creatinine, and ammonia are excreted. Also, some toxic substances are removed via the kidneys. Excess mineral salts such as calcium, chloride, magnesium, oxalate, phosphate, potassium, sodium, and sulfate are found in the urine. Thus the kidney regulates the internal chemistry of the body by reabsorbing substances that are needed and excreting those that are toxic and in excess.

Water balance is effected through the kidneys. The antidiuretic hormone (ADH), which is synthesized by the pituitary gland, promotes the reabsorption of water in the distal tubules of the nephron. It is postulated that there are osmoreceptors in the hypothalamus that are sensitive to changes in osmotic pressure, and these cause the release of ADH. Water balance is also mediated through the action of the hormone aldosterone. When serum sodium levels are low, the renal cortex releases an enzyme, renin, into the blood. The enzyme hydrolyzes angiotensinogen, a protein synthesized by the liver, into angiotensin I. Angiotensin I is converted to angiotensin II, which is a strong vasoconstrictor and stimulates the secretion of aldosterone from the adrenal cortex. Aldosterone causes the reabsorption of sodium and hence water. Potassium ions are lost in exchange for sodium ions. This is one of the means by which the kidney regulates blood pressure.

When the acidity of the blood is high, excess hydrogen ions are excreted; in alkalosis, excess bicarbonate ions are lost in the urine. Thus the blood pH can be maintained between 7.35 and 7.45. Hydrogen can be combined with phosphate and excreted as sodium dihydrogenphosphate. Glutamine can be broken down and the released ammonia converted to ammonium ion, which replaces either sodium or potassium ions.

The kidney also elaborates a hormone, erythropoietin, which stimulates red blood cell production. The kidney converts 25-hydroxycholecalciferol into the active vitamin D metabolite 1,25-dihydroxycholecalciferol.

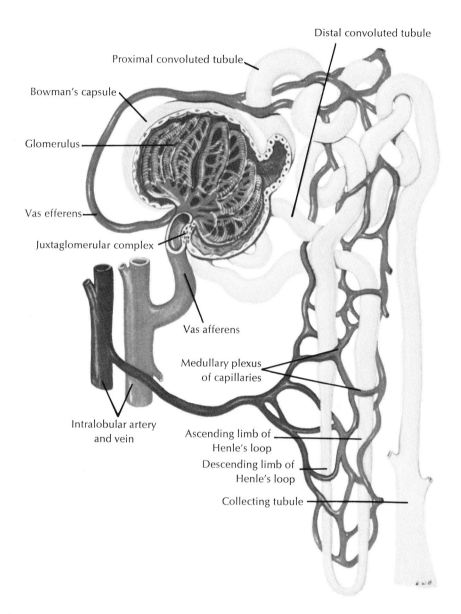

Fig. 6-1. Nephron and its associated blood supply. Wall of Bowman's capsule has been cut away to reveal detail of glomerulus. (From Schottelius, B. A., and Schottelius, D. D.: Textbook of physiology, ed. 18, St. Louis, 1978, The C. V. Mosby Co.)

Anatomy

Each kidney contains approximately 1,250,000 nephrons. The nephron is the basic structural unit, in which blood flows as follows: renal artery, vas afferens (afferent arteriole), glomerulus, vas efferens (efferent arteriole), peritubular capillaries, and finally to the renal vein. The fluid that filters through the glomerulus passes into Bowman's capsule, proximal convoluted tubule, Henle's loop, distal convoluted tubule, and lastly into the collecting tubule, which empties into the ureter and then into the bladder (see Fig. 6-1).

Each minute one fourth of the cardiac output passes through the glomeruli; therefore, in 4 to 5 minutes the entire blood supply has passed through the kidneys. Approximately 190 L of fluid are filtered per day, and normally only 1 to 2 L of urine are excreted. All except 1% of the glomerular filtrate is reabsorbed. For example, in 1 day, 270 g of glucose are filtered and totally reabsorbed, while only 15 to 25 g of urea of a total of 48 g are excreted. Glucose, amino acids, and most salts are reabsorbed. Potassium and hydrogen ions are secreted in the urine.

DIAGNOSIS OF RENAL DISEASE
Blood analysis

Elevation of the nitrogenous constituents of the blood such as urea and creatinine can indicate renal disease. Urea is measured as blood urea nitrogen (BUN) and is normally 10 to 20 mg/dl (Urea = BUN × 2.14); however, serum urea nitrogen (SUN) is also used. Normal creatinine levels are 0.7 to 1.5 mg/dl.

Urinalysis

The pH of normal urine is slightly acidic (pH 6). However, it varies slightly depending on the diet that is consumed. In the case of acidosis the pH of the urine will be much lower.

The specific gravity varies throughout the day and ranges from 1.008 to 1.030. This is the basis for the Mosenthal test. Urine samples are collected every 2 hours, and the specific gravity of each is measured. In renal dysfunction the values are nearly constant.

In renal disease, microscopic examination of the urine will reveal the presence of casts. These are made up of cells, fatty substances, and protein that have solidified in the kidney tubules and have been washed out by the urine.

Proteinuria (protein in the urine) and hematuria (blood in the urine) may be indicative of renal dysfunction.

Renal function tests

Phenolsulfonphthalein excretion test. The dye phenolsulfonphthalein (PSP) is injected intravenously, and urine is collected 15, 30, 60, and 120 minutes after the injection. In the normal individual the dye is excreted rapidly in the urine (60% by 1 hour), but the dye is retained when the kidneys are diseased.

Clearance tests. As kidney function is lost, the ability to excrete substances is diminished. The degree of kidney dysfunction can be ascertained by measuring clearance or glomerular filtration rate (GFR). The GFR is the number of milliliters of plasma completely cleared of a substance in 1 minute.

Substances that are filtered but not reabsorbed can be used to determine clearance. One such substance is the polysaccharide inulin. Since clearance varies with body size, GFR values should be corrected for surface area. Normal inulin clearance is approximately 120 ml per minute per 1.73 m.^{2} Creatinine clearance is also used since this substance is already present in the bloodstream and thus does not have to be injected. Normal values are 97 to 140 ml per minute per 1.73 m^2 for men and 85 to 125 ml per minute per 1.73 m^2 for women. Urea clearance (75 ml per minute) is not as accurate since it reflects in part protein intake. Diodrast and para-aminohippurate (PAH) are also used to determine clearance.

KIDNEY DISEASE
Nephrotic syndrome

Nephrotic syndrome may occur in conjunction with other diseases or following the ingestion of toxins. It appears frequently in children without any apparent cause. Characteristic symptoms are massive edema, albuminuria, hypoalbuminemia, hypercholesterolemia, hypertriglyceridemia, urinary casts, and hypertension.

Corticosteroids are useful in some cases. Diuretics are given to relieve the edema.

If the GFR is normal, the diet should contain adequate kilocalories and 100 g of protein. For patients with diminished kidney clearance the protein should be of high biological value and should compensate for the protein lost in the urine. Sodium intake should be restricted to 90 mEq or less per day to relieve edema and hypertension.

Nephrosclerosis

In older patients, sclerosis of the arteries is a result of arteriosclerosis and hypertension. The blood supply to the kidneys is diminished because of the narrowing of the lumen of the blood vessels. Death generally is due to cardiac failure or cerebral hemorrhage. This occurs before there is extensive damage to the kidneys. In younger patients, nephrosclerosis may lead to uremia and death. Treatment involves the reduction of blood pressure to prevent further damage to the kidneys.

Acute glomerulonephritis

Most cases of glomerulonephritis result from a streptococcal infection; the glomeruli become inflamed. Hematuria, albuminuria, oliguria (scanty urine), azotemia (nitrogenous compounds in the blood), edema, and hypertension are common symptoms.

Pencillin is administered for the treatment of the streptococcal infection. Diuretics and antihypertensive agents may be necessary.

Severe protein restriction is necessary when SUN levels are elevated. If oliguria is severe, the diet should at first be protein free. Then 0.5 g of protein of high biological value per kilogram of body weight is allowed. Calories should be provided mainly from carbohydrates. Sodium intake should be restricted to 0.5 to 1 g per day when edema and hypertension are present. Fluid consumption must be restricted when there is oliguria.

Chronic glomerulonephritis

Acute glomerulonephritis may be completely healed, or it may proceed to a latent or subacute phase and then become chronic. The glomeruli becomes fibrotic and hyalinized. Renal insufficiency is characterized by proteinuria, edema, hypertension, and nocturia (voiding of urine at night). Later, renal failure occurs.

Dietary treatment. Dietary treatment is aimed toward keeping the patient in good nutritional status. Generally 60 to 70 g of protein a day plus the amount lost in the urine is prescribed. When uremia develops, the protein restriction becomes more severe. Caloric requirements are met by 300 to 400 g of carbohydrate and 80 g of fat.

A mild salt restriction is generally followed even when edema is not present. This is to decrease the work load on the kidneys. Highly salted foods and salt in cooking or at the table should be avoided. To relieve the edema by diuresis, a 0.5 to 1 g sodium diet may be prescribed. The patient must be monitored to avoid sodium depletion.

Acute renal failure

Acute renal failure may result from acute glomerulonephritis, burns, injuries, infection, ingestion, of toxic agents such as heavy metals or carbon tetrachloride, shock due to injury, surgery, or myocardial infarction, obstructed blood flow to the kidney, or an obstructed flow of urine. The kidney shuts down and loses its excretory function. The result is either oliguria or anuria (no urine). The blood retains its excretory products such as urea, uric acid, and creatinine. Sodium, potassium, and water are also retained. If kidney function does not return within a week, dialysis is used to prevent the development of uremia.

When food cannot be taken by mouth, tube or parenteral feeding becomes necessary. At Massachusetts General Hospital, an intravenous solution consisting of eight essential amino acids and vitamins in a 47% dextrose solution was administered to 28 patients with acute renal failure.[1] Twenty-one patients survived, and their renal failure improved more quickly than the control patients who received only a glucose solution. The amino acid–glucose solution was used successfully with 200 additional patients. It is now used as standard therapy for acute renal failure.

In patients who are able to take food by mouth the intake of nitrogen, potassium, phosphate, and sulfate is limited by removing protein from the diet. A carbohydrate intake of 100 to 200 g per day prevents the breakdown of tissue proteins and ketosis. If fat is tolerated, commercial preparations of sugar and oil may be administered. Fluid intake should be restricted to 600 ml per day plus an additional amount for any unusual losses. Sodium is only given to replace that which is lost.[2]

The diet is liberalized when diuresis begins. Protein intake is gradually increased to the normal intake. The amount of protein given is based on SUN and serum creatinine levels. Sodium and potassium levels should be monitored since large amounts of these ions may be excreted.

Chronic renal failure

Symptoms. As the number of functioning nephrons diminishes, the kidney loses some if its ability to excrete nitrogenous metabolic products and to conserve or excrete water and electrolytes. The disease may progress slowly without any symptoms for years. Eventually the surviving nephrons are unable to keep up with the demand. This occurs when 90% of renal function is lost. The terminal stage is uremia, which means the presence of urinary constituents in the blood. Many symptoms are manifested in varying degrees.[3] The first uremic symptoms appear when creatinine clearance drops to 20 ml per minute.[4]

The glomerular filtration rate decreases, thus creatinine and urea clearance are diminished. The plasma SUN, uric acid, and creatinine levels are elevated. Both the urine concentrating and diluting abilities are lost. Sodium, phosphate, calcium, potassium, and glucose metabolism are altered. The net result is acidosis.

Proteinuria, pyuria (pus in the urine) cylindruria (tube casts in the urine), and broad casts are commonly found. The specific gravity of the urine is low.

The anorexia, nausea, and vomiting experienced by the patient in chronic renal failure make it difficult for him to ingest food. An ammoniacal or unpleasant taste in the mouth leads to an aversion to food. Hiccups are also common. Ulcerations of the gastrointestinal tract result in blood loss. The patients may experience constipation or diarrhea.

The uremic patient may either be drowsy or suffer from insomnia. Muscle twitching, overall weakness, and convulsions are experienced. Coma appears in the untreated individual.

Uremic patients usually have a deep, sighing respiration as a result of acidosis. The breath smells like urine. The uremic pneumonitis that develops is easily treated.

Hypertension is common to all uremic patients. Some individuals develop a serofibrinous pericarditis.

The normochromic, normocytic anemia develops as a result of a lack of the hormone erythropoietin, which is necessary for the synthesis of new red blood cells, and the decrease in the life span of the erythrocyte. Arteriosclerotic and hypertensive retinopathy may develop.

The skin assumes a pale yellow pallor because of the accumulation of urochrome pigments and anemia. Urea is excreted in sweat; after the sweat evaporates white deposits of urea crystals are formed. This is called uremic frost. It is rarely seen.

Pruritus (itching) can be relieved by a parathyroidectomy. Purpura (small pinpoint purplish red spots on the skin caused by hemorrhaging) and skin infections may develop.

Medical treatment

Transplantation. It has been feasible for several years to transplant kidneys from one individual to another. With the advent of equipment to maintain kidneys, immunosuppressant agents, and tissue matching, cadaver transplants are possible. However, the survival rate is not as great. Lowrie and co-workers have reported an 84.2% survival rate for parental transplants and an 89.5% survival rate for sibling transplants after 1 year.[5] The survival rate for cadaver allografts for the same period was only 68.7%. They suggest the need for further research in the area of tissue matching and prevention of transplant rejection.

Peritoneal dialysis. Peritoneal dialysis has been used to treat acute and chronic renal failure and water and electrolyte imbalance.[6,7] Older patients and those with systemic disease tolerate peritoneal dialysis better than hemodialysis.[8] The development of a permanent peritoneal catheter and a peritoneal dialysis machine has made the procedure simpler and safe. Generally, 2 L of dialysis fluid are instilled and removed after 30 minutes. The process is repeated 30 to 50 times. The dialysis solution contains dextrose, 1.5 g/dl; sodium, 13 mEq/L; chloride, 102 mEq/L; magnesium, 1.5 mEq/L; calcium, 3.5 mEq/L; and lactate, 35 mEq/L. The solution is hypertonic, 350 mOsm/L.

Home peritoneal dialysis is also possible. Some patients dialyze for 10 hours, four times a week.[8] Another method being used is continuous ambulatory peritoneal dialysis.[9] A plastic bag containing 2 L of dialysate fluid is connected to a permanent catheter in the peritoneal cavity. The fluid remains in the cavity for about 5 hours, with the plastic bag attached around the waist. Then the bag is lowered to drain off the fluid. Every day this process is repeated three times at 4- to 8-hour intervals.

The major difficulties associated with peritoneal dialysis are peritonitis and malnutrition due to the loss of nutrients in the effluent dialysate.[10] Protein losses have ranged from 20 to 200 g per dialysis. However, newer techniques have resulted in less protein's being lost.

It is important that patients undergoing peritoneal dialysis be maintained in an optimal nutritional state. An intake of 1 to 1.5 g of high biological value protein per kilogram of body weight per day is recommended.[10] Higher amounts are prescribed in cases of protein malnutrition. An energy intake of 35 kcal per kilogram of body weight per day is supplemented by the glucose absorbed from the dialysis solution. The hypertriglyceridemia often seen in uremics is reduced when the dietary intake of carbohydrate is reduced to 30% to 35% of calories, and the intake of polyunsaturated fats is increased. Clofibrate and activated charcoal can also be used to reduce hypertriglyceridemia. Daily supplements of ascorbic acid (100 mg), pyridoxine (10 mg), folate (1 mg), vitamin D (if needed), and the recommended allowances for the other vitamins are prescribed. Daily supplements of calcium (2 g) are necessary. Instead of an oral iron preparation iron-dextran is administered parenterally. Sodium (2 to 3 g) and potassium (3 to 3.5 g) are moderately restricted. Higher intakes of sodium necessitate more frequent dialysis. Hyperphosphatemia is prevented by decreasing the intake of dairy products and administering aluminum antacids that bind phosphate.

When the individual cannot be maintained enterally, parenteral nutrition is instituted. A solution containing 4.25% amino acids, 5% dextrose, and water-soluble vitamins is infused into a peripheral vein. Additional calories can be provided by the administration of 10% soybean oil (Intralipid). (See Chapter 9, Uncategorized Clinical Conditions.) Total parenteral nutrition has also been used. Animal research indicates that it might be beneficial to administer amino acids and dextrose into the peritoneal cavity.

Hemodialysis. The first artificial kidney was developed by Kolff in the Netherlands during World War II. Blood is passed from an artery into twin cellophane coils wound around a drum. The drum is rotated through a dialyzing solution to allow substances to diffuse in and out of the blood. Thus a portion of the waste materials not removed by the kidneys now can diffuse out into the dialysate. This process can be regulated to a certain degree by varying the concentrations of the substances in the dialyzing solution. A pump returns the blood to a vein.

A Kiil dialyzer was subsequently developed in which the blood is passed through cellophane sheets held in place by plastic plates. It functions in the same way as the Kolff artificial kidney except that dialysis takes longer.

The artificial kidney was originally used to treat acute episodes of renal failure of short duration. In 1960, a method was developed for repeatedly attaching and removing an individual from the machine. The techniques commonly used are an arteriovenus shunt or a fistula.

Patients are generally dialyzed two to three times a week for 6 to 8 hours on the coil-type machine or 10 to 14 hours on the plates.[11] This is an expensive procedure, and it is disruptive to the patient's life to report to the hospital for such long periods of time. Some of these difficulties have been overcome by the use of home dialysis.[12] For this method to be successful a member of the family must be able to operate the machine; thus the patient is able to undergo dialysis at his own convenience.

Fish and co-workers reported that 46 patients in chronic renal failure were trained for home dialysis.[13] A program of dialysis of three times a week for a total of 24 to 30 hours allowed them to consume a diet of 80 g of protein per day. Thirty-six patients were able to carry out their normal routines, while the remainder returned to part-time activity.

COST. The costs for dialysis vary.[14] Each hemodialysis costs from $146 to $259 in a hospital ($24,738 per year), $100 to $116 ($16,520 per year) in a limited care facility, and $33 to $66 ($6729) for home dialysis. The 1976 report of the National Institutes of Health Renal Transplant Registry indicated that 2.2% of patients were on peritoneal dialysis, 74.1% on facilities hemodialysis, and 23.7% on home hemodialysis (total number of patients 17,229). During that same year it was estimated that 3500 transplants were performed.

RESEARCH. Efforts are continuing on the development of a miniaturized artificial kidney that would allow the patient more mobility.[15-17] Other alternatives to hemo-dialysis are being studied. Hemofiltration has been successfully used to control blood pressure and reduce serum triglycerides.[18] Oxystarch and charcoal have been used as oral and intestinal bypass sorbents to increase fecal nitrogen excretion.[19] Gastrointestinal dialysis with a mannitol solution has also increased fecal nitrogen excretion.[20] Another aspect of research has been concerned with the oral administration of bacterial enzymes that would use waste substances in the gastrointestinal tract.[21]

Dietary treatment

Historical background. Borst in 1948 proposed a very restrictive diet for uremics.[22] The diet contained no protein or potassium and consisted solely of mixtures of butter, sugar, and starch made into soup, pudding, or butter balls.

In 1963 Giordano reported that uremic patients fed 2 g of essential amino acid nitrogen as the sole source of nitrogen with adequate calories, vitamins, and minerals showed lowered SUN levels.[23] Endogenous protein catabolism decreased and the individuals were kept in positive nitrogen balance. The nonessential amino acids were synthesized from endogenous urea.

Similar results were reported by Giovannetti and Maggiore.[24] A high-calorie, basal–protein deficient diet (1 to 1.5 g nitrogen) was fed first. Then a powdered mixture of essential amino acids (1.74 g nitrogen) or egg albumin (1.5 to 2.2 g nitrogen) was added. The SUN levels did not increase, and the patients were maintained in positive nitrogen balance.

Shaw and others modified the Giovannetti diet for British tastes.[25] Eighteen to twenty-one grams of protein from egg and milk provided the minimum daily requirement of essential amino acids. In addition, 500 mg of methionine and multivitamin and iron supplements were given. Bread and other special products made from low-protein flour were used to reduce the intake of nonessential amino acids and to increase the caloric content of the diet. Patients with a urea clearance greater than 3 ml per minute experienced relief of their uremic symptoms.

Bailey and Sullivan adapted the Giovannetti-Giordano diet for Americans.[26] The dietary treatment is successful for uremic patients with a creatinine clearance greater than 3 ml per minute. The essential amino acids are provided by one egg and 195 ml (6.5 oz) of milk for a total of 13.5 g of protein. Up to 22 g of protein are allowed. Meat is not permitted because of its high amounts of nonessential amino acids. Calories are provided from carbohydrate, fat, and alcohol. A low-protein bread is also recommended to reduce the intake of nonessential amino acids and to increase the caloric content of the diet.

Modifying dietary constituents.[27] In addition to protein intake, the fluid, sodium, and potassium levels of the diet for the uremic patient must be controlled. It is also important that an adequate amount of calories be consumed.

The primary problem in treating the uremic patient is to determine the ideal amount of protein and essential amino acids that will result in a positive nitrogen balance. Nitrogen balance is the difference between the nitrogen ingested in the diet and the nitrogen excreted from the body. Hence in positive nitrogen balance the amount of nitrogen ingested is greater than that lost from the body. Of the dietary intake of nitrogen, 70% is lost in the urine, 10% to 20% in the feces, and 5% from the skin. Since most of the ingested nitrogen is excreted in the urine, many nitrogen balance studies measure only the nitrogen lost via this route.

Negative nitrogen balance will occur when there is an inadequate intake of nitrogen or a lack of one or more essential amino acids. For the adult, eight amino acids are essential: isoleucine, leucine, lysine, methionine, phenylalanine, threonine, tryptophan, and valine. These amino acids cannot be synthesized in the body and so must be ingested in the diet. The nonessential amino acids (alanine, arginine, aspartic acid, cysteine, cystine, glycine, glutamic acid, histidine, proline, serine, and tyrosine) can be synthesized in the body, provided a source of nitrogen is available.

In renal dysfunction the normal amino acid catabolites excreted via the kidney—urea 86%, creatinine 4.6%, ammonia 3.0%, and uric acid 1.6% (percent of total nitrogen)—accumulate instead in the blood. If to correct this, dietary protein is restricted, endogenous body protein is catabolized, and nitrogen balance becomes negative. The uremic would then break down his own body or, in other words, lose lean body mass; therefore some protein must be supplied, namely, the essential amino acids. Rose and Dekker observed that endogenous urea was used to synthesize nonessential amino acids as long as the essential amino acids were provided.[28] This principle is made use of in treating uremics. The essential amino acids are provided in the diet, and the blood urea nitrogen is used to synthesize the nonessential amino acids. This is followed by an improvement of the uremic symptoms.

Uremic patients fed a diet containing 2.7 to 3 g nitrogen supplemented with essential amino acids either orally or intravenously went into positive nitrogen balance.[29] The addition of histidine, tryptophan, and human growth hormone further improved the nitrogen balance. When the amino acids were supplied via the oral route, protein synthesis occurred preferentially in the plasma, whereas intravenous administration favored protein synthesis in the muscle.

When Kopple and Swendseid fed a diet containing 21 g of eight essential amino acids to three uremic patients, nitrogen balance was negative for two patients and neutral for the other one.[30] Low plasma levels of histidine indicated that perhaps this amino acid is essential in renal failure. It was felt that the amount of nitrogen in this diet was too low and that a higher intake would have improved nitrogen balance. Although the essential amino acid requirements for uremics are not known, they may be twice that of normal individuals.[31] However, some essential amino acids may be needed in higher amounts than others.

Another approach has been to feed the amino acid precursors to reduce the toxic nitrogenous substances in the blood of uremic patients. The experiments that have been conducted were reviewed by Close.[32] Alpha-keto and alpha-hydroxy analogues of amino acids can be transaminated to synthesize both essential and nonessential amino acids. Therefore the renal patient could use his nitrogenous wastes to transaminate these analogues to make amino acids.

The keto or hydroxy analogues are used in conjunction with a protein-restricted diet; otherwise they would be oxidized.[33] The following mixture has been used by Walser: "keto-valine," "keto-leucine," "keto-isoleucine," phenyllactate, hydroxymethionine, lysine acetate, histidine, threonine, and tryptophan. The analogues of lysine and threonine cannot be transaminated; therefore, the amino acids must be provided. Histidine and tryptophan analogues can be transaminated, but the amino acids were used in some of the original studies.[34] The calcium salts of the acids are used, since renal patients have difficulty excreting sodium. Gastric irritation, hypophosphatemia, and hypercalcemia have been observed in some patients.[35]

Several studies have shown that the beneficial effects of the analogues that improve nitrogen balance are evidenced only when the dietary intake of protein is restricted to 30 g or less.[36-40] Giordano and his co-workers proposed a new formula of essential amino acids and keto acids for nutrition in uremia that was found effective in promoting a positive nitrogen balance.[41] The formula contains a higher content of tyrosine, since this amino acid is found in low concentrations in uremics. Methionine content is restricted since an excess would stimulate the formation of toxic substances. The amount of histidine is equivalent to the concentration found in human milk and egg protein.

In some instances the analogues have not been effective. It was found that infants and children grew better and showed more positive nitrogen balance when the amino acid formula was fed rather than formulas containing mixtures of keto acid and amino acids.[42] Patients on intermittent dialysis were supplemented with essential amino acids or a mixture of essential amino acids (lysine, threonine, tryptophan, histidine, and tyrosine), plus the keto analogues of the others.[43] Since these individuals were consuming a high level of protein (1 g/kg of body weight), the amino acids and amino acid–keto acid analogues were found to be ineffective.

It is not feasible to supply a synthetic essential amino acid mixture to a uremic individual; therefore, protein foods high in these amino acids must be selected. Biological value is a measure of the percentage of absorbed nitrogen retained for growth and maintenance. Biological values are determined by conducting nitrogen balance studies first on a protein-free diet and then with the test protein. Proteins with a high biological value contain a large percentage of the essential amino acids. The amount of each is approximately proportional to the minimum daily requirements. Table 6-1 lists some of the biological values of protein foods. Uremic patients are provided with proteins of high biological value such as found in eggs and milk, because these provide all of the essential amino acids and are low in nonessential amino acids.

The 1980 recommended daily dietary allowances propose the intake of 0.8 g protein per kilogram of body weight for adults. However, if protein of high biological value is consumed, the requirement is lower. The protein and essential amino acid requirements for uremics are not known. Protein intake is adjusted to the degree of renal failure. For a creatinine clearance (1 ml per minute per 1.73 m^2) of less than 5 the daily protein intake is 0.26 g/kg body weight; from 5 to 19 the intake is 0.38 g/kg

Table 6-1. Biological values*

Whole egg	94	Casein	73
Milk		Wheat, whole	67
Human	95	Potatoes, white	67
Cow	90	Corn, whole	60
Liver	77	Peas, dried	40
Meat, beef	76	Beans, dried	40
Fish	76	Gelatin	0
Rice, whole	75		

*Adapted from The Heinz handbook of nutrition, New York, 1965, McGraw-Hill Book Co.

body weight; and from 20 to 30 it is 0.5 to 0.7 g/kg body weight.[44] As the renal function decreases, a low level of dietary intake, namely, 18 g a day, is prescribed. This should be provided from protein of high biological value such as found in eggs and milk. It is difficult for the patient to adhere to the severely restricted diet in that well-liked foods, for example, meats, are not allowed. In addition, nausea, vomiting, and an unpleasant taste in the mouth further diminish the appetite.

Giordano recommended a protein intake of from 25 to 40 g a day for patients with a glomerular filtration rate (GFR) of 20 ml per minute or more and no clinical symptoms of uremia.[45] Those with symptoms and a GFR less than 20 ml per minute should ingest 25 g of protein per day. When the GFR falls below 10 ml per minute, the dietary prescription is less than 25 g of protein per day prior to dialysis or transplantation. Patients with a GFR of 3 ml per minute or less can be maintained for a short time on an essential amino acid diet. However, the caloric intake from carbohydrates and fats must be at least 45 kcal/kg of body weight or higher in order to achieve a positive nitrogen balance.

Recently diets containing 15 to 20 g of protein per day and a third of the calories provided by a carbohydrate and essential amino acid supplement have been prescribed.[31,46] In this way the patient is not restricted to a monotonous diet of high-quality protein but instead can choose from a variety of low-protein foods. The patients improved on this regimen. In severe renal insufficiency, salt retention may impose additional restrictions.

It is necessary to balance the intake and output of fluid in the uremic patient. In oliguria and anuria the allowance is based on the previous day's output plus 600 ml to compensate for insensible losses. The water present in the foods ingested must be taken into account. Food composition tables can be used to make these calculations.

Another source of water arises from the metabolism of foodstuffs. The burning of 100 g of fat, carbohydrate, and protein results in 107 g, 55 g, and 41 g of water, respectively.

It is difficult to provide an adequate caloric intake, since the uremic patient's appetite is diminished, and his selection of foods is severely restricted. An intake of 1800 to 3500 kcal primarily from carbohydrate sources should be consumed with

Table 6-2. Dietary supplements

Product	Manufacturer	Content
Cal-Power	Henkel Corporation	549 kcal/224 g (8 oz)—deionized glucose
Controlyte	Doyle Pharmaceutical Co.*	1,000 kcal/196 g (7 oz) hydrolysate of corn-starch and vegetable oil—powder
HYCAL	Beecham-Massengill Pharmaceuticals	295 kcal/112 g (4 oz)—demineralized glucose
Lipomul Oral	Upjohn Co.	90 kcal/10 g (0.35 oz)—corn oil emulsion
Polycose	Ross Laboratories	Powder, 100 g (3.5 oz) = 400 kcal; Liquid, 100 g = 200 kcal—glucose polymers

*Recipes available from Doyle Pharmaceutical Co., Highway 100 at West 23 Street, Minneapolis, Minn. 55416.

protein to achieve the protein-sparing action of carbohydrates. Since a 50 g protein diet provides approximately 1400 kcal, Cost suggested the use of desserts that are high in calories and low in proteins.[47] It is important that the patient consume an adequate caloric intake to prevent the breakdown of lean body mass.

Several commercial products are available to help increase the caloric intake of the diet. Henkel Corporation (formerly General Mills) supplies a dp low-protein baking mix and wheat starch. The dp low-protein bread can be purchased already baked and packaged in a can. Aproten products, which contain 0.5% protein, 20 mg sodium per 100 g, and 10 mg potassium per 100 g are also available. They may be obtained as Anellini (ring macaroni), Ditalini (short-ribbed macaroni), Rigationi (ribbed macaroni), Spaghettini (spaghetti), Taglialette (flat noodles), porridge, and rusks. Other products that can be purchased are dp low-protein, chocolate-flavored chip cookies and Prono, a low-protein gelled dessert mix.

Table 6-2 lists some of the other supplements, either powder or liquid, that can be purchased. They can be used in the preparation of a variety of foods or used to make desserts, sauces, or beverages.

Nonstarch supplements such as candy, popsicles, sugar, and honey are good sources of protein-free calories.

Sodium occurs in high concentrations outside of the cell, whereas potassium is found in greater amounts inside the cell. The ratio of sodium to potassium helps to maintain an exchange of ions across the semipermeable cell membrane. In the renal tubule, sodium maintains an electrochemical gradient that allows chloride, urea, and water to be passively diffused.

The dietary prescription for sodium is dependent upon the ability of the kidney to conserve and excrete sodium. The presence of large amounts of sodium in the blood contributes to edema, since sodium ions attract water molecules. The aim is to keep the body in sodium equilibrium. Since patients with renal disease cannot conserve sodium or adapt to a decreased intake, a reduction in dietary sodium may rapidly lead to sodium depletion. Dietary sodium levels must be reduced to extremely low levels in order to lower the hypertension in some patients. In these cases the diuretic furosemide increases sodium excretion so that sodium balance can be maintained on 40 mEq sodium per day without hypertension.[48]

Some patients with severe renal disease exhibit "salt wasting."[49] The increased excretion of sodium in the urine leads to extracellular fluid volume contraction. Danovitch et al. gradually reduced the sodium intake of patients with chronic renal disease who exhibited this salt-losing tendency.[50] When the reduction was gradual, the patients were able to stay in sodium balance. However when there was a large reduction in dietary sodium, the patients exhibited a salt-losing tendency. The researchers concluded that the salt-losing tendency is a result of the long-term adaptation for sodium excretion; it is reversible.

The amount of sodium excreted in the urine is used as the basis for the dietary allowance. The sodium balance may then be followed by daily weighing of the patient. A consistent weight gain of 0.9 kg (2 lb) or more per day indicates that there is too much sodium in the diet or that the patient has not adhered to the sodium restriction. The sodium consumed in medications must also be considered. Special precautions must be taken when diuretics are prescribed, since they cause excretion of both sodium and potassium.

The average dietary intake of sodium when food is salted liberally is about 5 g or 200 mEq per day. By avoiding heavily salted foods and salt in cooking or at the table, the sodium content of the diet may be reduced to 90 to 120 mEq per day or 2 to 3 g. In renal failure with edema and hypertension, 40 to 90 mEq sodium (1 to 2 g) are prescribed. When the edema is massive and the hypertension is severe, only 20 mEq of sodium are allowed.

After vomiting, diarrhea, or the administration of diuretics, the amount of sodium in the body may be very low. The intake may need to be increased to over 90 mEq per day.

For calculation of percentage of sodium and conversion to milliequivalents see below.

Percentage of sodium

Molecular weight of sodium chloride (NaCl) = 23 + 35.5 = 58.5 g
Percent of sodium in NaCl

$$\frac{Na}{NaCl} \times 100 = \frac{23}{58.5} \times 100 = 39.3\%$$

1 g NaCl = 0.393 g Na = 393 mg Na

Conversion to milliequivalents

SODIUM

$$1 \text{ mEq} = 23 \text{ mg}$$

$$\frac{460 \text{ mg}}{23 \text{ mg/mEq}} = 20 \text{ mEq}$$

$$20 \text{ mEq} \times 23 \text{ mg/mEq} = 460 \text{ mg} = 0.460 \text{ g}$$

POTASSIUM

$$1 \text{ mEq} = 39 \text{ mg}$$

$$\frac{7800 \text{ mg}}{39 \text{ mg/mEq}} = 200 \text{ mEq}$$

$$200 \text{ mEq} \times 39 \text{ mg/mEq} = 7800 \text{ mg} = 7.8 \text{ g}$$

The average intake for potassium is 80 to 200 mEq per day or 3 to 8 g. Potassium affects the acid-base balance and the contractility of muscles (skeletal and cardiac) and is needed for the excitation of nerves. The uremic patient may exhibit either hyperkalemia (elevated serum potassium > 5 mEq/L) or hypokalemia (low serum potassium < 3.8 mEq/L).

In hyperkalemia, cardiac arrhythmias, muscular weakness, cramps, increased nervous irritability, and mental disorientation appear. A twofold to threefold increase in serum potassium levels may result in death. Ion exchange resins (such as sodium polystyrene sulfonate [Kayexalate]) or an infusion of a glucose solution containing insulin and sodium bicarbonate can be administered to quickly reduce potassium levels. Dietary intake is restricted to approximately 1.5 g. This is difficult since potassium is found in large concentrations in meat, milk, eggs, fruits, and vegetables. The potassium content may be reduced by boiling for a long period of time in large amounts of water, which causes diffusion of potassium into the water. Orange and grapefruit juice, low in both sodium and potassium and with a satisfactory taste, have been prepared.[51] The juices were passed through two ion exchange resins.

On a potassium-restricted diet that is also restricted in sodium, low-sodium milk cannot be used. The milk is passed through a resin that exchanges sodium ions for potassium. Salt substitutes that contain potassium salts are contraindicated.

Hypokalemia may occur when more fluid is taken in than can be excreted by the kidney such as in oliguria or anuria. Adrenocortical steroids, mercurial diuretics, vomiting, and diarrhea can also reduce blood levels of potassium. Parenteral administration of potassium is necessary when the hypokalemia is severe. In other cases, foods high in potassium should be included in the diet, such as orange juice, tomato juice, milk, and bananas.

When the protein intake is less than 50 g per day, a multivitamin capsule plus an additional 5 mg of folic acid is recommended. A majority of uremic patients have been found to have a deficiency of vitamin B_6.[46,52] Since this vitamin functions as a coenzyme for many reactions in amino acid metabolism, a pyridoxine supplement is recommended. One of the complications of long-term chronic renal failure is renal osteodystrophy. This process can be slowed down by a high-calcium, low phosphorus diet.[53] This is difficult to achieve since a low-phosphorus diet would also result in a severe restriction of protein. Supplementation with calcium carbonate, calcium lactate, or calcium gluconate can provide the necessary calcium. Phosphorus can be reduced by the administration of aluminum hydroxide (Amphojel) or aluminum carbonate (Basaljel) gels, which bind phosphorus in the gastrointestinal tract and interfere with its absorption. Dietary restriction of 700 to 800 mg phosphorus per day is necessary when the GFR is less than 25 ml per minute.

The abnormal calcium metabolism could be corrected by the use of 1,25-dihydroxycholecalciferol (1,25-$(OH)_2D_3$), which is no longer synthesized in adequate amounts by the kidney. At present, sufficient amounts of this vitamin D metabolite are not available for testing. However, similar compounds such as 1-α-OH-D_3,5,6 transvitamin D_3 and dihydrotachysterol have been used successfully both in animals and humans.[46,53]

Dietary treatment for children. Children with uremia have a decreased muscle mass, reduced adipose tissue stores, and a low weight-for-height ratio.[54] This is a result of a dietary energy deficit and the catabolic state associated with uremia. Growth retardation is seen in uremic children who are on hemodialysis or who have had transplants.[55] Several factors have been implicated such as undernutrition, osteodystrophy, acidosis, hyposthenuria (decreased urinary osmolality), deficiencies of sodium, phosphate, magnesium, zinc, and potassium, chronic infection, hypertension, corticosteroids, and somatomedin. Uremic children have a higher than normal requirement for calories; the requirement for protein has not been determined. Anorexia and many other factors contribute to the decreased food intake.

Renal osteodystrophy also alters the growth rate. The factors involved in this syndrome are phosphorus, parathyroid hormone, acidosis, aseptic necrosis, calcium, and vitamin D. The treatment involves aluminum hydroxide for excess phosphorus, a correction of the acidosis, and administration of calcium and analogues of vitamin D.

Spinozzi and Grupe recommend a caloric intake of 80% or more of the recommended allowance, carbohydrate or fat supplements and 1.5 to 2 g of high biological value protein per kilogram of body weight per day.[55] However, anorexia makes dietary treatment difficult.

Berger recommends that the dietary prescription for protein, fluid, and electrolytes be based on laboratory data and clinical symptoms; the diet must be adapted to each child.[56] The most important dietary component is energy. Dietary instruction for children is difficult since they do not understand the need for all the restrictions. Yet, repeated attempts must be made to educate children and their parents.

Dietary treatment during dialysis. During dialysis, nitrogen-containing compounds, vitamins, and water-soluble nutrients are lost. Kopple and co-workers recommended that a dietary intake of 0.75 to 1.25 g of protein per kilogram of body weight is sufficient to maintain the dialysis patient in neutral or positive nitrogen balance.[57] The lower amount of protein is poorly tolerated, and the higher amount results in an increase in uremic symptoms. The amount can be lowered to 0.63 g/kg of body weight if the protein is of high biological value. This amount was also recommended by Smith and Hill for patients on intermittent dialysis.[58] Ginn and co-workers recommended 0.75 g/kg of body weight for patients undergoing dialysis twice a week.[59] The protein fed was a mixture of egg and beef. A requirement of 0.63 g/kg would be needed to keep the individual in positive nitrogen balance if only egg protein were fed. Burton recommended 1 g of protein per kilogram of body weight, of which 75% should come from protein of high biological value.[60] The energy needs should be met by providing 35 to 45 kcal per kilogram of body weight.

The Artificial Kidney–Chronic Uremia Program of the National Institutes of Health has started a cooperative study to determine whether dialysis time can be changed to 2 to 4 hours instead of 5 to 6 hours and whether patients can tolerate higher BUN levels.[61] Strict dietary control is being used to keep the subjects within the prescribed 1 g of protein per kilogram of body weight. A good control is set at a BUN of 80 ± 10 mg/dl and a protein catabolic rate of 1.1 ± 0.3 g/kg per 24 hours. These criteria were selected since it is assumed that the degree of dietary control is reflected by the BUN levels. Previous studies have shown a linear relationship between urea synthesis and protein catabolism; therefore the protein catabolic rate is also used as a guideline. Patients who are out of target range are seen by the dietitian for intensive counseling.

Potassium levels must be carefully monitored, since hyperkalemia can result in cardiac arrest or arrhythmias. It is difficult to restrict dietary potassium, since it is present in a variety of foods, in particular fruits, vegetables, and meats. The sodium intake should be restricted to 65 to 87 mEq per day to control hypertension and the retention of fluid.[60]

Dialysis dementia. Aluminum phosphate–binding gels have been prescribed for uremic patients on dialysis to control serum phosphate levels. It was thought that these gels were excreted with the bound phosphate in the feces with very little absorption of aluminum. A dialysis encephalopathy of unknown cause had been reported in several chronic hemodialysis patients. [67] Since the aluminum phosphate–binding gels had been administered for 2 years prior to this illness, the aluminum content of muscle, bone, and brain was measured. Higher aluminum levels were found in the trabecular bone and muscle of patients on dialysis as compared with control subjects. The aluminum levels in the brain gray-matter were higher in the patients who had died of the encephalopathy syndrome as compared to uremics who had died of other causes and in the control subjects. This suggested that the dialysis encephalopathy syndrome could be due to aluminum intoxication.

In another dialysis center an outbreak of dialysis dementia occurred when the city altered its water purification processes, resulting in higher water aluminum levels.[68] However, since this was a retrospective study, tissue levels of aluminum were not measured. The etiology still remains unknown, and other factors have also been implicated.

In chronic renal failure there is a decreased intake of dietary iron and synthesis of red blood cells. Aluminum hydroxide, which is administered to bind phosphate, can also bind iron in the gastrointestinal tract. Patients on hemodialysis show a decreased incorporation of iron into erythrocytes and a greater loss of iron from the body because of blood sampling and losses in the artificial kidney.[62] It is therefore recommended that supplemental iron be administered via the parenteral route to replenish bone marrow iron stores. Mirahmadi et al. have concluded that serum ferritin levels appear to reflect the level of bone marrow iron stores.[63] Patients with serum ferritin levels less than 120 ng/ml may need iron supplementation, while those with higher ferritin values should not be given iron.

Renal failure patients on long-term hemodialysis may be prone to vitamin deficiences. It is possible that water-soluble vitamins are lost in the dialysate. The loss of folic acid during hemodialysis has been reported.[64] Vitamin depletion may also occur from dietary restrictions; for example, a diet restricted in potassium may reduce the intake of water-soluble vitamins that are found in similar food sources. Sullivan and Eisenstein suggested that 1 g of ascorbic acid be added to the dialysate at the beginning and midpoint of dialysis to avoid the depletion of body stores of vitamin C.[65] Altered excretion, metabolic function, and drug administration also promote vitamin deficiency. Kopple and Swendseid suggested that amounts equivalent to the recommended daily dietary allowances for thiamine, niacin, pantothenic acid, and riboflavin are adequate for patients on hemodialysis.[66] Dietary supplements of vitamin B_6, folic acid (1 mg per day), and ascorbic acid (100 mg per day) should be prescribed. The fat-soluble vitamins A, E, or K do not need to be supplemented.

Hyperlipidemia. Hyperlipidemia has been observed in children and adults who are undergoing chronic hemodialysis and after renal transplantation.[69,70] Hypertriglyceridemia is commonly found; cholesterol levels are generally normal. Low levels of HDL cholesterol have been found in uremic patients.[71-73] Type II and type IV hyperlipoproteinemia occur;[71,72,74,75] however, a higher incidence of type IV is found in those on dialysis, whereas type II appears most often after renal transplantation. A decreased incidence of hyperlipidemia was found in those who had been on dialysis for more than 5 years.[75]

The pathogenesis of this disorder has not been elucidated. The hypertriglyceridemia could be due to an increased rate of hepatic synthesis or a decreased rate of removal from plasma. Decreased postheparin lipolytic activity has been found to be due to a decrease in hepatic triglyceride lipase, whereas lipoprotein lipase activity is normal.[69,71,76]

Since acetate is used in the dialysate, it was suggested that this might contribute to the hypertriglyceridemia. However, an infusion of acetate in dialysis patients and normal volunteers did not result in an increase in serum cholesterol or triglycerides.[77]

Activated charcoal and oxystarch (periodic acid oxidation product of soluble corn starch) have been used as intestinal sorbents to treat uremia. Charcoal absorbs uremic metabolites and oxystarch binds nitrogenous waste products. When both were administered to hemodialysis patients, there was a decrease in serum lipids, triglycerides, and cholesterol.[78] When the sorbents were discontinued, the values returned to the pretreatment levels. The lipid-lowering effect has been shown to be due to the activated charcoal and not to the oxystarch.[79] It has been postulated that the charcoal binds lipids in the gut.

Since the administration of lipid-lowering drugs may cause additional complications in uremic patients, further dietary modifications have been tested as a means of reducing the hyperlipidemia. Sanfelippo, Swenson, and Reaven fed two isocaloric formula diets to 12 patients with chronic renal failure.[80] The first diet approximated the patients' normal intakes and consisted of 10% of calories from protein, 50% from carbohydrates, and 40% as fat, 600 mg cholesterol, and a P/S ratio of 0.2. The second diet contained 10% of calories from protein, 35% from carbohydrates, and 55% from fat, 300 mg cholesterol, and a P/S ratio of 2.0. The latter diet resulted in a decrease in the fasting serum triglyceride levels in each subject; serum cholesterol levels were unchanged.

In a later study these researchers studied the effects of dietary modification on 12 patients on hemodialysis.[81] Three isocaloric formula diets were used: conventional diet—10% of calories as protein, 50% as carbohydrates, and 40% as fat, 600 mg cholesterol, and a P/S ratio of 0.2; low-carbohydrate, polyunsaturated fat diet—10% of calories as protein, 35% as carbohydrates, and 55% as fat, 300 mg cholesterol, and a P/S ratio of 2.0; low-carbohydrate, saturated fat diet—10% of calories as protein, 35% as carbohydrates, and 55% as fat, 600 mg cholesterol, and a P/S ratio of 0.2. Both low-carbohydrate diets resulted in a decrease in fasting serum triglyceride levels in 11 of 12 patients. A study of triglyceride kinetics in dialyzed and nondialyzed patients with renal failure suggested that there is a defect in triglyceride clearance.

In another study a modified fat diet consisting of 40% of calories from fat, 50% from carbohydrate, and 10% from protein, 275 mg cholesterol, and a P/S ratio of 1 was used.[82] Ten chronic hemodialysis patients who had type IV and 10 patients with type IIb hyperlipoproteinemia consumed this diet for 1 month as outpatients. Even though the carbohydrate content of the diet was higher than the diet previously prescribed, serum triglyceride and cholesterol levels decreased. However, after 12 patients returned to their previous diet, their serum cholesterol and triglyceride levels increased to the pretreatment values.

Dietary calculations—patient education. The diets for chronic renal failure patients are very restrictive and thus not very appealing. The restriction of protein, sodium, potassium, and fluid makes it extremely difficult for the individual to understand, let alone adhere to. In some instances, a system of priorities must be established in treating the patients. Geriatric patients on a 24 g protein diet are allowed 1 free day a month in which they can eat anything they want.[83] This has helped the patients to adhere to the diet for the rest of the month.

Several methods have been devised to assist with meal planning. Jordan and co-workers devised a basic meal pattern for controlled protein, sodium, and potassium diets.[84] A food exchange system similar to the diabetic exchange lists indicates the protein, sodium, potassium, and water content of foods classified into six categories, namely, meats, vegetables, fruits, cereals, rice, and sweets.

De St. Jeor, Carlston, and Tyler established protein equivalent groupings.[85] Their method takes into account the protein content of fruits, vegetables, and other foods low in protein. Eight protein groups were established on the basis of their protein, amino acid, sodium, potassium, and fluid content. The groups are (1) milk, (2) eggs, (3) meat, fish, poultry, (4) starches, (5) vegetables, (6) fruits, (7) fats, and (8) miscellaneous. Groups 1, 2, and 3 supply protein of high biological value. Minimum amino acid requirements are met, but vitamin and mineral supplements must be provided for most diets. A sample menu and dietary calculations for a 40 g protein (500 mg sodium, 2000 mg potassium, 500 ml fluid, 2000 kcal) diet are given. This system makes it easier for the dietitian to calculate the restricted nutrient content of the diet. Although it was used for hospital patients, the authors suggest that it could be used for outpatients.

To facilitate the dietary planning for hemodialysis patients, Robinson and Paulbitski devised three basic diets, types I, II, and III, that could easily be individualized for each patient.[86] The type I diet contains 60 g of protein, 1 g of sodium, and 2 g of potassium. The type II diet allows 40 g of protein, 0.5 g of sodium, and 1.5 g of potassium. In it the meat allowance is decreased from the 140 g (5 oz) of type I to 91 g (3¼ oz), and the intake of vegetable and cereal products is reduced. The sodium content of these two diets can be varied by either increasing or decreasing the amount of salt used at the table. Potassium levels are adjusted by varying the beverages, fruits, and vegetables. The type III diet provides 20 g of high biological value protein from eggs, milk, and milk products. The content of sodium is 0.5 g and potassium is 1.2 g. Fats, nonprotein bread, and desserts low in protein are used to maintain an adequate intake of calories. A sample menu for the type I diet was included as well as a sample of recipes. A booklet for patients supplied information about the dietary restriction for protein, sodium, and potassium. A sample menu pattern and a list of nine food groups with the calorie, protein, sodium, and potassium content of each was also included. Programmed instruction and sessions with the dietitian have proved helpful in educating the patient about his diet.

Another method for calculating diets for hemodialysis patients is based on a point system.[87] One point is equal to 1 mEq; therefore, one sodium point is the equivalent of 23 mg of sodium or 1 mEq. Dietary prescriptions generally call for 60 to 80 g protein (60 to 80 protein points), 1500 mg sodium (65 sodium points), and 3 g potassium (77 potassium points). A booklet was prepared based on food groups with the number of points of protein, sodium, and potassium. The groups were fats, fruits, juices, milk, protein foods, starchy foods, vegetables, miscellaneous, and miscellaneous fluids. Dietary instructions were also given to each patient.

Vetter and Shapiro developed a program in which lists of allowed foods plus alternate foods are grouped together on the basis of their protein, sodium, and potassium content.[88] The eight lists consist of milk; meat, eggs, fish, and cheese; bread and cereals; low-protein products; vegetables and soups; fruits and fruit juices; fats; and miscellaneous free foods. The number of servings of each food group is based on the dietary prescription. The patient is instructed as soon as dietary control is necessary. The person preparing the meals and other family members are also taught the diet.

At Southern California Medical Center a dietetic food store has been set up for patients on hemodialysis where low-sodium and low-protein products are sold.[89] Diabetic and weight-reduction products, low-cholesterol products, and allergy foods are also stocked. Twelve hemodialysis patients were provided with scales for use in their homes. A dietitian visited the patients to explain the use of the scales and to answer questions concerning dietary procedures. Ten of the patients showed less weight gain between dialyses and lower serum potassium levels. This improvement was attributed to the patients' adherence to their diets. While the patients were undergoing dialysis, they were equipped with headphones and a microphone which allowed them to ask questions of the dietitian and spend some of the time during dialysis in a useful way.

A novel approach to patient education was sponsored by the Illinois Council on Renal Nutrition.[90] Two gourmet-cooking workshops were held. At the first one, two complete meals were prepared, and at the second, four entrees and five special desserts were presented. The participants were able to sample all the foods. In addition, several displays were set up, recipes were distributed to the audience, and questions were answered. The workshop pointed out that there was much misinformation about renal diets and thus a great need for patient education.

Several self-instruction programs have been developed and found to be of assistance in teaching uremic patients.[91-98]

A selected bibliography on renal disease has been prepared by the Council on Renal Nutrition of the National Kidney Foundation.[99] Updates are published in the *Council on Renal Nutrition News.*

Dietary compliance. Fifty-three patients on chronic hemodialysis were studied as to their compliance to a renal diet order of 80 g of protein, 2 g sodium, and 2 g potassium.[100] Three compliance indicators were measured: serum potassium, serum phosphorus, and between-dialyses weight gains. Serum potassium levels of 3.5 to 5.0 mEq/L were considered acceptable. This parameter also indicates protein compliance and the restrictions placed on fruits, vegetables, and certain desserts. Acceptable serum phosphorus levels were established at 3.5 to 5.0 mg/dl. Compliance indicated the avoidance of a high intake of dietary phosphorus and the taking of the prescribed medication. In this dialysis center, phosphate is controlled by medication rather than by dietary restriction. A weight gain of 1.8 kg (4 lb) or less indicated compliance with a restricted intake of fluid and dietary sodium.

Compliance was defined as falling within the acceptable limits at least 50% of the examined times. It was found that 79% of the patients were potassium compliant, 62% were phosphorus compliant, and 49% were weight compliant. It was concluded that perhaps motivational techniques could be used with hemodialysis patients so that they would comply more closely with their treatment program.

Biller described her difficulties with dietary compliance prior to a kidney transplant.[101] In particular she described the unacceptability of the wheat starch bread and the repetition of each meal. She recommended that the diet be made more palatable and that patient education be more effective. This could be accomplished by individualizing the diet and taking into account the patient's food preferences; providing lower cost, special dietary products; providing recipes; educating hospital personnel; and better understanding the needs and desires of the renal patient.

Renal calculi[102,103]

Renal calculi (stones) may be found anywhere along the urinary tract. In many cases there are no symptoms.

Calcium stones. Most renal stones that are found contain, in part, calcium. Several conditions may lead to the excretion of large amounts of calcium in the urine, thus enhancing the possibility of stone formation. Primary hyperparathyroidism increases serum calcium and decreases serum phosphate. The excess calcium is excreted in the urine. An excessive intake of vitamin D or increased production of 1,25 dihydroxyvitamin D also results in hypercalciuria (elevated urinary calcium levels) as this leads to increased intestinal absorption of calcium. The milk-alkali syndrome, caused by an excessive intake of milk and alkali to treat a peptic ulcer, and the ingestion of calcium-based antacids cause an increase in the excretion of urinary calcium. Prolonged immobilization because of illness or destructive bone disease promotes the excretion of calcium. In the case of idiopathic hypercalciuria and renal tubular acidosis, serum calcium levels are normal, but urinary excretion is elevated.

Approximately 50% of the stones formed are composed of calcium oxalate. This may result from congenital or familial oxaluria or a high intake of food oxalate; in particular cabbage, spinach, tomatoes, citrus fruits, rhubarb, chocolate, and tea. Increased intestinal absorption can result in hyperoxaluria. Some individuals who have undergone ileal resection or intestinal bypass operations develop oxalate stones.

A high fluid intake is prescribed to dilute the urine and prevent the formation of new stones. A low-calcium diet may be helpful in some cases. An acid ash diet will render the urine acidic and thus decrease the precipitation of calcium salts, since they are most insoluble at alkaline pHs. If the stones contain oxalate, then the diet should not contain foods that have a high oxalate content.

Uric acid stones. A small percentage of renal calculi are uric acid. This is an end product of purine metabolism. Large amounts of uric acid are produced in gout, a metabolic disorder. Hyperuricosuria, low urine volume, and low urine pH contribute to stone formation. Low-purine diets were prescribed in the past; however, since these diets are very restrictive, only foods with a high purine content should be avoided. Increased fluid intake and alkaline agents are prescribed to prevent the formation of uric acid stones. The drug allopurinol is used when urinary uric acid levels are extremely elevated.

Cystine stones. Cystinuria is a rare inborn error of amino acid metabolism. Due to a defect in transport, cystine, arginine, lysine, and ornithine are not reabsorbed in the kidney tubules. When the urine is acidic, cystine precipitates out. A restriction of methionine reduces the excretion of cystine. However, this entails the restriction of dietary protein. Treatment involves a high fluid intake, alkaline agents to increase urinary pH, and an alkaline ash diet. If this is not successful then the drug D-penicillamine is used to complex and solubilize cystine.

REFERENCES

1. Able, R. M., et al.: Acute renal failure: treatment with intravenous amino acids and glucose, N. Engl. J. Med. **288**:695, 1973.
2. Lemann, J.: Acute renal failure, Am. Fam. Physician **18**(3):148, 1978.
3. Pullman, T. N., and Cole, F. L.: Chronic renal failure, Summit, N. J., 1973, Clinical Symposia of Ciba-Geigy Corp.
4. Hamburger, R. J.: The management of uremia, Am. Fam. Physician **16**(3):125, 1977.
5. Lowrie, E. G., et al.: Chronic hemodialysis and renal transplantation: survival rates, N. Engl. J. Med. **288**:863, 1973.
6. Smith, E. C., and Dunea, G.: Practical methods of renal dialysis, Am. Fam. Physician **2**(2):87, 1970.
7. Vaamonde, C. A., and Perez, G. O.: Peritoneal dialysis today, Kidney **10**:31, 1977.
8. Oreopoulous, D. G.: Renewed interest in chronic peritoneal dialysis, Kidney Int. **13**:S-117, 1978.
9. The body may be best, Time, Dec. 18, 1978, p. 82.
10. Blumenkrantz, M. J., et al.: Nutritional management of the adult patient undergoing peritoneal dialysis, J. Am. Diet. Assoc. **73**:251, 1978.
11. Dunea, G.: Peritoneal dialysis and hemodialysis, Med. Clin. North Am. **55**:155, 1971.
12. Muehreke, R. C., et al.: Home hemodialysis, Med. Clin. North Am. **55**:1473, 1971.
13. Fish, J. C., Remmers, A. R., Jr., Lindley, J. D., and Sarles, H. E.: Albumin kinetics and nutritional rehabilitation in the home dialysis patient, N. Engl. J. Med. **287**:478, 1972.
14. Friedman, E. A., Delano, B. G., and Butt, K. M. H.: Pragmatic realities in uremia therapy, N. Engl. J. Med. **298**:368, 1978.
15. Stephen, R. L., et al.: Combined technolog-

ical-clinical approach to wearable dialysis, Kidney Int. **13**:S-125, 1978.
16. Blackshear, P. L.: Two new concepts that might lead to a wearable artificial kidney, Kidney Int. **13**:S-133, 1978.
17. Klein, E.: A compound artificial kidney without dialysis: an analysis of remaining problems, Kidney Int. **13**:S-188, 1978.
18. Henderson, C. W.: Hemofiltration, Kidney Int. **13**:S-145, 1978.
19. Sinclair, A., et al.: Roux-Y intestinal bypass for administration of sorbents in uremia, Kidney Int. **13**:S-153, 1978.
20. Young, T-K, and Lee, S-C.: Gastrointestinal dialysis in the therapy of uremia, Kidney Int. **13**:S-185, 1978.
21. Setälä, K.: Bacterial enzymes in uremia management, Kidney Int. **13**:S-194, 1978.
22. Borst, J. C. G.: Protein katabolism in uraemia, effects of protein-free diets, infections and blood transfusions, Lancet **1**:824, 1948.
23. Giordano, C.: Use of exogenous and endogenous urea for protein synthesis in normal uremic subjects, J. Lab. Clin. Med. **62**:231, 1963.
24. Giovannetti, S., and Maggiore, Q.: A low nitrogen diet with proteins of high biological value for severe chronic uraemia, Lancet **1**:1000, 1964.
25. Shaw, A. B., et al.: The treatment of chronic renal failure by a modified Giovannetti diet, Q. J. Med. **34**:237, 1965.
26. Bailey, G. L., and Sullivan, N. R.: Selected protein diet in terminal uremia, J. Am. Diet. Assoc. **52**:125, 1968.
27. Burton, B. T.: Nutritional implications of renal disease. I. Current overview and general principles, J. Am. Diet. Assoc. **70**:479, 1977.

28. Rose, W. C., and Dekker, E. E.: Urea as a source of nitrogen for the biosynthesis of amino acids, J. Biol. Chem. **223**:107, 1956.

29. Bergstrom, J., Furst, P., Josephson, B., and Noree, L. O.: Factors affecting the nitrogen balance in chronic uremic patients receiving essential amino acids, intravenously or by mouth, Nutr. Metab. **14**:162, 1972.

30. Kopple, J. D., and Swendseid, M. E.: Nitrogen balance and plasma amino acid levels in uremic patients fed an essential amino acid diet, Am. J. Clin. Nutr. **27**:806, 1974.

31. Walser, M., and Mitch, W.: Dietary management of renal failure, The Kidney **10**:13, 1977.

32. Close, H.: Use of amino acid precursors in nitrogen-accumulation diseases, N. Engl. J. Med. **290**:663, 1974.

33. Walser, M.: Keto-analogues of essential amino acids in the treatment of chronic renal failure, Kidney Int. **13**:S-180, 1978.

34. Walser, M.: Keto acid therapy in chronic renal failure, Nephron **21**:57, 1978.

35. Walser, M.: Principles of keto acid therapy in uremia, Am. J. Clin. Nutr. **31**:1756, 1978.

36. Bergström, J., et al.: Metabolic studies with keto acids in uremia, Am. J. Clin. Nutr.**31**:1761, 1978.

37. Burns, J., et al.: Comparison of the effects of keto acid analogues and essential amino acids on nitrogen homeostasis in uremic patients in moderately protein-restricted diets, Am. J. Clin. Nutr. **31**:1767, 1978.

38. Ell, S., et al.: Metabolic studies with keto acid diets, Am. J. Clin. Nutr. **31**:1776, 1978.

39. Heidland, A., et al.: Evaluation of essential amino acids and keto acids in uremic patients on low protein diet, Am. J. Clin. Nutr. **31**:1784, 1978.

40. Bauerdick, H., Spellerberg, P., and Lamberts, B.: Therapy with essential amino acids and their nitrogen-free analogues in severe renal failure, Am. J. Clin. Nutr. **31**:1793, 1978.

41. Giordano, C., Desanto, N. G., and Pluvio, M.: Nitrogen balance in uremic patients on different amino acid and keto acid formulations—a proposed reference pattern, Am. J. Clin. Nutr. **31**:1797, 1978.

42. Giordano, C., et al: Amino acid and keto acid diet in uremic children and infants, Kidney Int. **13**:S-83, 1978.

43. Ulm, A., Neuhauser, M., and Leber, H. W.: Influence of essential amino acids and keto acids on protein metabolism and anemia of patients on intermittent hemodialysis, Am. J. Clin. Nutr. **31**:1827, 1978.

44. Anderson, C. F., et al.: Nutritional therapy for adults with renal disease, J. A. M. A. **223**:68, 1973.

45. Giordano, C.: The role of diet in renal disease, Hosp. Pract. **12**(11):113, 1977.

46. Swendseid, M. E.: Nutritional implications of renal disease. III. Nutritional needs of patients with renal disease, J. Am. Diet. Assoc. **70**:488, 1977.

47. Cost, J. S.: Diet in chronic renal disease: a focus on calories, J. Am. Diet. Assoc. **64**:186, 1974.

48. Ulvila, J. M., Kennedy, J. A., Lamberg, J. D., and Scribner, B. H.: Blood pressure in chronic renal failure: effect of sodium intake and furosemide, J. A. M. A. **200**:223, 1972.

49. Kassirer, J. P., and Gennari, F. J.: Salt wasting—consequence of functional adaptation, N. Engl. J. Med. **296**:42, 1977.

50. Danovitch, G. M., Bourgoignie, J., and Bricker, N. S.: Reversibility of the "salt-losing" tendency of chronic renal failure, N. Engl. J. Med. **296**:14, 1977.

51. Levy, N., Boxer, J., and Carter, A.: Citrus juice treated with exchange resins, N. Engl. J. Med. **289**:753, 1973.

52. Kopple, J. D., et al.: Amino acid and protein metabolism in renal failure, Am. J. Clin. Nutr. **31**:1532, 1978.

53. Schoolwerth, A. C., and Engle, J. E.: Calcium and phosphorus in diet therapy of uremia, J. Am. Diet Assoc. **66**:460, 1975.

54. Holliday, M. A., and Chantler, C.: Metabolic and nutritional factors in children with renal insufficiency, Kidney Int. **14**:306, 1978.

55. Spinozzi, N. S., and Grupe, W. E.: Nutritional implications of renal disease. IV. Nutritional aspects of chronic renal insufficiency in childhood, J. Am. Diet. Assoc. **70**:493, 1977.

56. Berger, M.: Dietary management of children with uremia, J. Am. Diet. Assoc. **70**:498, 1977.

57. Kopple, J. D., et al.: Evaluating modified protein diets for uremia, J. Am. Diet. Assoc. **54**:481, 1969.

58. Smith, E. B., and Hill, P. A.: Protein in diets of dialyzed and nondialyzed uremic patients, J. Am. Diet. Assoc. **60**:389, 1972.

59. Ginn, H. E., Frost, A., and Lacy, W. W.: Nitrogen balance in hemodialysis patients, Am. J. Clin. Nutr. **21**:385, 1968.

60. Burton, B. T.: Current concepts of nutrition

and diet in disease of the kidney, J. Am. Diet. Assoc. **65**:627, 1974.

61. Wineman, R. J., Sargent, J. A., and Piercy, L.: Nutritional implications of renal disease. II. The dietitian's key role in studies of dialysis therapy, J. Am. Diet. Assoc. **70**:483, 1977.

62. Iron metabolism in renal failure, Nutr. Rev. **30**:110, 1972.

63. Mirahmadi, K. S., et al.: Serum ferritin level. Determinant of iron requirement in hemodialysis patients, J. A. M. A. **238**:601, 1977.

64. Dialysis, renal failure and vitamin homeostasis. Nutr. Rev. **27**:75, 1969.

65. Sullivan, J. F., and Eisenstein, A. B.: Ascorbic acid depletion during hemodialysis, J. A. M. A. **220**:1697, 1972.

66. Kopple, J. D., and Swendseid, M. E.: Vitamin nutrition in patients undergoing maintenance hemodialysis, Kidney Int. **7**:S-79, 1975.

67. Alfrey, A. C., Le Gendre, G. R., and Kaehny, W. D.: The dialysis encephalopathy syndrome, N. Engl. J. Med. **294**:184, 1976.

68. Dunea, G., et al.: Role of aluminum in dialysis dementia, Ann. Intern. Med. **88**:502, 1978.

69. McCosh, E. J., et al.: Hypertriglyceridemia in patients with chronic renal insufficiency, Am. J. Clin. Nutr. **28**:1036, 1975.

70. Hussey, H. H.: Hyperlipidemia in children following long-term hemodialysis or renal transplantation, J. A. M. A. **236**:1387, 1976.

71. Mordasini, R., et al.: Selective deficiency of hepatic triglyceride lipase in uremic patients, N. Engl. J. Med. **297**:1362, 1977.

72. Bagdade, J. D., and Albers, J. J.: Plasma high-density lipoprotein concentrations in chronic hemodialysis and renal-transplant patients, N. Engl. J. Med. **296**:1436, 1977.

73. Norbeck, H. E., Orö, L., and Carlson, L. A.: Serum lipoprotein concentrations in chronic uremia, Am. J. Clin. Nutr. **31**:1881, 1978.

74. Ponticelli, C., et al.: Lipid abnormalities in maintenance dialysis patients and renal transplant recipients, Kidney Int. **13**:S-72, 1978.

75. Frank, W. M., et al.: Relationship of plasma lipid to renal function and length of time on maintenance hemodialysis, Am. J. Clin. Nutr. **31**:1886, 1978.

76. Heuck, C. C., et al.: Serum lipids in renal insufficiency, Am. J. Clin. Nutr. **31**:1547, 1978.

77. Port, F. K., Easterling, R. E., and Barnes, R. V.: Effect of acetate administration on blood lipids, Am. J. Clin. Nutr. **31**:1893, 1978.

78. Friedman, E. A., et al.: Reduction in hyperlipidemia in hemodialysis patients treated with charcoal and oxidized starch (oxystarch), Am. J. Clin. Nutr. **31**:1903, 1978.

79. Friedman, E. A., et al.: Charcoal-induced lipid reduction in uremia, Kidney Int. **13**:S-170, 1978.

80. Sanfelippo, M. L., Swenson, R. S., and Reaven, G. M.: Reduction of plasma triglycerides by diet in subjects with chronic renal failure, Kidney Int. **11**:54, 1977.

81. Sanfelippo, M.L., Swenson, R. S., and Reaven, G. M.: Response of plasma triglycerides to dietary changes in patients on hemodialysis, Kidney Int. **14**:180, 1978.

82. Gokal, R., et al.: Dietary treatment of hyperlipidemia in chronic hemodialysis patients, Am. J. Clin. Nutr. **31**:1915, 1978.

83. Carmena, R., and Shapiro, F. C.: Dietary management of chronic renal failure: experience at Hennepin County General Hospital, Geriatrics **27**:95, 1972.

84. Jordan, W.L., et al.: Basic pattern for a controlled protein, sodium and potassium diet, J. Am. Diet Assoc. **50**:137, 1967.

85. De St. Jeor, S. T., Carlston, B. J., and Tyler, F. H.: Planning low protein diets for use in chronic renal failure, J. Am. Diet. Assoc. **54**:34, 1969.

86. Robinson, L. G., and Paulbitski, A. H.: Diet therapy and educational programs for patients with chronic renal failure, J. Am. Diet. Assoc. **61**:531, 1972.

87. Stein, P. G., and Winn, N. J.: Diet controlled in sodium, potassium, protein and fluid: use of points for dietary calculation, J. Am. Diet. Assoc. **61**:538, 1972.

88. Vetter, L., and Shapiro, R.: An approach to dietary management of the patient with renal disease, J. Am. Diet. Assoc. **66**:158, 1975.

89. Card, B. K.: Dietetic food store for patients on hemodialysis, J. Am. Diet. Assoc. **62**:425, 1973.

90. Beto, J. A., and Myscofski, J. M. W.: Gourmet cooking workshops for dialysis patients, J. Am. Diet. Assoc. **70**:626, 1977.

91. Programmed instruction: potassium imbalance, Am. J. Nurs. **67**:343, 1967.

92. Freeman, R. M., and Bulechek, G. M.: Programmed instruction: an approach to dietary management of dialysis patients, Am. J. Clin. Nutr. **21**:613, 1968.

93. Freeman, R. M., and Bulechek, G. M.:

Programmed instructions for the dialysis patient, Iowa City, Iowa, 1968, University of Iowa Press.

94. Lawson, V. K., Traylor, M. N., and Gram, M. R.: An audio-tutorial aid for dietary instruction in renal dialysis, J. Am. Diet Assoc. **69:**390, 1976.

95. Kane, T. C., et al.: Self-instructional package for patients with kidney disease, Houston, 1973, Medical Illustration and Audiovisual Education.

96. Garron, M. S.: Dietary education program for renal failure, Los Angeles, 1974, California Dietetic Association (slides and cassette).

97. Ota, E. S.: Nutritional care in renal disease, New York, 1978, Communications in Learning, Inc. (audio tape and slides).

98. Heimbuch, L.: An orientation to principles of diet therapy in chronic renal failure, Detroit, 1978, Dietary Department, Harper-Grace Hospitals, (slide and tape).

99. Council on Renal Nutrition: Selected bibliography on renal disease 1978. National Kidney Foundation, 2 Park Avenue, New York, N.Y. 10016.

100. Blackburn, S. L.: Dietary compliance of chronic hemodialysis patients, J. Am. Diet. Assoc. **70:**31, 1977.

101. Biller, D. C.: Patient's point of view: diet in chronic renal failure, J. Am. Diet. Assoc. **71:**633, 1977.

102. Smith, L. H., Van Der Berg, C. J., and Wilson, D. M.: Nutrition and urolithiasis, N. Engl. J. Med. **298:**87, 1978.

103. Coe, F. L.: Nephrolithiasis, Kidney **12(1):**1, 1979.

7 Diabetes mellitus

CLASSIFICATION

Presently there are 4½ million diabetics in the United States. Diabetes mellitus is one of the earliest reported diseases known to man. Diabetes is the Greek word for siphon or passing. Mellitus is Latin for honey. Consequently, this disorder was very aptly described as the passing of honey. It is a chronic metabolic disorder that is the result of an abnormality of insulin metabolism, which gives rise to hyperglycemia, glycosuria, increased protein catabolism, ketosis, and acidosis. The discovery of insulin and antibiotics to treat infections lengthened the life of diabetics, but as a result, diabetics became subject to vascular and neural complications. For example, degenerative changes in the retina of the eye can lead to blindness, and renal failure and cardiovascular disorders occur more frequently and at a younger age in the diabetic.

Primary diabetes mellitus is an inherited disorder. At first there is a prediabetic stage in which no symptoms are evident; this proceeds to clinical diabetes, the stage in which the disorder is manifest. Clinical diabetes can occur either in childhood (insulin-dependent-youth onset) or in adulthood (insulin-independent-maturity onset). Secondary diabetes may be the result of a disorder of another endocrine gland such as the adrenal or pituitary glands. Destruction of the pancreas from inflammation, hemochromatosis, neoplasm, or pancreatectomy results in insulin deficiency. Stress reactions such as infection, surgery, pregnancy, drug therapy, low carbohydrate intake, and starvation can also create a diabetic state.

Fasting blood glucose levels, glucose tolerance test, and the cortisone glucose tolerance test are used to categorize diabetes into four stages—prediabetic, subclinical, latent, and overt. The prediabetic exhibits normal blood glucose levels, and glucose tolerance is normal. However, even though there are no clinical symptoms there is an inherited predisposition to the disease. In the subclinical or suspected stage the cortisone glucose tolerance test is abnormal. During periods of stress the glucose tolerance test may be abnormal. In latent or clinical diabetes both tolerance tests are abnormal, and fasting blood glucose levels may be elevated. The final stage is overt diabetes. Hyperglycemia obviates the need for performing a tolerance test.

Insulin-dependent diabetes usually appears quite suddenly in childhood or puberty. The child appears undernourished and exhibits the classic symptoms of polyphagia, polydipsia, polyuria, and nocturia. Blood glucose levels are difficult to control. A small change in insulin dosage or exercise or the presence of an infection results in a great fluctuation in blood glucose. Control is difficult and if the child does not eat properly or insulin is not administered, ketosis results. Dietary control is important. Insulin must be administered, for the beta cells of the pancreas have become hyalinized and replaced by fiber, and no insulin is produced. Oral hypo-glycemic agents are not useful since there are no pancreatic cells to stimulate. In a few years after diagnosis vascular complications become evident.

The insulin-independent diabetic presents a different syndrome. The disorder appears gradually after the age of 35 years. No symptoms are evident. The individual may just experience fatigue or ill-defined complaints. Most adult diabetics are obese. Rapid changes in blood glucose are not observed. Diet may be the only therapy necessary, and often after a reduction diet and attainment of normal weight, the individual is not diabetic. In the adult there may be a delayed response to glucose, or a decreased amount of insulin is secreted. Oral hypoglycemic agents that stimulate the pancreas are frequently used. Approximately 20% to 30% of the adult diabetics require insulin. Control is much easier in the older diabetic if the prescribed diet is followed.

METABOLISM

Before insulin can affect cellular metabolism it must bind to a specific protein receptor on the target cell.[1] Plasma insulin concentration inversely regulates the number of these receptors. Therefore the hyperinsulinemia associated with obesity leads to a decrease in the number of receptors and thus insulin resistance.

Insulin regulates its own receptors, but other factors may also play a role, namely, the relationship between insulin receptors, glucose transport, coupling between receptors and transport, and intracellular enzymatic reactions. It has been suggested that in obesity different mechanisms for insulin resistance may exist in different tissues. For example, it is possible that in the adipose cell there is an intracellular enzymatic defect, whereas in hepatic and muscle tissue there may be a decreased number of insulin receptors.

After digestion and absorption, approximately 70% of the ingested glucose is utilized by the liver. Insulin promotes the absorption of glucose by the hepatocytes. The hormone stimulates the synthesis of glycogen and glucose-6-phosphate. Glyco-genolysis and gluconeogenesis are inhibited. From 200 to 350 g of glucose are re-leased daily from the liver by the action of glucose-6-phosphatase.

In the diabetic state the liver continues to release glucose into the circulation. More amino acids are absorbed from the blood and are used for gluconeogenesis. Glycogenolysis is increased and glycogenesis is decreased. These all contribute to hyperglycemia.

Protein metabolism is also affected. The increase in amino acid catabolism leads to an increase in the synthesis of urea.

The increased breakdown of triglycerides by adipose tissue results in the excess fatty acids being taken up by the liver. Some fatty acids are deposited and contribute to the formation of a fatty liver. Catabolism of fatty acids results in the formation of an excess of the ketone bodies—acetone, acetoacetic acid, and β-hydroxybutyric acid.

Insulin is needed for the movement of glucose into the adipose cell. Glucose can be metabolized either into acetyl CoA for fatty acid synthesis or into α-glycerophosphate. Both of these metabolites can be converted into triglycerides. Insulin stimulates the enzyme lipoprotein lipase, which clears the blood of lipoproteins. The lipase in the fat cell is inhibited by insulin.

In the absence of insulin there is an increased breakdown of triglycerides. The resulting fatty acids are released into the blood. Since lipoprotein lipase is not activated, lipoproteins are not cleared from the circulation.

Muscle cells need insulin for the absorption of glucose. Excess glucose can be converted into glycogen for storage. When energy is needed, glucose is metabolized to lactate or to carbon dioxide and water if oxygen is available. The lactate is released into the blood and carried to the liver for metabolism. Pyruvate can be transaminated to alanine and released to the liver for resynthesis into glucose again. Insulin stimulates the uptake of amino acids into muscle and therefore promotes protein synthesis.

In the diabetic state there is an increased uptake of fatty acids and ketones by the muscle cell. Instead of amino acid uptake, the process is reversed, and the amino acids are released into the circulation.

The islet cells of the pancreas elaborate the hormone insulin, which increases glucose utilization, glycogenesis, and lipogenesis. Glucogenesis and glycogenolysis are inhibited; the net result is hypoglycemia. Growth hormone elaborated by the anterior pituitary gland contributes to hyperglycemia by stimulating glycogenolysis in liver and muscle. The prolonged elevation of blood sugar stimulates the pancreas to elaborate insulin.

The alpha cells of the islets of Langerhans manufacture glucagon. This hormone promotes hepatic glycogenolysis, lipolysis, ketogenesis, and gluconeogenesis; this leads to hyperglycemia. Insulin stimulates hepatic glycogenesis, lipogenesis, and protein synthesis or hypoglycemia. Some researchers have suggested that diabetes mellitus is due to a bihormonal abnormality—a lack of insulin and an excess of glucagon.[2,3] Others have stated that the primary abnormality in diabetes is due to a deficiency of insulin rather than hyperglucagonemia.[4] However, glucagon may worsen the situation.

The anterior pituitary gland produces thyrotropin, which in turn stimulates the release of thyroxine from the thyroid gland. Similarly, adrenocorticotropic hormone (ACTH) from the pituitary gland stimulates the production of glucocorticoids by the adrenal cortex. Thyroxine and the glucocorticoids promote gluconeogenesis and thus contribute to hyperglycemia.

Epinephrine is released in response to hypoglycemia. It promotes glycogenolysis in the liver and muscle and stimulates the pituitary gland to release ACTH, growth hormone, and thyrotropin.

The hormone somatostatin, a peptide, was first isolated from the hypothalamus.

It was later found in the D cells of the islets of Langerhans.[5,6] It inhibits the release of growth hormone, insulin, and glucagon. Since the hormone exhibits a hypoglycemic effect, it was tested in diabetic subjects. In one study with insulin-independent diabetics an infusion of somatostatin resulted in a decrease in plasma insulin and glucagon.[7] Plasma glucose levels decreased at first but then increased. Experimental evidence suggests that somatostatin interferes with or delays carbohydrate absorption. In addition, the plasma levels of β-hydroxybutyrate and the branched chain amino acids were elevated. Therefore the authors recommended that somatostatin not be used in insulin-independent diabetics.

SYMPTOMS

When the renal threshold (160 to 180 mg/dl) is exceeded, glucose spills over into the urine (glycosuria). The kidney attempts to keep removing glucose, and, as a result, large amounts of urine are excreted (polyuria). The kidneys become overwhelmed, and nitrogen, ketones, sodium, calcium, chloride, and phosphate are also excreted. The individual experiences excessive thirst (polydipsia).

In the untreated diabetic, dehydration may occur. This can lead to increased blood viscosity and decreased blood volume. The cardiac output falls off, and the blood flow through the muscles and kidneys slows down. The excess ketone bodies and ammonia are not removed by the kidney and thus contribute to acidosis. If treatment is not instituted, diabetic coma results.

ETIOLOGY

The beta cells of the islets of Langerhans synthesize the polypeptide insulin. At first the storage form, proinsulin, is elaborated, and then by removal of a peptide the active form is generated. An increase in blood glucose levels stimulates the release of insulin. When glucose comes in contact with the gut mucosa of the upper gastrointestinal tract, the hormones secretin, gut glucagon, and cholecystokinin act on the pancreas and initiate the production of insulin. Amino acids also cause the release of this hormone.

It has been suggested that the action of insulin is mediated through the activity of adenyl cyclase. This enzyme increases the synthesis of cyclic AMP, the intracellular messenger substance, which in turn produces the release of insulin.

Several different theories have been proposed for the etiology of diabetes mellitus.[8] The most obvious defect is the inability to synthesize insulin in the beta cells of the pancreas. This situation exists in the insulin-dependent diabetic where the beta cells undergo hyalinization and fibrinization and lose their capacity to elaborate insulin. Some have suggested that insulin is rapidly destroyed in the diabetic, but the rate of insulin disappearance in the diabetic is the same as in the nondiabetic. Obese individuals show a resistance to insulin action; there is a delayed response, and insulin is not released immediately after glucose ingestion. Some researchers have suggested that diabetes is an autoimmune disease and that the diabetic makes antibodies against his own insulin. Plasma proteins could bind insulin and render it inactive. The protein synalbumin has been found to inhibit the action of insulin. It is also possible that diabetes mellitus might arise because of the increased action of other hormones. Growth hormone, corticosteroids, glucagon, and epinephrine all cause hyperglycemia and may overwhelm the hypoglycemic effect. A deficiency of the trace minerals zinc and chromium may contribute to the inactivity of insulin. Epidemiological studies have shown a relationship between viral infections and the onset of diabetes.[9] Virologists have devised model systems in which viruses seem to produce diabetes in animals. Much controversy exists as to all of these theories, and at present no agreement as to which one is correct has been reached.

DIAGNOSIS

In diabetes mellitus, excess glucose is found in the urine. Benedict's reagent can be used to test urine; however, a positive test indicates the presence of a reducing sugar and is not specific for glucose. Strips of paper impregnated with the enzyme glucose oxidase and a chromogen test only for glucose (Diastix, Ames Company, and Tes-Tape, Eli Lilly & Company). The resulting color is dependent upon the concentration of glucose and is estimated by comparison with a color chart.

Ketone bodies (ketonuria) may be present in the urine of the untreated diabetic or of an individual in poor control. Treated paper strips can be used to test for the presence of ketones in the urine (Ketostix, Ames Company). Tablets can be used to test either blood or urine samples (Ace test, Ames Company). One strip can be used to test both for urinary glucose and ketone bodies (Keto-Diastix, Ames Company). The tests can be used in screening the population for diabetes mellitus or for determining whether a diabetic is under control.

The volume of urine excreted daily is approximately 1.5 L. The diabetic excretes large volumes of fluid in an attempt to decrease blood glucose levels. The specific gravity of the urine will be 1.030 or higher because of the presence of the sugar.

If diabetes mellitus is suspected, a standard glucose tolerance test is performed.[8] For 3 days prior to the test a diet consisting of at least 200 g of carbohydrate should be consumed. Drugs that affect blood glucose levels should not be ingested. After an overnight fast a blood sample is drawn. Then 100 g of glucose are administered orally. Various carbonated beverages are available that contain this amount of glucose and are palatable to drink. Blood samples are then taken at ½, 1, 1½, 2, and 3 hours after the administration of the test dose.

In the normal individual, fasting blood glucose levels are below 100 mg/dl, reach a peak of 160 mg/dl or lower between ½ and 1 hour, and return to normal levels 2 or 3 hours after the administration of the test dose. Diabetics may have a normal fasting blood glucose level or it may be elevated. After the initiation of the test, levels may exceed 160 mg/dl and then start to decline to 120 mg/dl at 2 hours. After 3 hours, the levels may return to those found in the fasting state. Borderline diabetics show blood glucose levels somewhere between the normal and diabetic values.

The glucose tolerance test should not be performed on individuals with infections, liver disorders, or when dietary carbohydrate intake has been severely restricted.

An intravenous glucose tolerance test is performed when the absorption of glucose from the intestine is abnormal.[8] A solution containing 0.5 g of glucose per kilogram of body weight is administered intravenously. A blood sample is drawn before the test and ½, 1, 2, and 3 hours after the glucose is given. In the normal individual, blood glucose levels return to normal after 2 hours, whereas in the diabetic individual they are still elevated.

A glucose cortisone tolerance test is used to detect the potential for diabetes in a person with a family history of the disorder.[8] This test detects the disturbance in carbohydrate metabolism earlier than the normal load test. The procedure is the same, but in addition, cortisone acetate is administered 8½ hours before the ingestion of glucose. Normal individuals have a fasting blood glucose of less than 140 mg/dl, which at ½ to 1 hour peaks at 180 mg/dl and at 2 hours returns to the initial value. On the other hand, persons with diabetic potential have blood sugar levels greater than 200 mg/dl throughout the test.

A tolbutamide tolerance test is performed to determine whether the beta cells of the pancreas will respond to stimulation.[8] Tolbutamide is administered, and a blood sample is taken. Then 20 minutes and again at 30 minutes after the glucose load, an additional blood sample is taken. The blood glucose levels in normal individuals will drop to less than 75% of the pretest values, while in diabetics they will be in excess of 89% of the original value.

TREATMENT

Insulin must always be used for insulin-dependent diabetics and for individuals who are prone to ketoacidosis. Since insulin is a polypeptide, it must be injected subcutaneously to avoid the action of digestive enzymes.

Regular or crystalline insulin is the active hormone that acts quickly. It is used to treat diabetic coma and acidosis. In order to parallel the body's release of insulin upon ingestion of glucose, it would be necessary to inject insulin before every meal. To avoid the need for multiple injections, the duration of action of insulin is modified either by the addition of a protein or zinc; therefore, it is possible to have intermediate and prolonged action.[10]

Protamine zinc insulin (PZI) is insoluble because of the addition of the protein protamine. It is released slowly from the tissues and is active for 36 hours. When this insulin is used, it is necessary to ingest a bedtime snack to avoid hypoglycemia. NPH insulin (neutral, protamine, Hagedorn) or isophane insulin also contains the protein protamine, but it exhibits an intermediate type of action.

Globin insulin contains the protein globin, and it shows an intermediate type of action. The duration of the action of insulin can be modified by the addition of zinc and an acetate buffer to form the lente insulins. Two forms of the zinc-insulin com-

Table 7-1. Insulin preparations

Type	Action	Onset (hours)	Peak (hours)	Duration (hours)
Regular	Rapid	½-1	2-4	6-8
Semilente	Rapid	½-1	2-4	8-10
Globin	Intermediate	1-2	6-8	12-14
NPH	Intermediate	1-2	6-8	12-14
Lente	Intermediate	1-2	6-8	14-16
Protamine zinc	Prolonged	4-6	18±	36-72
Ultralente	Prolonged	4-6	8-12	24-36

Table 7-2. Oral hypoglycemic agents

Generic name	Trade name	Approximate duration of action (hours)
Sulfonylureas		
Tolbutamide	Orinase	6-10
Chlorpropamide	Diabinese	40-72
Acetohexamide	Dymelor	10-16
Tolazamide	Tolinase	10-16

plex can be made. The amorphous form is quickly soluble, and the crystalline form takes longer to dissolve. By varying the concentrations of these two forms, a rapid (semilente), intermediate (lente), and prolonged (ultralente) type of insulin can be made (see Table 7-1).

Various combinations of insulins can be used to meet the need of the individual. Since insulin must be injected, research continues for a physiologically active compound that can be ingested orally.

Two forms of oral hypoglycemic agents have been used. However, the Food and Drug Administration banned the use of the phenylethylbiguanides (phenformin), and currently only the sulfonlyureas are prescribed (see Table 7-2). These drugs are useful for insulin-independent diabetics who cannot be controlled solely by diet.

The sulfonylurea-type compounds stimulate the beta cells of the pancreas to secrete insulin. Hypoglycemia is also promoted by inhibiting the breakdown of glycogen.

In 1961 the University Group Diabetes Program (UGDP) was established.[11] It consisted of 12 university clinics and a coordinating center. The objectives were to evaluate the effect of the hypoglycemic agents in the development of vascular disease in diabetes, to collect information on the natural history of diabetes and the relationship of blood glucose levels to vascular disease, and to develop methods for other long-term trials. Five different treatment groups were established: (1) insulin dosage adjusted to maintain normal blood glucose levels; (2) standard insulin dose of 10 to 16 units depending upon body surface area; (3) tolbutamide 1.5 g per day divided dose; (4) phenformin 100 mg per day divided dose (this group was added 18 months after the study was initiated); and (5) placebo consisting of lactose. The patients who were not insulin dependent were randomly assigned to a group. The study was completed in 1966, and approximately 200 patients were in each group of the study.

No evidence was found that the control of blood glucose levels would prevent vascular complications. A higher incidence of cardiovascular mortality was found in the patients treated with tolbutamide. A review of the findings for nonfatal cardiovascular disease also indicated that there was no benefit associated with the long-term use of tolbutamide.[12] The combination of diet and tolbutamide was no more effective than diet alone in the treatment of diabetes. It was recommended that insulin-independent diabetics be treated first with a diet. If this did not establish control then insulin should be used, since it is most effective in controlling hyperglycemia.

Many patients on diet and oral agents can be controlled by diet alone.[13] Those who cannot should be treated with insulin to avoid the possible risk of increased cardiovascular disease. Oral hypoglycemic agents may be prescribed for patients who are allergic to insulin or who cannot inject themselves.[14]

The results of the UGDP generated interest in the development of new oral hypoglycemic agents. Fenfluramine is an anorectic agent similar in structure to amphetamine.[15] This drug also has a hypoglycemic effect in that it increases the uptake of glucose by muscles. The mechanism of action is similar to that of phenformin. Maximum activity is observed when the fenfluramine is administered immediately before a meal. Blood glucose levels were lowered in insulin dependent diabetics, but a greater effect was observed in insulin-independent diabetics.

A few transplants of the total or subtotal pancreas have been attempted in humans.[16,17] Usually these individuals have also had a kidney transplant and are receiving immunosuppressant agents. This pancreatic allograft corrects the metabolic deficiency of diabetes mellitus; however, most of the transplants have been rejected because the islet cells are highly immunogenic. Thus better immunosuppressive techniques are needed before pancreatic transplantation will be feasible.

Another approach has been to transplant pancreatic islet cells intramuscularly, intraperitoneally, or into the portal vein of patients who had previously received renal transplants.[18] In some patients there was a transient decline in insulin requirements. One of the difficulties associated with this technique is the inability to prepare enough islet tissue that is not contaminated with exocrine tissue digestive enzymes. However, the use of tissue cultured cells could obviate this difficulty.

Automation has been used to manage diabetic patients.[19] The nurse-clinician uses a computer for automated consultation. The patient's clinical data is coded into the computer. A printout recommends the doses of insulin and time of administration for four types of insulin (regular, lente, semilente, and ultralente). The diet prescription states the number of kilocalories and grams of carbohydrate, fat, and protein.

Albisser and his colleagues devised an artificial pancreas that was used successfully in depancreatized dogs.[20] Blood sugar was continually monitored, and the results were fed to a minicomputer that was programmed to deliver either insulin or glucose in response to the present level. Thus insulin can be administered as it is in the normal individual in response to the ingestion of glucose. Three human subjects were tested for 2 days.[21] On the first day the usual doses of insulin were administered subcutaneously. On the second day the insulin was given intravenously as programmed by a computer. A comparison of the blood sugar patterns between the 2 days showed a significant improvement in glucose homeostasis on the second day.

The authors commented that no major advances in therapy for diabetes have been made since the discovery of insulin 50 years ago. Since insulin is not administered on the basis of physiological demand, the effects of the periods of hyperglycemia tend to be cumulative and contribute to the vascular complications.

In a later experiment the artificial pancreas monitored blood glucose levels continually, and a computer was programmed to respond to the degree of glycemia by releasing the appropriate hormone.[22] Diabetics often develop hypoglycemia due to inadequate levels of glucagon. Since the normal individual responds by releasing glucagon, the hypoglycemia in these diabetics was treated with glucagon rather than, as in the previous experiment, with a dextrose infusion. Nine diabetic subjects were controlled by the artificial pancreas for 10 to 12 hours. Blood glucose values were maintained in the normal range in most instances; however, the artificial pancreas must be modified and miniaturized before it can be used other than by the bedside.

For 2 weeks nine adult diabetics were treated with a preprogrammed 5-hour pulse of insulin at each meal to approximate the normal diurnal pattern of insulin.[23] During this time the subjects consumed 600 kcal meals three times a day and a bedtime snack of 300 kcal. At the end of the experimental period, six of the diabetics showed improved glucose tolerance while being maintained only with diet therapy. Eight subjects increased their output of endogenous insulin. The authors suggested that the administration of the exogenous insulin allowed the beta cells to rest, and afterwards these cells were able to produce more insulin. Thus a longer period of treatment might lead to a longer remission of diabetes.

COMPLICATIONS

The short-term complications observed in diabetics are insulin reaction and diabetic coma.

Insulin reaction producing hypoglycemia can be a result of unusual exercise, decrease in the amount of food eaten, overdose of insulin, vomiting, or diarrhea. Blood sugar levels drop to about 35 mg/dl very rapidly. Sugar should be consumed immediately, preferably as glucose. The hormone glucagon or epinephrine (Adrenalin) can be injected. If the patient is unconscious, glucose must be given intravenously.

Diabetic coma is brought on by a lack of insulin, excess of food, or reduced utilization of carbohydrates. The onset is slow. Hyperglycemia, glycosuria, ketonuria, and acidosis are some of the clinical manifestations. The treatment involves the administration of insulin.

Diabetics are more prone to infections that tend to be severe and difficult to control. Impaired leukocyte function and vascular disease may be involved.[24]

Since the advent of insulin therapy, diabetics have become more prone to the chronic complications of neuropathy, retinopathy, nephropathy, and atherosclerosis.[25,26] Neuropathy has been found to be due to a segmental demyelinization of the nerve cells. This may be brought about by the increased activity of the polyol pathway.[27,28] The following metabolic reactions take place in nerve cells that are fully permeable to glucose.

$$\text{D-glucose} + \text{NADPH} + \text{H}^+ \rightarrow \text{Sorbitol} + \text{NADP}^+$$
$$\text{Sorbitol} + \text{NAD}^+ \rightarrow \text{D-fructose} + \text{NADH} + \text{H}^+$$

Both sorbitol and fructose cannot leave the cell, and as a result the osmotic pressure increases. Water moves into the cell and swelling results. Amino acids, ATP, and myoinositol leave the cells. The first evidence of neuropathy is a decrease in nerve conduction velocity. Data from rats with experimental diabetes suggested that this was related to the decrease in nerve myoinositol concentration.[29] In humans with controlled diabetes, excessive amounts of myoinositol are excreted in the urine.[28]

The neuropathy can be improved by reducing the hyperglycemia either by means of medical or diet therapy. The degeneration of the axons of the nerve fiber that appears in severe neuropathy cannot be reversed or improved by reducing the hyperglycemia.

Atherosclerotic vascular disease is found in the diabetic at an earlier age than in the normal population.[25,26] Hyperglycemia is one of the many risk factors found in epidemiological studies to contribute to atherosclerosis. A direct effect is exerted on metabolism in the aorta. The polyol pathway also operates in aortic tissue. In addition, large amounts of growth hormone are secreted in uncontrolled diabetics. It has been suggested that this hormone can increase platelet aggregability and increase arterial medial cell proliferation in vitro.

A thickening of the basement membrane of the capillaries in tissues has been observed in diabetics. This is due to the accumulation of a glycoprotein in the membrane. It is possible that this comes from the entrance of glucose into the glucuronic acid pathway and the eventual synthesis of mucopolysaccharides and glycoproteins.[30] The resulting thickened basement membrane leads to neuropathy, retinopathy, and kidney disease.

Glycosylated hemoglobin is a form of hemoglobin in which glucose is joined to the terminal amino acid of the β chain.[31] Higher concentrations (10% to 28%) of this compound are found in blood samples from diabetics, whereas normal subjects have approximately 7% of this type of hemoglobin. As the erythrocyte ages, the amount of glycosylated hemoglobin that forms is dependent upon the blood glucose concentration. Therefore, repeated measurements would be indicative of the degree of blood glucose control. Repeated elevated levels of glycosylated hemoglobin would be seen in diabetics who are poorly controlled. This test would be more useful for monitoring diabetics than the current procedure of measuring blood glucose levels.

DIETARY TREATMENT

Through the years different proportions of carbohydrate, protein, and fat have been prescribed for diabetic diets. These have been reviewed by Wood and Bierman[32] and Kay.[33] Dietary prescriptions have ranged from low, normal, and high carbohydrate combined with low- and high-fat intakes. Even protein has been restricted. Many researchers have advocated a restriction of caloric intake, some even to near starvation. Other diets have prescribed certain foods such as skim milk, rice, potatoes, or oatmeal.

In 1971 the Committee on Food and Nutrition of the American Medical Association made recommendations for patients with diabetes mellitus.[34] The aim of diet therapy is to avoid the harmful effects of the metabolic imbalances caused by diabetes mellitus and to reduce the risk factors associated with the complications. Caloric intake should be just sufficient to maintain ideal body weight. A reduction diet for obese diabetics is necessary to lessen the risk of complications. Meals should be on a regular basis and spaced according to the prescribed insulin dosage and the amount of physical activity. The aim is to maintain normoglycemia. Simple sugars should not be consumed, since they lead to hyperglycemic peaks.

Since recent evidence has shown that the ingestion of large amounts of carbohydrates does not increase the insulin requirement, it was proposed that the diabetic diet should include a normal amount of carbohydrate, 45% or more of the total caloric intake. The only exception is the individual who has carbohydrate-sensitive endogenous hypertriglyceridemia. No recommendation was made for the restriction of fat and cholesterol and the increase of polyunsaturated fats. However, an increase in carbohydrate intake results in a decrease in fat intake. Serum lipids can be lowered by restricting calories, saturated fat, and cholesterol.

The committee also stressed the fact that the diet must be planned for the individual. In addition, they suggested that there is a need for a dietary study in young diabetics to determine the proportions of fat to carbohydrate that would aid in the prevention of neuropathy and microangiopathy.

Anderson, Herman, and Zakim studied the effect of high intakes of glucose and sucrose on the glucose tolerance of normal men.[35] The initial diet consisted of 40% calories as carbohydrates, 43% as fat, and 17% as protein. The other diets were liquid and contained 15% of calories as calcium caseinate and 20%, 40%, 60%, or 80% as glucose, and the remaining calories were supplied by corn oil. The two sucrose diets contained 40% or 80% of calories from sucrose, 45% or 5% of calories from corn oil, and 15% of calories as sodium caseinate. Oral and intravenous glucose tolerance tests were performed on the 13 subjects. The low-glucose diet (20%) resulted in an abnormal glucose tolerance test. Improvement was seen as the percentage of glucose calories increased to 80%. Improvement in the glucose tolerance test was seen in the subjects on the diet with 80% of calories from sucrose. Plasma insulin values were slightly decreased. The ingestion of a diet high in sucrose did not impair glucose tolerance, but serum triglyceride levels were increased significantly by this treatment.

The proportion of dietary fat and carbohydrate for diabetics was studied by Weinsier and his co-workers.[36] Eighteen diabetics not on insulin therapy were tested for 20 weeks on a 40% carbohydrate, 45% fat, and 15% protein diet and for 20 weeks on a 60% carbohydrate, 25% fat, and 15% protein diet. Diabetic control was evaluated by determining the following parameters: fasting and 1-hour postprandial blood sugar levels, the presence of sugar in the urine collected when the fasting and postprandial blood samples were taken, and a 24-hour urine sugar level. A system to quantify control was scored on these values. The patients maintained diabetic control on the high-carbohydrate diet. Oral and intravenous glucose tolerance tests, fasting blood glucose, and insulin levels were not altered by the increased carbohydrate. Triglyceride levels were not significantly elevated by the increased carbohydrate intake.

A more severe dietary modification was tested by Brunzell and his co-workers.[37] Nine normal patients and 13 mild diabetics were tested on two formula diets for 8 to 10 days. The control diet contained 40% fat, 45% carbohydrate, and 15% protein. The test diet contained 85% carbohydrate and 15% protein. The high-carbohydrate diet caused a decrease in fasting blood glucose levels and fasting insulin levels. The insulin response to glucose did not change. Glycosuria was present in only one person with mild diabetes when he was on the high-carbohydrate intake. Glucose tolerance showed improvement on the 85% carbohydrate diet. It was suggested that the high-carbohydrate diet improved glucose tolerance by increasing the sensitivity of peripheral tissues to insulin.

However, when the diabetics were treated with insulin or oral hypoglycemic agents, the high-carbohydrate diet resulted in a significant decrease in fasting blood glucose. Hypoglycemia developed in two subjects, and the insulin dosage was decreased. One subject was tested with diets containing 5%, 25%, 45%, and 85% carbohydrate. The fasting plasma glucose levels were lower on the high-carbohydrate intake. These diets with a concomitant reduction in fat intake would prove useful for reducing plasma lipids and aid in the prevention of atherosclerosis.

Low-carbohydrate diets (44% calories from carbohydrate and 55% of these calories as oligosaccharides) and a high-carbohydrate diet (75% calories from carbohydrates and 47% of these calories as oligosaccharides) were fed to 14 men with chemical diabetes.[38] After 1 week on the high-carbohydrate diet, plasma glucose and insulin responses were lower. Oral and intravenous glucose tolerance tests were improved. It was suggested that this was due to the increased insulin sensitivity. This same effect is not seen in normal individuals on high-carbohydrate diets. Fasting triglyceride levels were higher on the 75% carbohydrate diet than on the 44% carbohydrate diet. The reverse situation was observed when postprandial triglyceride levels were measured. Additional studies are needed to determine the long-term effect of high-carbohydrate diets.

Impaired glucose tolerance on a low-carbohydrate diet is not understood. Jackson and his co-workers measured forearm glucose uptake of normal subjects before and after a low-carbohydrate diet.[39] They found that glucose tolerance was impaired and the rise of serum insulin was delayed. Uptake of glucose by the forearm was normal; therefore the impairment of glucose intolerance was not the result of a decrease in peripheral glucose utilization. The authors suggested that the defect was a delay in glucose uptake by the liver due to low levels of glucokinase.

Simple sugars such as glucose and sucrose have been restricted in diabetic diets. It was assumed that these simple sugars are absorbed quickly and thus produce a more rapid postprandial increase in plasma glucose and insulin levels. The complex carbohydrates such as starch would take longer to digest, and thus they would not be as rapidly absorbed. However, conflicting results have been reported.

Crapo et al. administered glucose, sucrose, and various starches either as a drink or as a meal in combination with other nutrients.[40] Glucose, either alone or in a meal, resulted in higher plasma insulin and glucose levels than did the starch. Sucrose caused a greater plasma insulin response than did the glucose. When glucose, sucrose, and starch were consumed with meals, there was a lower glucose response than when these compounds were administered alone, as in a drink. Plasma insulin responses were not changed. Another interesting finding was that lower plasma glucose and insulin levels resulted from the ingestion of rice starch rather than potato starch.

The same investigators studied the effects of four different kinds of starch—potato, rice, corn, and bread—on plasma glucose and insulin levels in normal subjects.[41] The results indicated that there are different rates of digestion and absorption for the starches. Potato starch and glucose gave similar plasma glucose and insulin responses; lower responses were given by rice, corn, and bread. Additional studies are needed to determine whether diabetic patients would give more marked responses. If this were the case, then the type of complex carbohydrate that is prescribed for a diabetic diet should be considered.

Normal subjects and insulin-dependent and insulin-independent diabetics were fed four isocaloric breakfasts containing 45% of calories from carbohydrate.[42] The amounts of oligosaccharides varied in each diet as follows—5%, 30%, 45%, and 65% of the carbohydrate calories. In the adult subjects the breakfasts containing 45% and 65% of the carbohydrates as oligosaccharides resulted in the smallest rise in blood glucose levels. The results with the insulin-dependent diabetics were variable. This study showed that the complex carbohydrates were not digested and absorbed more slowly than the oligosaccharides. However, some of the subjects who ate the meals with a high concentration of oligosaccharides showed symptoms of hypoglycemia and requested additional food. Diets high in oligosaccharide content are therefore not recommended since this can lead to excessive consumption of calories.

Several studies have shown that by increasing the fiber content of the diet, decreased postprandial serum glucose[43-47] and insulin levels result.[43,44,47] Jenkins and his co-workers observed this effect when guar flour, pectin, or both, were consumed by normal and diabetic subjects.[43,44] Guar and pectin have the ability to form gels. These carbohydrates may exert their effect by reducing the rate of diffusion of glucose to the mucosal lining of the small intestine. The uptake of glucose by the tissues is assisted by the slower rate of intestinal absorption. Guar and pectin may exert their influence on the release of gastrointestinal hormones and the hormones of the pancreas. Miranda and Horwitz fed diets containing either 3 or 20 g of crude fiber to insulin-requiring diabetics for 10 days.[45] Plasma glucose levels were lower on the high-fiber diet, but serum insulin levels were unchanged. However, serum glucagon levels were significantly lower on the high-fiber diet. The differences in plasma glucose levels were not due to a change in insulin levels. Therefore the researchers suggested that the fiber may alter the secretion of gastrointestinal hormones or may act directly on the alpha cells of the pancreas to reduce plasma glucose levels.

High-fiber and high-carbohydrate diets have been found to improve glucose tolerance in diabetics.[46,47] After 2 weeks of therapy on a diet containing 75% of the kilocalories from carbohydrate and 15 g of crude fiber, lower plasma glucose levels were observed in 10 of the 13 subjects. Fasting triglyceride levels also decreased in 10 of the diabetic subjects; serum cholesterol levels were reduced in all the patients. The diabetics who required more than 40 units of insulin per day did not respond to diet therapy.

Additional studies with the high-carbohydrate (75% kilocalories from carbohydrate, of which 75% are from polysaccharides), high-fiber diets (20.9 g crude fiber and 70.6 g dietary fiber) have resulted in improved glucose tolerance and lower fasting serum cholesterol and triglyceride levels.[47] Bran is the major source of fiber in the diets. Since insulin levels were lower on the high-carbohydrate diet, the improvement in glucose metabolism may be due to an increased sensitivity to the available insulin. These high-carbohydrate, low-fat, high-fiber diets are of benefit to diabetics taking oral hypoglycemic agents or less than 20 units of insulin per day. The reduction in serum cholesterol and triglyceride levels may assist in preventing the long-term vascular complications.

Wall, Pyke, and Oakley studied the effect of carbohydrate restriction in 200 obese diabetic patients.[48] One diet was limited to 1000 kilocalories, and the other diet restricted the carbohydrate intake to 100 to 150 g per day. Diabetic control was determined from the symptoms, blood glucose levels, and the degree of glycosuria. Good control was achieved in 159 of the 200 patients solely by means of dietary treatment. The remaining 41 patients were given oral hypoglycemic agents. Only 34 of the patients were able to reach 10% of their expected weight, while only three attained their normal weight. Even though dietary studies were not carried out, the authors concluded that carbohydrate restriction was an important factor. Control of the diabetic state was attained without a significant weight reduction.

A protein-sparing modified fast was used to treat seven insulin-requiring, obese adult diabetics.[49] Positive nitrogen balance was attained on an intake of 1.2 to 1.4 g of animal protein per kilogram of ideal body weight. The insulin dosage was gradually reduced and then discontinued. Serum glucose, insulin, cholesterol, and triglyceride levels decreased, while free fatty acid and ketone body concentrations increased. It has been suggested that the elevated levels of ketone bodies induce protein conservation by decreasing the oxidation of the branched chain amino acids in the muscles. On the protein modified fast, men lose 0.3 kg (0.7 lb) of fat per day, and women lose 0.2 kg (0.4 lb) of fat per day while being in positive nitrogen balance.

Since diabetics are prone to atherosclerosis, the dietary treatment of hyperlipidemia is important. Studies in the past have excluded diabetics, and hence the effect of dietary treatment in preventing the atherosclerotic vascular complications is unknown. Weight reduction in the obese diabetic with hyperlipidemia will not only lower blood lipids but will also improve glucose tolerance.[50] Individuals with hypercholesterolemia should consume a diet low in cholesterol (<300 mg) and saturated fat (20%). Some polyunsaturated fats should be included. Low-fat diets are prescribed for exogenous hypertriglyceridemia. There is no consensus of opinion as to the dietary treatment for endogenous hypertriglyceridemia. A diet low in carbohydrates (40%) has been used. Others prescribe a low-fat (35%) and a high-carbohydrate (50%) diet. The type of carbohydrate included in the diet is important. Sugar may predispose the individual not only to diabetes but to obesity and hypertriglyceridemia as well. If dietary treatment is not successful in reducing the plasma cholesterol and triglyceride concentration, then drugs such as clofibrate, cholestyramine, d-thyroxine, and nicotinic acid are prescribed.[50]

The incidence of hyperlipidemia was studied in 73 Japanese diabetics.[51] Those who were uncontrolled had twice the incidence of hyperlipidemia than those who were controlled. Yet 30% of the controlled hyperlipidemia group had hypertriglyceridemia. Most controlled hypertriglyceridemic patients consumed significantly greater amounts of sucrose, alcohol, and total calories than did the patients who had normal triglyceride levels. The dietary reduction of sucrose, alcohol, and total calories and the regulation of blood glucose levels were effective in reducing serum triglyceride levels.

Hypertriglyceridemia is the lipid abnormality observed most often in diabetics.[52] Type IV hyperlipidemia is seen most often in insulin-dependent diabetics with ketoacidosis. When the plasma glucose levels are controlled with insulin, the serum lipids generally return to normal. In insulin-independent diabetics there is no consistent type of hyperlipidemia; the secretion of insulin may be abnormal, decreased, or increased. These diabetics can be divided into two categories—the diabetic-hypertriglyceridemic syndrome or the hypertriglyceridemic-diabetic syndrome.[52] In the diabetic-hypertriglyceridemic syndrome the hypertriglyceridemia is a result of the diabetes. This hypertriglyceridemia of the type IV pattern is reduced when glucose levels are controlled. For obese diabetics a weight reduction diet is necessary. Carbohydrate has been limited to 20% to 30% of the total caloric intake; however, Kissebah recommended 50% carbohydrate, 30% fat, and 20% protein.

In the hypertriglyceridemic-diabetic syndrome the reduction of plasma glucose levels does not reduce the marked hypertriglyceridemia. The initial treatment involved intravenous fluids for 2 to 3 days. This was followed by the ingestion of 600 to 800 kcal per day with less than 20 g of fat. The carbohydrate intake was restricted. After diet therapy for 4 to 6 weeks, drug therapy may be indicated.

Type II and III hyperlipidemia is seen in some insulin-independent diabetics. A low-cholesterol (300 mg), low–saturated fat, and high–polyunsaturated fat diet is prescribed. Caloric restriction is necessary for obese diabetics. Drug therapy is instituted if plasma lipid concentrations remain elevated.

DIETARY CALCULATIONS

In order to help diabetic patients plan their menus, food exchange lists were published in 1950.[53] The system was developed by the American Diabetes Association and The American Dietetic Association in cooperation with the Chronic Disease Program—Public Health Service, Department of Health, Education, and Welfare. Foods are divided into six basic categories, and the servings of food are adjusted so that they contain equivalent amounts of carbohydrates, proteins, and fats. See Table 7-3 and Appendix B.

The exchange lists were revised in 1976[54] (see Table 7-4 and Appendix C).

In the new exchange lists there is an emphasis on caloric reduction. Information is also given as to the nutrient content of the foods included in each particular exchange list. The following are some of the differences found in the 1976 exchanges. Nonfat milk is used as the milk exchange rather than whole milk. The lists of vegetable groups A and B have been discontinued. Since the carbohydrate and caloric content of the starchy vegetables approximate those of the bread exchange, these vegetables are now included in the list. The bread exchanges include bread, cereals, starchy vegetables, and prepared foods. Meat exchanges have been divided into three categories. All contain 7 g of protein per ounce (28 g) but differ in the amount of fat: lean meat, 3 g; medium fat, 5.5 g; and high fat, 9 g. Dried peas and beans are also included in the meat exchange. Fats high in polyunsaturates are printed in boldface in the fat exchange list.

A guide was also published to assist professionals with diet counseling of diabetics based on the new exchange system.[55] However, it is important that the diet be individualized for each patient.

Thus from the diet prescription and a dietary interview of the individual to ascertain a meal pattern, a diet can be planned. For example, if the dietary prescription calls for 2000 kcal, 225 g carbohydrate, 90 g protein, and 82 g fat, the diet

Table 7-3. Composition of food exchanges

List	Food	Measure	Carbohydrate (g)	Protein (g)	Fat (g)	Kilocalories
1	Milk	0.24 L (1c)	12	8	10	170
2A	Vegetable	As desired	—	—	—	—
2B	Vegetable	0.12 L (½c)	7	2	—	36
3	Fruit	Varies	10	—	—	40
4	Bread	Varies	15	2	—	68
5	Meat	28 g (1 oz)	—	7	5	73
6	Fat	5 ml (1 tsp)	—	—	5	45

Table 7-4. Composition of new food exchanges*

List	Food	Measure	Carbohydrate (g)	Protein (g)	Fat (g)	Kilocalories
1	Milk, nonfat	0.24 L (1 c)	12	8	—	80
	Milk, 1% fat	0.24 L (1 c)	12	8	2.5	103
	Milk, 2% fat	0.24 L (1 c)	12	8	5	125
	Milk, whole	0.24 L (1 c)	12	8	10	170
2	Vegetable	0.12 L (½ c)	5	2	—	28
3	Fruit	Varies	10	—	—	40
4	Bread	Varies	15	2	—	68
5	Meat, lean	28 g (1 oz)	—	7	3	55
	Meat, medium fat	28 g (1 oz)	—	7	5.5	78
	Meat, high fat	28 g (1 oz)	—	7	8	100
6	Fat	Varies	—	—	5	45

*The exchange lists are based on material in the *Exchange Lists for Meal Planning* prepared by Committees of the American Diabetes Association, Inc., and the American Dietetic Association in cooperation with the National Institute of Arthritis, Metabolism and Digestive Diseases and the National Heart and Lung Institute, National Institutes of Health, Public Health Service, U.S. Department of Health, Education, and Welfare.

plan can be worked out by using the exchange system. First, the amount of fruit, milk, vegetable, and bread exchanges are selected according to the person's food preferences to meet the carbohydrate prescription:

EXCHANGES	CARBOHYDRATE	PROTEIN	FAT
7 fruit	70	—	—
2 whole milk	24	16	20
2 vegetable	10	4	—
8 bread	120	16	—
Total (g)	224	36	20

Second, the amount of protein from the carbohydrate exchanges is subtracted from the total protein and divided by 7 to get the number of meat exchanges:

$$90\,g - 36\,g = 54\,g \qquad\qquad 54/7 = 8 \text{ exchanges}$$

EXCHANGES	CARBOHYDRATE	PROTEIN	FAT
fruit, milk, vegetable, bread	224	36	20
6 lean meat, 2 medium fat meat	—	56	29
Total (g)	224	92	49

The amount of fat already used is subtracted from the total and divided by 5 to get the number of fat exchanges:

$$82\,g - 49\,g = 33\,g \qquad\qquad 33/5 = 7 \text{ exchanges}$$

EXCHANGES	CARBOHYDRATE	PROTEIN	FAT
fruit, milk, vegetable, bread, meat	224	92	49
7 fat	—	—	35
Total (g)	224	92	84

The carbohydrate distribution is dependent upon the type of insulin administered (see Table 7-5). A bedtime snack must be provided with the intermediate and prolonged acting insulins to prevent hypoglycemia.

Table 7-5. Carbohydrate distribution

Type of insulin	Breakfast	Lunch	Dinner	Bedtime
None	$1/3$	$1/3$	$1/3$	
Rapid*	$2/5$	$1/5$	$2/5$	
Intermediate	$1/5$	$2/5$	$2/5$	20-40 g
Prolonged	$1/5$	$2/5$	$2/5$	20-40 g
Prolonged	$1/7$	$2/7$	$2/7$	$2/7$

*Before breakfast and dinner.

Table 7-6. Meal plan for a diabetic diet based on exchanges

Exchange	Carbohydrate (g)
Breakfast (1/5 total = 40 g)	
1 fruit	10
2 meat (medium fat)	—
2 bread	30
2 fat	—
Coffee or tea	—
Lunch (2/5 total = 92 g)	
2 meat (lean)	—
3 bread	45
1 vegetable	5
2 fat	—
1 milk	12
3 fruit	30
Dinner (2/5 total = 77 g)	
3 meat (lean)	—
2 bread	30
1 vegetable	5
2 fat	—
1 milk	12
3 fruit	30
Snack (15 g)	
1 meat (lean)	—
1 bread	15
1 fat	—

Table 7-7. Sample menu for a diabetic diet

Breakfast	Dinner
Orange juice—½ c	Roast chicken—3 oz
Eggs—2	Mashed potato—½ c
Toast—2 slices	Green peas—½ c
Margarine—2 tsp	Tomatoes—½ c ⎱ salad
Coffee	Lettuce ⎰
Lunch	Mayonnaise—1 tsp
Loin lamb chops—2 oz	Margarine—1 tsp
Rice—1 c	Milk, whole—1 c
Roll—1	Apple juice—⅔ c
Carrots—½ c	Peach—1 medium
Margarine—2 tsp	**Snack**
Milk, whole—1 c	Tuna—¼ c
Grapefruit juice—½ c	Bread—1 slice
Applesauce—1 c	Mayonnaise—1 tsp

After the number of exchanges has been determined, they are then distributed according to the meal pattern of the individual including the snacks. Table 7-6 illustrates a distribution of carbohydrate for breakfast ($^1/_5$), lunch ($^2/_5$), and dinner ($^2/_5$), plus a bedtime snack according to the exchanges just calculated.

Then the individual can select the foods from the exchange list after the menu is planned. In this way even though the diet is restricted, some selection of foods can be made each day, thus allowing some variety in meal planning. A sample menu is given in Table 7-7.

The diabetic patient needs much instruction by the dietitian in how to plan his diet with the aid of the exchange lists. Since diabetes cannot be cured, the person must accept the prescribed routine for the rest of his life. Dietary treatment becomes an important aspect of the total program. In view of the other restrictions imposed on the patient, it is difficult to also accept dietary restrictions and the reason for them.

Several surveys have indicated that diabetics do not understand their diet.[56-60] Williams and his co-workers asked 61 patients attending a university metabolic clinic to do a 24-hour recall.[56] The surveys were scored as to the food intake and meal regularity. Only 12% of the patients achieved a maximum score. Over half the patients missed at least one meal; some even did not consume two meals a day. Only one person out of eight followed his diet, and only one out of every six patients had any satisfactory spacing of meals. In a second study 17 diabetic patients were asked to keep a 7-day food record. Similar results were found in that 75% of the patients were not meeting their dietary prescription. Almost 50% were not following their diet every day. When foods were categorized according to exchange groups, it was found that less than the amounts prescribed were eaten—for fruits on 73% of patient days, nonstarchy vegetables 53%, meats 46%, and milk 45% respectively. Caloric intake varied from day to day as did the amount of carbohydrate, protein, and fat. Irregularity of meals was also noted. The authors suggested that observation of food practices and dietary counseling should be done at home. The physician should prescribe drug therapy to more closely match the patient's customary eating habits.

The Diabetes Supplement of the National Health Survey (1964-1965) reported that 53% of diabetics followed their diet (group A), 25% (group B) did not, and 22% (group C) had never been given a diet.[57] Additional questions tested their dietary knowledge. Of the patients in group A, 52% correctly gave two meat substitutes, 50% two low-calorie vegetables, and 32% two low-calorie drinks. The correct responses in group B were 40%, 40%, and 27% and group C 43%, 45%, and 29% respectively. Only 9% of the diabetics had attended classes, and 19% had received the booklet *Meal Planning with Exchange Lists*. The results of the survey indicated that the patient does not have a basic knowledge of how to follow a diet.

In the Diabetes Supplement of the National Health Survey, 1800 respondents were interviewed to ascertain their knowledge of the food exchanges.[58] They were asked if their diet included a list of food exchanges. If the answer was no, the individual was included in the inadequate knowledge group. Those who answered yes were asked the number of bread exchanges allowed in the diet and the number from the other food groups—vegetables, fruits, milk, meat, and fat. The caloric intake was also determined. Of the total population surveyed, 77% were on a diet, but 75% had been taught how to follow it. Fifty-three percent followed their diets, but only 20% could answer how many bread exchanges they were allowed. Approximately 25% of these individuals were classified as having good knowledge of their diet. Of the patients who had been instructed in their diet by a dietitian, 20% scored in the good knowledge group, while 13% of those taught by physicians and 14% of those taught by nurses were in this category. The results show the need for more instruction in the use of food exchanges. This would best be done by dietitians.

In 1968 a 7-day food record was collected for 63 diabetic patients in Leeds, England.[59] Of the total patients, 30% were found to have satisfactory control (actual intake was within dietary prescription), 38% tolerable (actual intake deviated 11% to 20% from the prescription), and 32% were classed as hopeless. Diabetic control was determined and considered satisfactory if blood glucose levels were between 50 to 200 mg/dl, there was no ketonuria, and weight was maintained. Those who had satisfactory diabetic control were 42% of those judged satisfactory by dietary control, 33% of those who were tolerable, and 40% of the hopeless group. No relationship existed between dietary and diabetic control. It was also found that the cost of the diabetic diet was higher than that of the general population.

West proposed some of the major causes that contribute to failure in diet therapy.[60] These include a diet prescription that does not fit the patient's needs as regards cultural, sociological, economic status, intelligence, education, incentive and self-discipline; inability of the insulin-dependent diabetic to have frequent scheduled meals with the same amounts of carbohydrate, protein, and fat; misunderstanding by the patient of the aims of diet therapy and the mechanics of the diet such as the food exchange system; lack of knowledge of principles, strategies, practices, and methodology of diet therapy by the physician, nurse, or dietitian; and lastly, an ineffective patient-education system. In the insulin-independent diabetic generally obesity leads to insulin insensitivity and a decrease in beta cell function. The most important aspect of therapy is weight reduction, which in the past has not been very successful. Confusion has existed as to the proportion of carbohydrate in the diabetic diet. The change from a low- to high-carbohydrate intake has been accepted slowly. In particular in the obese diabetic it is important to provide only the amount of carbohydrate that can be tolerated. All simple concentrated sugars must be avoided.

West suggested that the clinician must consider the role of diet therapy in the prevention of the vascular complications of the diabetic.[60] Accumulating evidence shows that a diet that prevents one type of vascular complication might cause another type. Research is needed as to the dietary modifications that will aid in the prevention of the various complications. Some doctors do not consider diet therapy important for several reasons such as restrictions only do harm, the traditional diabetic diet may promote atherogenesis, the prescription will not be followed, control of blood glucose is unimportant, and, primarily, there may be lack of dietary knowledge on the part of the physician.

Weinsier and his co-workers reported a program that was successful in obtaining dietary control in a group of 23 diabetics.[61] The subjects were placed on either a low-carbohydrate (40% kcal) or a high-carbohydrate diet (60% kcal) for 40 weeks. Instruction was given on the use of the food exchange lists. The diabetics were seen at the beginning of the study and on weeks 2, 4, 6, 8, 12, 16, and 20. Group sessions with three to four diabetics were led each time by a physician and nutritionist. Instruction and group discussion were conducted during breakfast. Teaching materials were distributed, and then each subject was seen individually by the physician and nutritionist. The laboratory results were discussed with the patient, and a dietary interview was taken. It was found that the mean level of intake was 42% of carbohydrate kilocalories on the low-carbohydrate diet and 56% on the high-carbohydrate diet. There was no significant change in body weight. It was felt that the successful adherence to the diet was because of the group learning process, in which the subjects learned to interact to the extent that they met outside of the sessions to discuss their problems. The group method of teaching was more successful than individual dietary instruction. The frequent follow-up and explanation of laboratory data, prescriptions based on individual dietary habits, and family involvement were important parts of the program. The authors suggested that it might be possible to form groups similar to Weight Watchers or Alcoholics Anonymous to provide continual support and education for the diabetic patient.

Hassell and Medved found that dietary instruction was more effective in a class using audiovisual techniques rather than by the bedside with the patient.[62] It was felt that class sessions were more effective since there was an exchange of ideas, and patients interacted with each other. They also stressed that individualization of the diet was very important. The dietitian was able to instruct eight patients per class per hour, whereas 15 minutes per patient was needed for bedside instruction. Therefore another advantage to classroom teaching is the amount of dietitian's time saved.

It has been estimated that it takes a minimum of 6 to 12 hours to effectively educate a patient about his diabetic diet. Therefore new teaching techniques such as programmed instruction, teaching machines, and slide/tape self-teaching methods are being used.

A seminar on diabetes mellitus was held in a rural area in the state of Utah.[63] In the morning information was presented on diabetic diets. This was followed by a buffet luncheon in which the dishes were labeled with exchange values. A bingo game based on the exchange list was used to present more dietetic information. Weight reduction was also discussed. The second part of the seminar was devoted to nursing management. Responses from a questionnaire sent to the participants indicated that this method of teaching had been successful. It was suggested that future seminars be devoted to weight reduction, hypertension, heart disease, low-cholesterol diets, and arthritis.

Another successful method for patient education was a family day for juvenile diabetics and their families that was sponsored by the Kishwaukee Hospital in DeKalb, Illinois.[64] A seminar with a health care team was held for the parents, while the children participated in a day camp. The children in camp played games such as diabetic bingo and Olympic games and watched a film on diabetes. A picnic lunch buffet with all foods labeled with exchange values was served to the whole family. Participation in a seminar given by physicians, pharmacists, nurses, podiatrists, and dietitians allowed the parents to discuss problems they experienced with their diabetic children. The seminar was evaluated positively by the adults. Several months later some of the families who attended the family day organized a club for diabetics.

REFERENCES

1. Olefsky, J. M.: The insulin receptor: its role in insulin resistance of obesity and diabetes, Diabetes 25:1154, 1976.
2. Gerich, J., et al.: Abnormal pancreatic glucagon secretion and postprandial hyperglycemia in diabetes mellitus, J.A.M.A. 234:159, 1975.
3. Unger, R. H., and Orci, L.: Role of glucagon in diabetes, Arch. Intern. Med. 137:482, 1977.
4. Felig, P., et al.: Insulin, glucagon, and somatostatin in normal physiology and diabetes mellitus, Diabetes 25:1091, 1976.
5. Unger, R. H.: Diabetes and the alpha cell, Diabetes 25:136, 1976.
6. Gerich, J. E.: Somatostatin, Am. Fam. Physician 15(3):149, 1977.
7. Tamborlane, W. V., et al.: Metabolic effects of somatostatin in maturity-onset diabetes, N. Engl. J. Med. 297:181, 1977.
8. Bondy, P. K., and Felig, P.: Disorders of carbohydrate metabolism. In Bondy, P. K., and Rosenberg, L. E., editors: Duncan's diseases of metabolism, ed. 7, Philadelphia, 1974, W. B. Saunders Co.
9. Diabetes: epidemiology suggests a viral connection, Science 188:347, 1975.
10. Bressler, R., and Galloway, J. A.: The medical treatment of diabetes, Nutr. Today 6(4):14, 1971.
11. Klimt, C. R.: The university group diabetes program, Diabetes 19(suppl. 2):1103, 1970.
12. University group diabetes program. A study of the effects of hypoglycemic agents as vascular complications in patients with adult-onset diabetes. VI. Supplementary report on nonfatal events in patients treated with tolbutamide, Diabetes 25:1129, 1976.
13. Prout, T. E.: A prospective view of the treatment of adult-onset diabetes: with special reference to the university group diabetes program and oral hypoglycemic agents, Med. Clin. North Am. 55:1065, 1971.
14. Bierman, E. L.: The oral antidiabetic agents, Am. Fam. Physician 13(1):98, 1976.
15. Turtle, J. R., and Burgess, J. A.: Hypoglycemic action of fenfluramine in diabetes mellitus, Diabetes 22:858, 1973.
16. What do you know about the "new cures" for diabetes? J. Am. Diet. Assoc. 66:127, 1975.
17. Matas, A. J., Sutherland, D. E. R., and Najarian, J. S.: Current status of islet and pancreas transplantation in diabetes, Diabetes 25:785, 1976.
18. Success of islet cell transplants raises hope of a diabetes cure, J.A.M.A. 236:2033, 1976.
19. Bolinger, P. E., Price, S., and Kyner, J. L.: Experience with automation as an aid in the management of diabetes, Diabetes 22:480, 1973.
20. Albisser, A. M., et al.: An artificial endocrine pancreas, Diabetes 23:389, 1974.
21. Albisser, A. M., et al.: Clinical control of diabetes by the artificial pancreas, Diabetes 23:397, 1974.
22. Marliss, E. B., et al.: Normalization of glycemia in diabetics during meals with insulin and glucagon delivery by the artificial pancreas, Diabetes 26:663, 1977.
23. Genuth, S., and Martin, P.: Control of hyperglycemia in adult diabetics by pulsed insulin delivery, Diabetes 26:571, 1977.
24. Thorton, G. F.: Infections and diabetes, Med. Clin. North Am. 55:931, 1971.
25. Fajans, S. S.: Current unsolved problems in diabetes management, Diabetes 21 (suppl 2): 678, 1972.
26. Gerich, J. E.: Diabetic control and the late complications of diabetes, Am. Fam. Physician 16(2):85, 1977.
27. Gabbay, K. H.: The sorbitol pathway and the complications of diabetes, N. Engl. J. Med. 288:831, 1973.
28. Anderson, J. W.: Metabolic abnormalities con-

tributing to diabetic complications. II. Peripheral nerves, Am. J. Clin. Nutr. **29**:402, 1976.

29. Winegrad, A. I., and Greene, D. A.: Diabetic polyneuropathy: the importance of insulin deficiency, hyperglycemia and alterations in myoinositol metabolism in its pathogenesis, N. Engl. J. Med. **295**:1416, 1976.

30. Anderson, J. W.: Alterations in the metabolic fate of glucose in the liver of diabetic animals, Am. J. Clin. Nutr. **27**:746, 1974.

31. Blood test may start new era in diabetes therapy evaluation, J.A.M.A. **237**:847, 1977.

32. Wood, F. C., Jr., and Bierman, E. L.: New concepts in diabetic dietetics, Nutr. Today **7**(3):4, 1972.

33. Kay, R.: Nutrition in the aetiology and treatment of diabetes mellitus, Nutrition **28**:97, 1974.

34. Bierman, E. L., et al.: Principles of nutrition and dietary recommendations for patients with diabetes mellitus: 1971, Diabetes **20**:633, 1971.

35. Anderson, J. W., Herman, R. H., and Zakin, D.: Effect of high glucose and high sucrose diets on glucose tolerance of normal men, Am. J. Clin. Nutr. **26**:600, 1973.

36. Weinsier, R. L., et al.: High and low carbohydrate diets in diabetes mellitus. Study of effects on diabetic control, insulin secretion and blood lipids, Ann. Intern. Med. **80**:332, 1974.

37. Brunzell, J. D., et al.: Effect of a fat free high carbohydrate diet on diabetic subjects with fasting hyperglycemia, Diabetes **23**:138, 1974.

38. Anderson, J. W.: Effect of carbohydrate restriction and high carbohydrate diets on men with chemical diabetes, Am. J. Clin. Nutr. **30**:402, 1977.

39. Jackson, R. A.: Dietary diabetes. The influence of a low-carbohydrate diet on forearm metabolism in man, Diabetes **22**:145, 1973.

40. Crapo, P. A., Reaven, G., and Olefsky, J.: Plasma glucose and insulin responses to orally administered simple and complex carbohydrates, Diabetes **25**:741, 1976.

41. Crapo, P. A., Reaven, G., and Olefsky, J.: Postprandial plasma-glucose and -insulin responses to different complex carbohydrates, Diabetes **26**:1178, 1977.

42. Lenner, R. A.: Studies of glycemia and glucosuria in diabetics after breakfast meals of different composition, Am. J. Clin. Nutr. **29**:716, 1976.

43. Jenkins, D. J. A., et al.: Unabsorbable carbohydrates and diabetes: decreased postprandial hyperglycaemia, Lancet **2**:172, 1976.

44. Jenkins, D. J. A., et al.: Decrease in postpran-

dial insulin and glucose concentrations by guar and pectin, Ann. Intern. Med. **86**:20, 1977.

45. Miranda, P. M., and Horwitz, D. L.: High fiber diets in the treatment of diabetes mellitus, Ann. Intern. Med. **88**:482, 1978.

46. Kiehm, T. G., Anderson, J. W., and Ward, K.: Beneficial effects of a high carbohydrate, high fiber diet on hyperglycemic diabetic men, Am. J. Clin. Nutr. **29**:895, 1976.

47. Anderson, J. W.: High polysaccharide diet studies in patients with diabetes and vascular disease, Cereal Foods World **22**:12, 1977.

48. Wall, J. R., Pyke, D. A., and Oakley, W. G.: Effect of carbohydrate restriction on obese diabetics: relationship of control to weight loss, Br. Med. J. **1**:577, 1973.

49. Bistrian, B. R., et al.: Nitrogen metabolism and insulin requirements in obese diabetic adults on a protein-sparing modified fast, Diabetes **25**:494, 1976.

50. Albrink, M. J.: Dietary and drug treatment of hyperlipidemia in diabetes, Diabetes **23**:913, 1974.

51. Maruhama, Y., et al.: Dietary intake and hyperlipidemia in controlled diabetic outpatients, Diabetes **26**:94, 1977.

52. Kissebah, A. H.: Management of hyperlipidemia in diabetes, Am. Fam. Physician **19**(4):144, 1979.

53. American Diabetes Association and American Dietetic Association and Chronic Disease Program, U. S. Public Health Service: Meal planning with exchange lists, Chicago, 1950, The American Dietetic Association.

54. American Diabetes Association and American Dietetic Association: Exchange lists for meal planning, New York, 1976, American Diabetes Association.

55. American Diabetes Association and American Dietetic Association: A guide for professionals: the effective application of "exchange lists for meal planning," New York, 1977, American Diabetes Association.

56. Williams, T. G., Anderson, E., Watkins, J. D., and Coyle, V.: Dietary errors made at home by patients with diabetes, J. Am. Diet. Assoc., **51**:19, 1967.

57. Holland, W. M.: The diabetes supplement of the National Health Survey. III. The patient reports on his diet, J. Am. Diet. Assoc. **52**:387, 1968.

58. Stulb, S. C.: The diabetes supplement of the National Health Survey. IV. The patients' knowledge of the food exchanges, J. Am. Diet. Assoc. **52**:391, 1968.

59. Tunbridge, R., and Witherill, J. H.: Reliability

and cost of diabetic diets, Br. Med. J. **2**:78, 1970.

60. West, K. M.: Diet therapy of diabetes: an analysis of failure, Ann. Intern. Med. **79**:425, 1973.

61. Weinsier, R. L., et al.: Diet therapy of diabetes. Description of a successful methodologic approach to gaining diet adherence, Diabetes **23**:669, 1974.

62. Hassell, J., and Medved, E.: Group/audio-visual instruction for patients with diabetes. Learning achievements and time economics, J. Am. Diet. Assoc. **66**:465, 1975.

63. Gines, D.: Diabetes seminar for the public in a rural area in Utah, J. Am. Diet. Assoc. **69**:651, 1976.

64. Koukal, S. M., and Parham, E. S.: A family learning experience to serve the juvenile patient with diabetes. J. Am. Diet. Assoc. **72**:411, 1978.

8 Cardiovascular disease

TERMINOLOGY

Heart attack, stroke, and high blood pressure are the terms commonly used by the lay public in connection with heart disease. Coronary occlusion, cerebrovascular accident, and hypertension are the respective terms used by health professionals. The terminology used concerning cardiovascular disease is extensive and complex. On occasion terms are used interchangeably when in fact these terms have a somewhat different connotation. For example, confusion exists over the terms "hyperlipemia," and "hyperlipidemia," and "hyperlipoproteinemia." As an aid to the discussion of cardiovascular disease, some of the terms used frequently are defined in the glossary at the end of this chapter rather than in the text.

ATHEROSCLEROSIS

Cardiovascular disease is the leading cause of death in the United States. The morbidity in the United States has not been studied, but it is assumed to be high. Although the incidence increases with age, atherosclerosis has been reported in young individuals. Autopsies of 15 to 19 year olds showed fatty streaks in 71% to 83% of the group.[1] Evidence of atherosclerosis was found in 77% of soldiers killed in the Korean War[2] and in 45% of those who died in the Vietnam War.[3] Atherosclerosis is uncommon in young females, but it has been reported in women aged 40 years and younger.[4]

Normal arteries consist of three layers. The innermost layer, the intima, is lined on the lumen side with a single layer of endothelial cells. These cells form a barrier that prevents the passage of the blood constituents into the artery wall. The media, or middle layer, is composed of smooth muscle cells surrounded by collagen, small elastic fibers, and mucopolysaccharides. The outer layer, or adventitia, contains fibroblasts mixed with smooth muscle cells set between bundles of collagen and surrounded by mucopolysaccharides. Atherosclerosis is a disease that involves the intimal lining of the larger arteries. There are three types of lesions that develop, namely, the fatty streak, fibrous plaque, and the complicated lesion.[5-7] Fatty streaks consist of a small number of intimal smooth muscle cells that contain, and are surrounded by, cholesterol and cholesteryl esters. The fibrous plaque contains the smooth muscle cells with cholesterol and cholesteryl ester. These cells are surrounded by lipid, collagen, elastin, and mucopolysaccharides. A fibrous cap covers the plaque and protrudes into the wall of the lumen.[8] The complicated lesion is a fibrous plaque that has been altered by hemorrhage, ulceration, mural thrombosis, calcification, and cellular necrosis. This is often seen when the artery becomes occluded.

Several theories had been proposed for the origin of atherosclerosis. It is now generally assumed that the lesion begins with the accumulation of smooth muscle cells in the intima of the artery. The current controversy centers around what initiates this process. The response to injury hypothesis is based on the fact that several factors could injure the endothelium and make it permeable to blood constituents.[9] Such factors are hyperlipidemia, hypertension, hormone dysfunction, and antibodies to carbon monoxide from cigarette smoke. If the injury is sustained, the smooth muscle cells continue to proliferate and amass lipids and connective tissue. A "derived growth factor" that is released from platelets aggregating at the site of injury may cause proliferation.[10] It has been shown in animals that if the injury is not repeated the lesion regresses. However, if the injury is sustained by one of the factors such as elevated plasma, low-density lipoproteins in humans, then the lesion continues to grow, and atherosclerosis results.

The response to injury hypothesis developed from results derived from animal experimentation, and it is not known whether plaques in humans develop in the same manner. On the other hand, the monoclonal hypothesis is based on evidence from human plaques. This theory suggests that the lesion arises from a single muscle cell that has been altered by some factor and continues to proliferate. Thus the plaque is considered a benign tumor.

Texon stated that atherosclerosis begins in utero as soon as blood starts to flow.[11] The severity of the lesion is not related to age but rather to the local hydraulic forces in the artery. The lesions occur primarily in the large and medium-size arteries, particularly the coronary and cerebral arteries.[12]

During the first 10 years of life fatty streaks develop most frequently in the proximal aorta and the thoracic segment.[12] The plaques that develop later in life appear most often in the distal aorta. The initial lesion, the fatty streak, only slightly narrows the lumen of the blood vessel. The streaks are found in the aorta of almost all children by age 3 and increase in number until 25 years of age.[13] Between 10 and 15 years of age the streaks appear in the coronary arteries and lastly in the cerebral arteries at age 35. A controversy exists as to whether these fatty streaks precede plaque formation.[12,13] Some fatty streaks turn into plaques, but others do not.

The effect of the atherosclerosis is caused by a narrowing of the lumen of the vessel.[14] When this occurs in the coronary arteries, angina pectoris develops on exertion or after stress. When the vessel is totally blocked, there is a myocardial infarction, cerebrovascular accident, or, if the affected area is large, sudden death. Gangrene develops when the block is in the extremities. The vessel can be plugged either by a thrombus or embolism. The process of plaque formation can also weaken the wall of the artery, and an aneurysm can form. This can very easily rupture, and hemorrhage ensues.

Plaque formation is a slow process, and an individual may be asymptomatic for years. Clinical symptoms may develop, or in some instances, the first myocardial occlusion or cerebrovascular accident is fatal; thus it is important that tests be developed to detect the asymptomatic stage. Hypercholesterolemia may be indicative of atherosclerosis. An electrocardiogram at rest and after exercise may be a valuable aid to the physician. The new technique of angiography can be used to detect atherosclerosis. A radiopaque dye is injected, and x-ray films are taken of the arteries. However, this is not a routine procedure as the individual must be hospitalized, and complications have sometimes developed.

The three major risk factors associated with premature atherosclerosis, especially coronary heart disease, are hypercholesterolemia, hypertension, and cigarette smoking.[15] The other associated factors that have been identified are diabetes mellitus, asymptomatic hyperglycemia, obesity, lack of exercise, psychosocial tensions, and family history. As many as 37 different factors have been cited in the literature as risk factors.[16] Some of the newer factors currently under investigation are the role of dietary fiber, minerals, trans-fatty acids, and stress.

Diet

Kannel has pointed out that no one has conclusively proved that the nutrient composition of the diets consumed by persons who suffer from coronary artery disease is different from those who do not.[17] The relationship has not been established between the nutrient composition of the diet and serum cholesterol values from one individual to another. Yet many studies have shown that saturated fat, cholesterol, and refined carbohydrate result in high blood lipids and thus are atherogenic. Diets can be modified to either produce or regress atherosclerotic lesions.

The relationship of cholesterol to atherosclerosis has been the subject of extensive research. No direct evidence exists that shows cholesterol causes coronary artery disease; however, research indicates that high blood levels of cholesterol are one of many factors that place one at high risk. Experiments with animals have demonstrated that feeding high levels of cholesterol will produce atherosclerosis. Epidemiological studies throughout the world have shown a higher incidence of coronary artery disease in populations with elevated blood cholesterol levels. When the plaques found in arteries are analyzed, large amounts of cholesterol are found to be present. Although atherosclerosis is associated with aging, individuals with inborn errors of cholesterol metabolism show evidence of plaque formation at a very young age.

Controversy exists as to the effect of dietary cholesterol on serum cholesterol. Some population groups consume large quantities of cholesterol, yet they do not exhibit hypercholesterolemia. Others have reported only a slight decrease in serum levels with dietary restriction. Serum cholesterol levels are also high when the intake of saturated fat is high. The replacement by polyunsaturated fats results in a decrease in serum cholesterol. Monounsaturated fatty acids such as oleic acid have no effect on cholesterol levels. The same response is found with the short-chain (less than 12 carbons) fatty acids. Even the response of the saturated fatty acids differs, and the hypercholesterolemic effect is due to lauric, myristic, and palmitic acids.[18,19] Whyte and Havenstein estimated the plasma cholesterol contribution of foods that are regularly eaten.[20]

The hydrogenation of polyunsaturated fats results in more saturated fats and a change in some unsaturated fats from the cis to the trans form. When a diet containing 40% trans-fatty acids was fed to swine, total plasma lipids and cholesterol levels were higher than in other groups fed tallow, corn oil, used fat, butterfat, egg yolk, whole egg powder, or crystalline cholesterol.[21] The significance of this for humans is not known.

Some researchers question the use of polyunsaturated fats, since the effects of long-term usage are not known. Reports have implicated polyunsaturated fats in gallstone formation,[22] colonic cancer, and increased vitamin E requirements.[16]

Controversy also exists as to the relationship between carbohydrate intake and coronary heart disease. Some studies have reported that individuals with coronary artery disease consume more sucrose as compared with starch.[23-26] The high-sucrose diets increase serum cholesterol and triglycerides, but this hypertriglyceridemia is only a transient effect.[23] Fructose exerts a lipogenic effect.[23,25,26] The mechanism by which these effects occur is not known.

The relationship of diet and coronary heart disease is extremely complex. Many studies have been carried out with animals and humans, with normolipidemic and hyperlipidemic subjects, and with a variety of diet modifications. Since the literature in this field is extensive, the reader is referred to two review articles.[27,28] Glueck and Connor described "animal experiments, human metabolic data, primitive people and vegetarians, migrants, between population data, within homogeneous population data, limitations on methodology, genetic factors, therapeutic diets, influences of dietary fat, cholesterol and protein, high-density lipoprotein cholesterol and coronary heart disease, and changes in the food intake of the U.S. population."[27] Truswell summarized the effect of the following on plasma total cholesterol or LDL: fatty acid pattern of glycerides, dietary sterols, carbohydrates, proteins and amino acids, dietary fiber, vitamins, minerals and trace elements, meal frequency and drinks, factors affecting plasma HDL and diets, and the tendency to thrombosis.[28] He concluded that diets should be modified to reduce LDL, increase HDL, and reduce the tendency to thrombosis in order to prevent or delay coronary heart disease. Additional research is needed with humans as to the factors affecting HDL and thrombotic tendency, and overall long-term effects. Truswell stated that it is more scientific to examine the effects of a whole food in the amounts normally consumed on plasma lipids rather than looking at its biochemical composition, for example, fat composition. More attention must be paid to the fact that individuals react differently to foods. For example, some individuals who consume eggs show an increase in plasma cholesterol, but others show no effect.

After many years of research with, in some cases, conflicting results, the diet-heart controversy has arisen, and some investigators question the relationship between diet and coronary artery disease. Mann stated that no studies to date have proved that dietary treatment is effective in preventing or modifying coronary heart disease.[29] Four reasons were presented to demonstrate that the diet-heart hypothesis is invalid. First, the data from the Framingham and Tecumseh studies that involved a large number of people did not prove any relationship between diet and blood cholesterol levels. Second, the mortality rates have not changed over the past 27 years; therefore Mann concluded that dietary changes could not have had any effects. The food consumption data from 1950 showed an increase in the intake of polyunsaturated fats, but there was no change in the amount of saturated fat and cholesterol. Third, clinical trials with subjects both free of coronary heart disease and those with disease have not shown that diet therapy is effective either in the prevention or treatment of coronary heart disease. Fourth, drugs are more effective than diet in lowering serum cholesterol levels; yet after 5 years of use the incidence of heart disease has not been reduced. Also it has been shown that the risk factors do not count after age 55, yet dietary studies are run with middle-age subjects; treatment for hypercholesterolemic children is more relevant. Mann further stated that hypercholesterolemia is not due to high dietary intakes of cholesterol, increased synthesis of cholesterol, or decreased excretion of sterols, but rather it is a result of a defect in the conversion of cholesterol to bile acids. Therefore research should be devoted to seeking out the reason why this reaction does not take place. Another area to be studied is the effectiveness of exercise in preventing heart disease. Many investigators, however, have disagreed with the above mentioned statements of Mann.

Reiser also examined the relationship between diet and heart disease.[30] He concluded that it is not necessary for the whole population to modify their food habits, since a majority of normolipidemic people would then be deprived of traditional and desirable foods such as eggs, dairy products, liver, beef, and pork. In addition, he feels that the information from food manufacturers and the American Heart Association implies that anyone who eats meat, eggs, and dairy products is in danger of developing coronary heart disease, and it thus appears that cholesterol is toxic. Reiser stated that the modified foods such as meat substitutes, egg substitutes, and margarine should be sold on their own merit and not promoted as medicines.

Another point raised by Reiser is the fact that not all people with atherosclerosis have heart disease. Much research has been carried out, but there is still a controversy over the relationship between cholesterol and other lipids and atherosclerosis and coronary heart disease. Some studies conclude that dietary cholesterol affects serum cholesterol, and others state that it has no effect. Recent research indicates that other factors in the diet such as pectin and phytosterol may have an effect. There is the possibility that other natural food constituents may have a hypocholesterolemic effect. Reiser indicated that individuals with cholesterol levels below the risk level should be studied to see whether the addition or removal of cholesterol from their diet has an effect on the incidence of coronary heart disease. On the basis of the experimental evidence now available, Reiser concluded that only individuals with hypercholesterolemia should be treated.

Hyperlipoproteinemia. In hyperlipoproteinemia the digestion of exogenous triglycerides in the intestine produces fatty acids and glycerol. The long-chain fatty acids are combined with glycerol, and triglycerides are again synthesized. This core is coated with protein, cholesterol, cholesteryl esters, and the phospholipid lecithin. These particles, called chylomicrons, enter the lacteals and are at peak concentrations 3 to 6 hours after the ingestion of a fatty meal. The chylomicrons are cleared from the blood within 6 to 8 hours by the enzyme lipoprotein lipase. Most of the fatty acids are taken up by adipose tissue, and the glycerol is released into the circulation.

The very-low-density lipoproteins (VLDL) are synthesized primarily in the liver and in small amounts in the intestine. VLDL are composed mainly of triglycerides, and thus their function is to transport these endogenous lipids of hepatic origin that are mostly derived from carbohydrates. High-carbohydrate diets produce a transient hypertriglyceridemia. The triglycerides in chylomicrons and VLDL are hydrolyzed by the enzyme lipoprotein lipase. The low-density lipoproteins (LDL) are synthesized in the liver from the breakdown products of VLDL. The LDL are involved in the transport of cholesterol. Much interest has been shown recently in the high-density lipoproteins (HDL) that are synthesized in the liver. The HDL may be able to carry cholesterol from the peripheral tissues back to the liver for catabolism. The composition of the lipoproteins is given in Table 8-1.

Total serum cholesterol levels have been used to predict the risk of coronary heart disease. Data from five study populations participating in the Cooperative Lipoprotein Phenotyping Study showed that persons with coronary heart disease had lower levels of HDL cholesterol than did those who were free of disease.[31] Therefore high levels of HDL cholesterol protect against coronary artery disease, while high levels of LDL cholesterol indicate a greater risk. The average serum HDL cholesterol level for men is 45 mg/dl and for women it is 55 mg/dl.[32] Heparin manganese is added to the HDL serum to cause precipitation. The HDL cholesterol remains in the supernatant, and thus it can be easily measured. In newborn infants approximately 50% of the total cholesterol is found in the HDL fraction, and in adults this drops to about 25%. Exercise, a moderate intake of alcohol, some drugs, and a change to a typical Asian diet have been shown to increase HDL levels.

It has been estimated that on the average diet, 100 g per day of exogenous fat are converted into chylomicrons and intestinal VLDL.[33] In the same period of time approximately 100 to 200 g of hepatic VLDL are transported. The lipoproteins serve as a means of lipid transport between tissues.

The cholesterol in blood is distributed between the lipoproteins as follows: low density (LD) 50% to 75%, high density (HD) 15% to 25%, and VLDL 6% to 12%.[34] This accounts for approximately 11 g or 10% of the total body cholesterol. Exogenous

Table 8-1. Plasma lipoproteins

	Chylomicrons	VLDL	LDL	HDL
Density g/ml	0.95	0.95-1.006	1.006-1.063	1.063-1.21
% Composition				
Protein	0.5-1	5-15	25	45-55
Triglycerides	85	50-70	5-10	2
Cholesterol	2-5	10-20	40-45	18
Phospholipid	3-6	10-20	20-25	30

and endogenous cholesterol mix in the intestinal lumen and are absorbed into the mucosal cell in a mixed micelle. Cholesterol is esterified and released in chylomicrons and VLDL. Dietary cholesterol inhibits the synthesis of hepatic cholesterol but not intestinal cholesterol. About half the average dietary cholesterol intake of 600 mg is absorbed. About 1 g of this compound is excreted daily in the feces as bile acids and sterols. Most cholesterol is metabolized into the bile acids—cholic, chenodeoxycholic, deoxycholic, and lithocholic acid. This pathway prevents the excessive accumulation of cholesterol in the tissues, because this sterol cannot be metabolized completely to carbon dioxide and water. Some cholesterol serves as a precursor for the synthesis of adrenal steroid hormones (cortisol, aldosterone, and corticosterone), the male sex hormones (testosterone and androstenedione), the female sex hormones (progesterone and estrogen), and vitamin D.

Primary hyperlipidemia may be caused by environmental or genetic factors.[34] Epidemiological studies that relate cholesterol levels and the incidence of coronary heart disease formed the basis for environmentally induced hyperlipidemia. This evidence indicated that the American way of life, in particular the diet, contributed to hypercholesterolemia and thus to the increased incidence of heart disease. Clinical and laboratory studies indicate that hypercholesterolemia, hypertension, and cigarette smoking increase the risk of coronary heart disease and may be possible causes. Other secondary risk factors are also involved. These factors can be modified, and so individuals with high-risk characteristics should be treated. A mass preventive program should help to reduce the incidence of cardiovascular disease.

Fredrickson, Levy, and Lees investigated the genetic basis of the lipid disorders, the so-called hyperlipoproteinemias.[35]

The cholesterol and triglyceride levels in Americans without evidence of coronary artery disease were measured, and those with levels in the top 5% were considered to be of genetic origin. These individuals with hyperlipoproteinemia had relatives with the same disorder. The lipid disorders of absorption, synthesis, circulation, and deposition of lipids and lipoproteins are considered genetic defects.[34] Some are affected by diet. Therapy for these hyperlipoproteinemias involves not only diet but drugs and in some instances surgery. The proponents of this view feel that it is useless to change the American way of life, and this should only be attempted for those at high risk. It is felt that the control of atherosclerosis in the future will be the result of research related to lipid metabolism, transport, and an understanding of the deposits in the artery wall.

Elevation of blood lipoproteins increases the risk of heart disease. The measurement of blood lipids determines which fractions, if any, are abnormal, and then proper treatment can be initiated. Generally for the majority of patients, hyperlipidemia can be detected by measuring blood cholesterol and triglyceride levels. Fasting samples are needed to measure triglycerides but not cholesterol.

Two methods are available for lipoprotein typing to detect the genetic disorders.[33] Ultracentrifugation separates the lipoproteins on the basis of their densities. The particles ranging in size from the lightest to the heaviest are chylomicrons, VLDL, LDL, and HDL. The values for the lipoprotein flotation rates are reported in Svedberg units. Blood lipoproteins can be separated by electrophoresis on filter paper or on agarose gel. A drop of blood is placed on the paper or gel in a buffer solution. On application of an electric current, the lipoproteins separate into bands. These bands may be stained with a dye. The intensity of color indicates the amount of lipoprotein present. The chylomicrons do not move from the origin. The alpha fraction moves the farthest followed by the pre-beta and then beta bands.

Either plasma or serum may be used for these determinations. The individual must fast for 12 to 16 hours before a blood sample is drawn. These tests should not be performed during weight reduction or periods of stress, as the lipid levels will be affected.

Confusion exists since different values are used to determine hyperlipidemia. Epidemiological data suggest that the upper limit of normal serum cholesterol is 220 mg/dl. As the levels increase, the risk increases. Table 8-2 shows that the cholesterol values for genetic disorders range from 230 to 330 mg/dl. Both cholesterol and triglyceride values increase with age, although there is no evidence that these values should increase with age. The values used to determine hyperlipidemia from genetic

Table 8-2. Lipid levels for establishing genetic abnormalities (suggested upper limits)*

Age	Cholesterol mg/dl	Triglycerides mg/dl
1-19	230	150
20-29	240	200
30-39	270	200
40-49	310	200
50-	330	200

*From The dietary management of hyperlipoproteinemia. A handbook for physicians and dietitians, Bethesda, Md., National Heart and Lung Institute, National Institutes of Health (reprinted 1974), DHEW Publication No. (NIH) 75-110.

causes are significantly higher than the levels based on epidemiological data. It should be emphasized that these are normal limits and not safe limits.

Lipoprotein profiles. In 1967 Fredrickson, Levy, and Lees identified five major types of hyperlipoproteinemias (I to V).[35] Later group II was subdivided into type IIa and IIb. Primary hyperlipoproteinemia is inherited or the result of dietary intake. Secondary hyperlipoproteinemia is associated with the following disorders: hypothyroidism, dysproteinemia, nephrotic syndrome, obstructive liver disease, and uncontrolled diabetes mellitus.[36] When the basic disorder is alleviated, the lipoprotein levels return to normal. The therapy for the primary hyperlipoproteinemias is dependent upon the type.[37]

Type I or hyperchylomicronemia is extremely rare. It is induced by exogenous fat. Since lipoprotein lipase is deficient, chylomicrons are not cleared from the plasma. Triglyceride levels are extremely high (over 5000 mg/dl), and cholesterol levels are normal or slightly elevated. LDL and VLDL levels are normal. Lipemia retinalis, hepatosplenomegaly, eruptive xanthomas, abdominal pain, and occasionally, pancreatitis are associated with this defect.

Type II (hyperlipoproteinemia) is subdivided into type IIa, which is indicated by normal triglycerides, increased LDL, and normal VLDL. Type IIb is characterized by hypertriglyceridemia and increased LDL and VLDL. In both types cholesterol levels are elevated (300 to 600 mg/dl). The most characteristic symptoms are extensor tendinous, xanthomas on the hands and Achilles tendon, premature corneal arcus, and early atherosclerosis of the coronary and other large arteries. This type may be found after excessive ingestion of cholesterol and saturated fats.

Type III is relatively rare and is called broad beta or floating beta disease. A pattern of both elevated triglycerides and cholesterol (both 350 to 800 mg/dl) is unique to this group. The clinical manifestations are accelerated atherosclerosis of the coronary and peripheral blood vessels, pain in the legs on walking, and xanthomas. The conversion of VLDL to LDL is defective.

Endogenous hyperlipemia or type IV is very common. It may be of genetic origin or caused by the ingestion of the typical American diet. Cholesterol levels are normal or slightly elevated. VLDL are increased, and LDL levels are either normal or increased. Triglycerides are elevated and may reach 1000 mg/dl. There are no clinical symptoms, but type IV is generally associated with diabetes mellitus, hyperuricemia, and premature atherosclerosis. Stress and excessive calories, carbohydrate, and alcohol lead to the type IV pattern.

Type V or mixed hyperlipemia is uncommon. Chylomicrons and VLDL are increased. LDL may be slightly increased. Cholesterol levels are high. Triglyceride levels may reach 6000 mg/dl. The clinical symptoms are eruptive xanthomas, abdominal pain, hepatosplenomegaly, and, occasionally, pancreatitis. Hyperglycemia and hyperuricemia are frequently found with type V.

The lipid levels in the various types of hyperlipoproteinemias are summarized in Table 8-3.

Table 8-3. Lipoprotein levels in hyperlipoproteinemias

Type	Chylomicrons	VLDL	LDL	Cholesterol	Triglycerides
I	Increased	Normal	Normal	Increased	Increased
IIa	None	Normal	Increased	Increased	Normal
IIb	None	Increased	Increased	Increased	Increased
III	None	Increased	Increased	Increased	Increased
IV	None	Increased	Normal or increased	Normal or increased	Increased
V	Increased	Increased	Normal or increased	Increased	Increased

Table 8-4. Summary of diets for types I-V hyperlipoproteinemia*

	Type I	Type IIa
Diet prescription	Low fat 25-35 g	Low cholesterol; polyunsaturated fat increased
Calories	Not restricted	Not restricted
Protein	Total protein intake is not limited	Total protein intake is not limited
Fat	Restricted to 25-35 g Kind of fat not important	Saturated fat intake limited Polyunsaturated fat intake increased
Cholesterol	Not restricted	As low as possible; the only source of cholesterol is the meat in the diet
Carbohydrate	Not limited	Not limited
Alcohol	Not recommended	May be used with discretion

*From The dietary management of hyperlipoproteinemia. A handbook for physicians and (reprinted 1974), DHEW Publication No. (NIH) 75-110.

Treatment.[37] In type I, chylomicrons cannot be cleared from the plasma, so dietary fat must be severely restricted to 25 to 35 g. Medium-chain triglycerides can be used. The fatty acids from these triglycerides are absorbed directly into the portal vein and thus do not form chylomicrons. The medium-chain triglycerides help to make the diet more palatable and decrease the amount of calories supplied from carbohydrate and protein. No drug therapy has been found useful for type I.

The diet prescription for type IIa calls for low cholesterol (300 mg per day), a decrease in saturated fats, and an increase in polyunsaturated fats. The only source of cholesterol in the diet should be from meat. Egg yolks, organ meats, whole milk, cream, and cheese should be avoided. The highly polyunsaturated vegetable oils should be used. In nonfamilial type IIa, dietary treatment alone may be successful. Drug therapy is generally necessary for familial type IIa.

The diet therapy for types IIb and III is the same. A reduction diet is prescribed

Type IIb & Type III	Type IV	Type V
Low cholesterol Approximately: 20% cal pro. 40% cal fat 40% cal CHO	Controlled CHO Approximately 45% of calories Moderately restricted cholesterol	Restricted fat 30% of calories Controlled CHO 50% of calories Moderately restricted cholesterol
Achieve and maintain "ideal" weight, i.e., reduction diet if necessary	Achieve and maintain "ideal" weight, i.e., reduction diet if necessary	Achieve and maintain "ideal" weight, i.e., reduction diet if necessary
High protein	Not limited other than control of patient's weight	High protein
Controlled to 40% calories (polyunsaturated fats recommended in preference to saturated fats)	Not limited other than control of patient's weight (polyunsaturated fats recommended in preference to saturated fats)	Restricted to 30% of calories (polyunsaturated fats recommended in preference to saturated fats)
Less than 300 mg —the only source of cholesterol is the meat in the diet	Moderately restricted to 300-500 mg	Moderately restricted to 300-500 mg
Controlled—concentrated sweets are restricted	Controlled—concentrated sweets are restricted	Controlled—concentrated sweets are restricted
Limited to 2 servings (substituted for carbohydrate)	Limited to 2 servings (substituted for carbohydrate)	Not recommended

dietitians, Bethesda, Md., National Heart and Lung Institute, National Institutes of Health until ideal weight is achieved. The maintenance diet should contain isocaloric amounts of fat and carbohydrate (40%). Cholesterol intake should be restricted to 300 mg per day. The polyunsaturated fat intake should be increased. Most often dietary treatment is successful, and drug therapy is not necessary.

A reduction diet is prescribed for type IV until ideal weight is achieved. The maintenance diet should contain approximately 45% of calories from carbohydrate. Excessive intakes of carbohydrate and alcohol will increase the synthesis of endogenous triglyceride. Cholesterol should be restricted to 300 to 500 mg per day. Polyunsaturated fats should be substituted for the saturated fats.

Type V individuals who are overweight must follow a reduction diet. When ideal weight is reached, blood lipid levels may be normal. The maintenance diet consists of fat, 30% of calories, and carbohydrate, 50% of calories. Polyunsaturated fats should be substituted for saturated fats. Medium-chain triglycerides may be used. Cholesterol intake should be held to 300 to 500 mg per day. The protein intake is higher than the recommended allowance and should be at least 1.5 to 2 g/kg of body weight. Alcohol is not recommended since it increases plasma triglyceride levels.

The diet therapy for types I to V hyperlipoproteinemia is summarized in Table 8-4. Table 8-5 summarizes the foods that are allowed and restricted in the five types of hyperlipoproteinemia according to food groupings.

When blood lipid levels do not return to normal with dietary restriction, then drug therapy must be instituted. The drugs commonly used to lower serum cholesterol levels are cholestyramine, colestipol, dextrothyroxine, sitosterol, and probucol.[38,39] Nicotinic acid and clofibrate reduce both serum cholesterol and triglyceride levels. Cholestyramine (Cuemid, Questran) and colestipol (Colestid) are ion exchange resins that bind bile acids in the intestine and are excreted in the feces. These compounds are used for type IIa hyperlipidemia. Dextrothyroxine (Choloxin) is an isomer of the thyroid hormone that lowers serum cholesterol levels. This drug is primarily used in young patients without any signs of cardiovascular disease. It is no longer used in the coronary drug project, since there was a high incidence of cardiac arrhythmias and new myocardial infarcts in patients taking this drug. Sitosterol (Cytellin) lowers serum cholesterol levels by interfering with its absorption in the intestine. Type IIa hyperlipidemia is treated with this drug. Nicotinic acid (Nicalex) reduces both serum cholesterol and triglyceride levels. The exact mechanism of its action is not understood. It has been used in the treatment of types IIa, b, III, IV, and V hyperlipidemia. Clofibrate (Atromid S) affects lipid metabolism in several ways: it inhibits hepatic triglyceride synthesis, decreases synthesis of VLDL, inhibits hepatic and intestinal synthesis of cholesterol, decreases the body pool of cholesterol, promotes fecal excretion of neutral sterols, and inhibits lipolysis in the adipocytes. It is indicated for types IIb, III, IV, and V hyperlipidemia.

The newest drug that has been used to lower serum cholesterol levels is probucol (Lorelco).[40] Its mechanism of action is not known. It is most effective when used in conjunction with a low-cholesterol, low–saturated fat diet for type IIa hyperlipopro-

Table 8-5. Specific diets according to type of hyperlipoproteinemia*

Type of food	Foods included	Foods excluded
Beverages (nondairy)	I, II—Coffee, tea, carbonated beverages, fruit, and vegetables juices III, IV, V—Same as above, but only unsweetened beverages allowed	I, II—None III, IV, V—Sweetened beverages
Breads and cereals	I, II, III, IV, V—Enriched varieties of all breads except egg bread, saltines, and graham crackers. Baked goods containing no whole milk or egg yolks (angel food cake). All cereals and grain products (rice, macaroni, noodles, spaghetti) I—4 servings per day allowed II—4 or more servings per day III, IV, V—Number of servings specified for weight control	I, II, III, IV, V—Biscuits, muffins, corn bread, pancakes, waffles, French toast, hot rolls, sweet rolls, corn or potato chips, flavored crackers
Dairy products	I—Skim milk, nonfat buttermilk, evaporated skim milk, dried skim milk, uncreamed (no fat) cottage cheese, cheese made from skim milk II—Same as for I, plus specially prepared cheese high in polyunsaturated fat ¼ cup creamed cottage cheese may be substituted for 1 oz meat III, V—Same as for I, plus 1 cup yogurt made from skim milk may be substituted for 1 teaspoon fat IV—Same as for I, except that 2 oz of any type cheese is allowed per week	I—Fresh, dried evaporated, or condensed whole milk; sweet or sour cream; yogurt; ice cream or ice milk; sherbert; commercial whipped toppings; cream cheese and all other cheese, except skim milk cheese; nondairy or other cream substitutes II, III, IV, V—Same as for I, with exceptions shown under foods included
Desserts	I—Angel food cake, puddings, or frozen desserts made with skim milk, jello, meringues, fruit ices or whips II, III, IV, V—Same as above, plus desserts made with allowed fats	I—All cake and cookie mixes, except angel food mix; any pies, cakes, cookies containing whole milk, fat, or egg yolks II, III, IV, V—Same as above, except allowed fats not excluded

*From Murphy, B. F.: Management of hyperlipidemias, J.A.M.A. **230:**1688, 1974.

Continued.

Table 8-5. Specific diets according to type of hyperlipoproteinemia—cont'd

Type of food	Foods included	Foods excluded
Fat	I—None except medium-chain triglycerides II—Safflower oil, corn oil, soft safflower margarine, commercial mayonnaise III, IV, V—Any liquid vegetable unsaturated fat (safflower, corn, cottonseed, olive, and peanut oils), commercial mayonnaise, commercial salad dressings containing no sour cream or cheese	I—All fats and oils, gravies and cream sauces containing fats, salad dressings, and mayonnaise II—Butter, lard, hydrogenated shortening, and margarine; coconut oil and other oils not listed; salt pork, suet, bacon, and meat drippings; gravies and sauces unless made with allowed fats and skim milk III, IV, V—Same as for II, except margarine made from unsaturated fat permitted
Fruits	I—Any fresh, frozen, canned, or dried fruit or juice (except avocado) of which 1 serving per day should be citrus fruit; 2 servings per day II—Same as for I, except small amounts of avocado allowed III, IV, V—Same as for I, except 3 servings per day, and small amounts of avocado allowed	I—Avocado II, III, IV, V—Small amounts of avocado allowed
Meat	I—Lean meat with fat trimmed off. Beef (ground round or chuck hamburger, roasts, pot roast, stew, steak, dried chipped beef), lamb, pork, ham, veal. Organ meats (liver, heart, brains, kidney, sweetbreads). Limit to 5 oz cooked per day, or 7 oz a day if eaten only 3 times weekly II—Same as for I, except organ meats not allowed. Limit to 9 oz cooked per day, including fish and poultry. Limit beef, lamb, ham, and pork to 3 oz portion 3 times per week III—Same as for I except organ meats not allowed. Limit to 6-9 oz cooked per day IV, V—Same as for I except limit to 6-9 oz cooked per day	I, IV, V—Fried meats, fatty meats such as bacon, cold cuts, hot dogs, luncheon meats, sausage, canned meats (e.g., Spam); corned beef, pork and beans, spareribs; commercially sold ground beef or hamburgers; meats canned or frozen in sauces or gravy; frozen or packaged prepared products II, III—Same as above, plus all organ meats (kidney, hearts, brains, liver, sweetbreads)

Table 8-5. Specific diets according to type of hyperlipoproteinemia—cont'd

Type of food	Foods included	Foods excluded
Poultry, fish, and eggs	I—Skinned turkey, chicken, or cornish hen; fish, water-packed tuna or salmon, limited amounts of shell fish (crab, clams, lobster, oysters, scallops, shrimp); egg white. Egg yolks limited to 3 per week, each of which may be substituted for 1 oz meat II, III—Same as for I, except no shrimp allowed, no egg yolks allowed IV, V—Same as for I, except the permitted 3 egg yolks per week may be substituted for 2 oz shell fish or 2 oz organ meats	I, IV, V—Poultry skin, fish canned in oil, goose, duck, fried poultry or fish, fish roe, including caviar II, III—Same as above, plus egg yolks and shrimp
Soups	I, II, III, IV, V—Bouillon, clear broth, any fat-free soups, cream soup made with skim milk, packaged broth-base dehydrated soups	I, II, III, IV, V—All others
Sweets	I, II—Hard candies, jams, jelly, honey, sugar III, IV, V—Most concentrated sweets eliminated	I, II—Chocolate, all other candy III, IV, V—All candy, chocolate, jams, jelly, syrups, honey, sugar
Vegetables	I—2 to 4 servings per day of any vegetable (at least one dark green and one deep yellow vegetable daily) prepared without fat II—Same as for I, except may be prepared with allowed fats III, IV, V—Same as for I, except limit amounts to medium-sized servings and limit amounts of potato, corn, lima beans, dried peas, and beans	I—Buttered, creamed, or fried vegetables II—Same as for I, except when prepared with safflower or corn oil III, IV, V—Same as for I, except when prepared with unsaturated fats
Miscellaneous	I—Pickles, salt, spices, herbs, vinegar, mustard, soy sauce, Worcestershire sauce II, III, IV, V—Same as for I, plus nuts except those excluded, cocoa, peanut butter, olives	I—Nuts, olives, peanut butter, coconut, chocolate II, III, IV, V—Coconut, cashew and macadamia nuts, chocolate

teinemia. In one study serum cholesterol levels of patients with familial type IIa hyperlipoproteinemia were lowered 13% (mean value) by a low-cholesterol, modified fat diet, and were lowered another 13% when probucol was administered along with the diet.[41] The drug also lowered serum cholesterol levels in those who previously had not responded to diet therapy.

When patients with highly elevated serum cholesterol levels have not responded to diet and drug therapy, a partial ileal bypass has been performed.[38] This procedure interferes with intestinal reabsorption of bile acids, and, as a result, serum cholesterol levels are lowered by 25% to 35%.

Hypertension

Hypertension is a major risk factor in cardiovascular, cerebrovascular, and renal disease. Treatment is effective in reducing morbidity and mortality. Although blood pressure is easily measured by means of a sphygmomanometer, millions of cases go undetected. Many individuals have no symptoms and are unaware of the potential danger they face. Blood pressure increases with age and fluctuates widely for even one individual. Thus it has been difficult for physicians to agree as to what values indicate hypertension and what necessitates treatment. Finnerty suggested that every patient whose diastolic pressure is over 100 mm Hg should be treated.[42] Patients younger than 45 years of age with levels over 80 mm Hg and a family history of hypertension should be treated. On the other hand, Aagaard suggested the following criteria should be used for treatment: under 30 years of age if diastolic pressure is over 85 mm Hg, over 90 mm Hg between 30 and 50 years old, and 95 mm Hg in those over 50.[43]

According to a survey of family physicians a systolic pressure of 140 mm Hg and a diastolic pressure of 90 mm Hg is considered normal.[44] Treatment is initiated when the blood pressure is higher than 160 mm Hg systolic and 100 mm Hg diastolic. It is not known whether therapy is beneficial for individuals whose blood pressure falls between these ranges. It has been estimated that approximately 20% of the American population is hypertensive.[45]

Hypertension is seen much more frequently and is manifest at a younger age in blacks. Prior to 40 years of age females have less incidence than males, but after this the situation is reversed. Obesity and diabetes mellitus contribute to hypertension. Salt intake may be involved. In rats salt has been found to induce a fatal hypertension.[46] In humans it is difficult to measure salt intake because of its ubiquitous nature. The levels of urinary sodium output do not always correlate with hypertension.

Two classifications are used to describe hypertension. Primary or essential hypertension accounts for 85% of the patients and has no known cause. It results from an abnormality in the systems that regulate peripheral vascular resistance.[45] A physiological basis has been found for secondary hypertension. Renal disease, tumors of the adrenal gland, brain disease, coarctation of the aorta, toxemia of pregnancy, and other conditions can result in hypertension.

Hypertensive patients retain sodium and water. This may result from the excessive secretion of the hormone aldosterone by a tumor in the adrenal glands. This hormone regulates the renin-angiotensin system. A decrease in oxygenated blood supply or a low concentration of sodium ion in the kidney tubule at the site of reabsorption may initiate the system. Renin, which is synthesized in the kidney, converts angiotensinogen to angiotensin I and then to an octapeptide, angiotensin II. Angiotensin II constricts arteries and stimulates the adrenal cortex to elaborate aldosterone. This in turn promotes sodium reabsorption and water retention. In some renal diseases an excess of renin is produced and hypertension results.

In addition to drug therapy, Aagaard suggested that hypertensive patients engage in exercise.[43] Relaxation is important for tense individuals. The role of weight reduction as part of the treatment for hypertension has been the subject of much debate.[47] Some researchers have stated that the decrease in blood pressure results from a reduced intake of salt rather than a caloric restriction. Twenty-four obese hypertensive subjects who did not receive drugs and 57 subjects who were not adequately controlled by drugs took part in a weight reduction program for 6 months.[47] A control group of 26 subjects on inadequate therapy did not participate in the weight reduction program. All the subjects were instructed to maintain their normal salt intake. Of 81 patients, only eight lost from 3 to 5 kg, while the others all lost more than 5 kg. Only two of the subjects in the weight reduction groups did not have a significant reduction in their blood pressure. Therefore, the authors concluded that weight reduction without restriction of salt intake can lead to a decrease in blood pressure.

It has been found that salt increases blood pressure in some susceptible individuals.[48] Potassium exerts a protective effect against sodium toxicity. American diets are high in sodium and low in potassium. Hypertension can be controlled in some individuals by restricting sodium intake. This is difficult to accomplish because of the preference for foods high in salt and the addition of salt in cooking or at the table.

In 1944 Kempner prescribed the rice-fruit diet for the treatment of hypertension.[49] Only rice, fruits, and sugar are allowed; thus the sodium, protein, and fat content is low. It has been recommended that hypertensive patients should restrict their salt intake.[45,50] No salt is added in cooking, and foods high in sodium are avoided. If a sufficient diuretic response is not attained, then drugs must be prescribed. However, in some instances a sodium restricted diet may decrease the dosage of the antihypertensive drugs and thus reduce the risk of side effects.

Every day about 20,000 mEq of sodium are filtered through the glomeruli of the kidney.[51] Only 1% of this is excreted. Normally 70% of the sodium is reabsorbed in the proximal tubule and 15% to 30% in the ascending loop of Henle and the distal tubule. The body is able to adjust to wide ranges of intakes of sodium and water. In disease states this cannot be done, and edema results. Diuretics increase the excretion of sodium and water by blocking the tubular reabsorption of sodium; as a result, the amount of sodium and water excreted is greater than the intake. The edema is reversed as diuresis is initiated.

A variety of diuretics are used as antihypertensive agents.[42,51-55] The thiazide type of diuretics blocks absorption of sodium in the proximal portions of the distal tubule.[51] This not only increases the excretion of sodium but also water, chloride, and potassium. Furosemide (Lasix) and ethacrynic acid (Edecrin) differ chemically but have similar pharmacological properties. They are more potent than the thiazides and interfere with sodium reabsorption both in the proximal portion of the distal tubule and in the ascending portion of the loop of Henle. Sodium, potassium, and chloride are excreted. Furosemide also slightly increases the output of bicarbonate. Two types of drugs that produce sodium excretion without the concomitant loss of potassium are spironolactone (Aldactone) and triamterene (Dyrenium).[42] The former drug inhibits the hormone aldosterone. Both act at the end of the distal tubule and the beginning of the collecting tubule. These antihypertensive agents cannot be used in renal disease. Another drug, reserpine, acts by interfering with the cellular storage of norepinephrine; it cannot be used in patients who are depressed or have a peptic ulcer, chronic sinusitis, or who are overweight. The drug methyldopa (Aldomet) is metabolized to methyl norepinephrine.[53] The latter compound acts as a false neurotransmitter by substituting for norepinephrine. The result is vasodilation. This compound cannot be used in patients with liver disease. Hydralazine (Apresoline) acts by decreasing peripheral arterial resistance and elevating cardiac output. Tachycardia can occur after the administration of this drug, so it is contraindicated in individuals with angina and congestive heart failure. Guanethidine (Ismelin) is a potent drug which may cause hypotension. The drug inhibits the release of norepinephrine and also prevents its storage.

A fairly recent drug, diazoxide (Hyperstat), is a nondiuretic thiazide derivative. The compound acts by reducing the peripheral resistance of arteries and increasing the cardiac output. Other diuretics must be administered concurrently since sodium and water are retained. However, it is a safe and effective antihypertensive agent. The drug sodium nitroprusside can only be given intravenously. It acts immediately to produce vasodilation, but it is of short duration. Another drug, propranolol (Inderal), has been approved for use by the FDA in only three specific conditions.[53] Reports from other countries indicate that it has been effective in treating essential hypertension. The reduction in blood pressure is the result of a decrease in cardiac output, inhibition of renin release, and an inhibition of centrally mediated functions.

In instances where the blood pressure is not reduced, a larger drug dose may be given, or a second diuretic is administered. The use of these antihypertensive agents may result in some undesirable side effects.[52-56] The administration of a diuretic to a patient with extensive edema may result in excessive diuresis. Excessive amounts of sodium chloride and water are excreted, and blood volume decreases. Sodium chloride must be given. Hyponatremia may develop after the use of thiazides. Hypokalemia may appear when the thiazides, furosemide, or ethacrynic acid is given. Potassium is needed for the action of the skeletal and heart muscle. The particularly lethal condition of digitalis intoxication can occur in hypokalemia, and potassium supplementation becomes necessary. Hyperuricemia is another side effect that can appear after the use of thiazides, furosemide, and ethacrynic acid. Blood urate levels may be controlled by the use of a uricosuric drug, probenecid (Benemid) or allopurinol (Zyloprim), which inhibits the synthesis of uric acid. Furosemide, ethacrynic acid, and triamterene increase urinary calcium excretion. The thiazides have the opposite effect in that the amount of calcium excreted in the urine is decreased, but serum calcium increases. Thiazide and diazoxide therapy can also affect carbohydrate metabolism. It is thought that the hyperglycemia is caused by decreased release of insulin from the pancreas and inhibition of glucose utilization by the peripheral tissues. Thiocyanate toxicity may develop in patients treated with sodium nitroprusside for a long period of time. The use of methyldopa may result in a hemolytic anemia, somnolence, gastrointestinal disturbances, and orthostatic hypotension.

Many hypertensives are poorly controlled because of the lack of compliance to their treatment program. In an attempt to improve compliance a physicians' tutorial program in hypertension was instituted at one clinic.[50] Physicians were assigned either to a tutorial group or a nontutorial group. Those in the tutorial group attended teaching sessions dealing with hypertensive therapy, patient compliance, and the need for changing their handling of patients. After the program was completed, patients treated by both groups of physicians were interviewed. It was found that 69% of the patients of the tutored physicians had adequately controlled blood pressure, whereas only 36% of the patients in the other group were adequately controlled. Patients of the tutored physicians had more knowledge about diet and drug therapy for hypertension. However, there was no significant difference between the two groups as to dietary compliance. The physicians in the tutorial program had been instructed about diet therapy. Since the physician has limited training in nutrition, better dietary compliance may be achieved by having a dietitian counsel the patients in this aspect of treatment. The study indicated that the physician could improve patient compliance to drug therapy. Further studies are needed as to whether dietitians would be successful in getting hypertensive patients to adhere to their dietary prescriptions.

Smoking

Many epidemiological studies have shown a higher incidence of myocardial infarction and coronary atherosclerosis in smokers.[57] The younger age group has a higher coronary heart disease mortality ratio. The mortality increases with the increased intensity of smoking. The incidence decreases when smoking is discontinued. However, it may take 10 years before the level of risk of the nonsmoker is reached. The mechanism by which cigarette smoking increases the risk of cardiovascular disease has not been completely elucidated. It is known that nicotine increases the release of catecholamines, and in turn the heart rate is increased.[8] An increase in blood pressure, cardiac output, stroke volume velocity of contraction, myocardial oxygen consumption, and arrhythmias has been observed. Carbon monoxide in smoke may have a toxic effect.[57] Cigarette smokers have higher levels of carboxyhemoglobin than do nonsmokers. The vascular changes may come about as a result of the decreased oxygen supply.

Data from the Framingham (Mass.) heart study indicated that there was a decrease in HDL levels in smokers.[58] The HDL levels decreased an average of 3 to 4 mg/dl in men and 5 to 6 mg/dl in women; the greatest decrease was seen in those who had smoked the greatest number of cigarettes daily. The cessation of smoking resulted in an increase in HDL levels but only after a period of time.

Minerals

Recent interest has been expressed in the role of certain trace elements in cardiovascular disease. Initial studies several years ago began with an investigation into the quality of water. The major ions in water are sodium, calcium, and magnesium. Several epidemiological studies showed that the number of cardiovascular deaths was inversely related to the hardness of the water.[59-62] It is not known whether there is a protective substance in hard water or a toxic substance in soft water. Schroeder suggested that the toxic substance in water is cadmium.[61] Soft water, as it passes through the pipes, dissolves trace elements such as cadmium, cobalt, and lead. The calcium in the hard water inhibits the absorption of these trace elements from the pipes and also into the body and thus acts as a protective agent.[59]

Water and urine samples collected during the Texas nutrition survey were analyzed for their calcium, magnesium, potassium, lithium, strontium, and silicon content; these values were then compared to the annual mortality rates for cardiovascular disease in individuals over 45 years of age.[63] The data suggested that calcium, magnesium, lithium, strontium, and silicon may protect against cardiovascular mortality by interfering with sodium and potassium intestinal transport, by increasing urinary excretion of sodium, or by other means.

Others have suggested that magnesium affords protective action against atherosclerosis.[64] Magnesium salts administered after a myocardial infarction have been reported to increase the chances of survival. Others have reported decreased beta lipoproteins, increased alpha lipoproteins, and decreased cholesterol after administration of magnesium salts. Magnesium increases fibrinolysis and inhibits coagulation and thus is effective in treating ischemic heart disease. The relationship of a decreased incidence of cardiovascular disease in hard water areas may be due to the fact that magnesium aids in maintaining normal heart rhythms. Abraham et al. found no differences in the serum magnesium levels of normal subjects and those who had had an acute myocardial infarction 6 months previously.[65]

Cadmium is purported to play a role in hypertension.[61,62] The ingestion of high levels in rats caused hypertension. The amount of cadmium found in the kidneys of these rats was approximately equal to that found in human adults. Hypertensive patients have been found to have abnormally large amounts of renal cadmium. These individuals also excreted cadmium in their urine; normally, little cadmium is found.

Some interesting results have been reported with cobalt.[16] The effects of this element depend on the method of administration. Cobalt had a hypercholesterolemic effect when it was injected into rabbits and chickens, and the degree of atherosclerosis increased. However, when the cobalt was given orally, the incidence of atherosclerosis decreased. In humans cobalt taken orally has a hypocholesterolemic effect.

The trace mineral chromium is necessary for carbohydrate and lipid metabolism. An autopsy of individuals who had died from coronary heart disease showed no chromium in their aortas. Schroeder suggested that carbohydrate and lipid metabolism become abnormal, and as a result, plaques develop.[61] Perry stated that there is an indirect relationship between chromium and atherosclerosis.[62] The direct relationship is between the higher incidence of atherosclerosis in adult onset diabetes.

The effect of different concentrations of zinc and copper on the plasma cholesterol levels was studied by Kelvay.[66] Two groups of rats were given identical diets. One group received water with a ratio of zinc to copper of 40, whereas the ratio in the other group was 5. The first group had higher plasma cholesterol concentrations. Other factors that have been implicated in coronary heart disease also cause an increase in the zinc and copper ratio. These factors are increased intake of sugar, decreased intake of fiber, drinking soft water, and lack of exercise. This high ratio of zinc to copper is maintained after absorption from the intestinal tract. This is followed by an abnormal distribution of these two elements in many important organs. Therefore Kelvay proposed that a metabolic imbalance of copper and zinc results in hypercholesterolemia and is the major factor in the etiology of coronary heart disease.[67]

Fiber

Experiments with both animals and humans have shown that fiber has a hypocholesterolemic effect.[16,68-71] The type of fiber that is fed also influences the results. Less atherosclerosis and a greater hypocholesterolemic effect was observed when rabbits were fed wheat straw in place of cellulose.[72] In vitro experiments indicated that all natural nonnutritive fibers (alfalfa, wheat straw, sugar cane pulp, bran, and oat hulls) had a greater capacity for binding bile salts than did synthetic nonnutritive fibers (cellophane spangles and cellulose).[73] Alfalfa bound the most bile salts. Ingested fiber then binds bile acids that are excreted via the feces.[68,69,71] This is the major pathway for cholesterol excretion. This increased excretion reduces the body cholesterol pool and lowers blood levels. This same type of action is exhibited by the drugs cholestyramine and colestipol that are used as hypocholesterolemic agents.[71]

Other experiments with animals have suggested another mechanism for the action of fiber. Baboons were fed a cholesterol-free test diet containing 40% carbohydrate (either as glucose, fructose, sucrose, or starch), 14% hydrogenated coconut oil, and 15% cellulose for one year.[74] A control group received bread, fruits, and vegetables. Fatty streaks developed in the aortas of the baboons fed the test diets. Serum cholesterol, triglycerides, and beta lipoprotein cholesterol levels were elevated. The test animals also showed a lower ratio of primary (cholic and chenodeoxycholic) to secondary (Deoxycholic and lithocholic) bile acids. Thus cholesterol was synthesized on the test-free diet, but less was metabolized to bile acids, and the excess then appeared in the serum. The experiment was repeated with rabbits, and similar results were obtained.[71] This suggested that on low-fiber diets less endogenous cholesterol is converted to bile acids.

In experiments with humans, rolled oats, Bengal gram, guar gum, and pectin have been found to lower blood cholesterol levels, whereas wheat fiber, cellulose, and lignin do not. Nine postgraduate students were fed 15 g of citrus pectin per day for 3 weeks.[75] The average decrease in plasma cholesterol was 13% (range −5% to −26%); plasma triglyceride levels were not affected. The fecal fat excretion increased on the average by 44%, neutral steroids by 17%, and fecal bile acids by 33%. Kay et al. summarized the results of other investigators and found that in most experiments pectin did reduce serum cholesterol levels.[76]

Fourteen patients with type IIa hyperlipoproteinemia were treated with a high-fiber diet for 6 months.[77] The fiber was provided by bread containing powdered cellulose and cocoa cookies made from soy hull fiber. Eight of the patients were treated for an additional 6 months with cholestyramine. The high-fiber diet resulted in only a small decease in serum cholesterol levels and a slight increase in serum triglyceride levels. It was of interest that 40% of the patients on the high-fiber diet had a mean decrease of 13% in serum cholesterol levels. The drug cholestyramine had a greater effect. However, the authors concluded that a high-fiber diet might be beneficial to type IIa hyperlipoproteinemia patients even though drug therapy results in a more dramatic decrease in serum cholesterol. For more details on fiber see Chapter 4, Gastrointestinal Disorders.

Protein

Much research has centered around the relationship between dietary lipids and atherosclerosis. Epidemiological data also indicates that the incidence of coronary heart disease is higher in populations consuming animal protein. In addition, plasma lipid levels are lower in vegetarians than in the rest of the American population. Recently there have been studies both with animals and humans to determine the relationship between dietary protein and atherosclerosis.[78]

In experiments with animals, casein has a hypercholesterolemic effect, while soy protein isolate is hypocholesterolemic. The mechanism by which this occurs is not known. Amino acid hydrolysates of both these proteins exert the same effect as the intact protein. Similar results have been observed with humans. In one study six young women were fed a mixed protein diet (70% animal protein) and a plant protein diet in which soy protein meat analogues and soy milk were substituted for animal protein.[79] The subjects started on the mixed protein diet, then the plant protein diet, and concluded with the mixed protein diet. Plasma cholesterol levels were lower on the plant protein diet. In a second study a crossover design was used, and the subjects were fed a mixed protein diet with 58% animal protein and a plant protein diet for a total of 78 days. The results indicated that plasma cholesterol levels were significantly higher on the mixed protein diet as compared to the plant protein diet. Thus the substitution of plant protein for animal protein resulted in lower plasma cholesterol levels. Additional studies are being carried out to determine which amino acids are hypocholesterolemic.

Stress

Coronary patients exhibit a definite behavior pattern. Rosenman and Friedman characterized persons with coronary heart disease as the type A behavior pattern.[80] The type A individual is ambitious, competitive, aggressive, impatient, and always meeting deadlines. The type B noncoronary individual does not exhibit this same sense of urgency. The coronary patient tends not to enjoy his leisure time and spends it in activities that do not provide much recreation.[81]

Some epidemiological studies of different population groups have shown a low incidence of coronary heart disease even though the fat intake is high. Persons living in high-stress geographic areas on low-fat diets also have a low incidence of the disease. Stressed animals in a laboratory develop atherosclerosis only on a high-fat diet; therefore, Russek stated that a high-fat diet and stress are a lethal combination, and both factors are involved in the pathogenesis of atherosclerosis.[81]

Although atherosclerosis has been associated with aging in Western civilizations, it is appearing at a much younger age. Emphasis has been placed on the American diet and coronary heart disease, but little has been said about the educational stress to which children are subject for many years.[81] Childhood for many is no longer happy and carefree but is as competitive as the adult world both in school and play. For many students school has become a traumatic experience making them more prone to coronary heart disease.

RECOMMENDATIONS

The Food and Nutrition Board of the National Research Council and the Council on Foods and Nutrition of the American Medical Association recommendations were made in view of the fact that plasma lipid levels of most Americans are elevated.[82] As cholesterol levels increase over 220 mg/dl, the incidence of coronary heart disease increases progressively with each increment of cholesterol elevation. These levels can be reduced by partial replacement of saturated fats with fats high in polyunsaturated fatty acids and by decreasing the intake of foods high in cholesterol content. Triglycerides also increase the risk of coronary heart disease but are not always associated with hypercholesterolemia. Plasma triglyceride levels can be reduced, but there is no evidence that this will reduce the risk for coronary disease. The committee recommended that (1) physical examinations should include a lipid profile; (2) persons in risk categories should receive dietary counsel to decrease their intake of saturated fat and cholesterol, and those who are obese should reduce their caloric intake and increase physical activity; (3) diet should meet the recommended daily allowances; (4) modified and ordinary foods should be labeled and made available;

and (5) further studies on modification of lipids and other risk factors should be initiated.

The American Heart Association[83] and the Inter-Society Commission for Heart Disease Resources[15] made some similar dietary recommendations. Reduction diets are advocated for obese individuals, since a loss of weight results in a reduction of serum lipids, blood pressure, and blood glucose. The average daily intake of 600 mg of cholesterol should be decreased to 300 mg. Even lower levels may be necessary for persons with severe hypercholesterolemia. Since most cholesterol is synthesized endogenously, only a severe dietary restriction will decease plasma levels; however, levels may be decreased by modifying the fat intake. Normal American diets provide 40% to 45% of calories from fat. The recommendation calls for no more than 35% of calories with approximately less than 10% from saturated fat and 10% or more from polyunsaturated fats and the remainder from monounsaturated fats. A high-fat meal at any time should be avoided.

The American Heart Association made additional dietary recommendations. As the fat content of the diet is decreased, carbohydrate intake is increased. This additional carbohydrate should be provided by vegetables, fruits, and cereals and not from refined sugar sources that provide only concentrated empty calories. This slight increase in carbohydrate content should not produce hypertriglyceridemia in most individuals. It is suggested that excessive salt intake be avoided since current experimental data implicate it as one of the factors in the etiology of hypertension. No recommendations were made as to other dietary factors such as trace minerals, hardness of water, vitamin intake, fiber, and coffee because of inconclusive evidence. Individuals should be concerned about the amount of alcoholic beverages they consume, since alcohol can supply a large quantity of calories that can contribute to the development of obesity and hyperlipidemia.

In 1975 the American Heart Association recommended that children along with the general public should modify their diets in order to prevent atherosclerosis.[84] Some investigators have suggested that dietary restrictions of fat and cholesterol should be prescribed only for children with hyperlipidemia. However, at present it is not feasible to screen the entire population to detect these children. Still others feel that since atherosclerosis begins in childhood, preventive measures must be instituted at an early age. Others question the safety of these diets. No immediate harmful effects of a diet low in cholesterol and fat and high in polyunsaturated fats have been observed in children. However, an increased incidence of gallstones has been reported in adults. Cholesterol is necessary for the myelination of the central nervous system, and thus low-cholesterol diets could result in neurological disorders. This has not been observed in children who normally eat low-cholesterol diets.

The British panel cited the following risk factors that predispose one to the development of ischemic heart disease: hypercholesterolemia, hypertriglyceridemia, hypertension, excessive cigarette smoking, physical inactivity, diabetes mellitus, obesity, inherited predisposition, and emotional stress.[85] The possible dietary risks discussed were overconsumption of food, fat, cholesterol, sucrose, and salt, low P/S ratio, fiber deficiency, and water softness. Because of insufficient evidence, no recommendations were made about the following: fiber, excess of vitamin B_{12}, thiamine, ascorbic acid, and cobalt, deficiency of chromium, imbalance of other trace elements, heated milk-protein food, and excessive intake of coffee and alcohol.

The panel recommended that obesity should be avoided in children and adults. The amount of saturated fat from both plant and animal sources should be reduced. No recommendations were made to increase the dietary intake of polyunsaturated fatty acids, since the panel felt that present evidence was unconvincing. The consumption of sucrose in foods and drinks should be reduced to aid in the prevention of obesity. The softening of water should be carefully considered because of the relationship between the death rate for ischemic heart disease and the degree of water softness.

The differences in recommendations by these three groups illustrate that the current research evidence is still inconclusive and subject to much interpretation.[86,87] The recommendations by the Food and Nutrition Board and the American Medical Association apply only to high-risk patients and not to the general population. The American Heart Association recommends dietary changes for the entire American population, since elevated blood lipids are so prevalent. The British panel did not advocate an increase in polyunsaturated fatty acid intake, since they felt that the evidence was still inconclusive; however, they did recommend that the intake of sucrose be curtailed even if this would only prevent obesity.

Further controlled dietary studies are obviously needed. However, these studies are fraught with difficulties. First of all the expenditure is great. Controlled experiments with humans are difficult. They must be long term and should probably be initiated in the young. As one dietary component is modified in a study, one or more nutrients may have to be altered. To what are the results attributed? In order to have valid results, a large population is needed, but then it is difficult to find a homogeneous group so that other risk factors are not introduced that would interfere with the factor being studied. Possibly, if the conditions of the experiment become too restrictive, the factor of stress is superimposed on the original factor being observed. The experimental design must be carefully planned.

MULTIPLE RISK FACTOR INTERVENTION TRIAL

The Multiple Risk Factor Intervention Trial (MRFIT) is supported by the National Heart and Lung Institute.[88,89] The objective of the MRFIT is to evaluate methods used to prevent heart attacks and deaths from cardiovascular disease by reducing blood cholesterol, hypertension, and cigarette smoking. There are 20 clinical centers that are presently enrolling 600 men between the ages of 35 to 57. These selected men do not have clinical coronary heart disease but are above average coronary heart disease risk because of hypercholesterolemia, hypertension, or cigarette smoking.

The program runs for 6 years. Two groups are established at each center. One group will return to the center each year for a cardiovascular examination and will use their own physicians for medical care. The second group will be entered into a special intervention program to reduce blood cholesterol levels, lower elevated levels of diastolic pressure, and eliminate smoking. At each clinical center the services of a cardiologist, nutritionist, behavioral scientist, and physician are available. The procedures have been in operation successfully in Baltimore and New York City MRFIT clinics since November 1973.

The intervention program consists of a balanced diet with 30% to 35% of calories from fat (less than 10% from saturated fats and 10% to 13% from polyunsaturated fats) and 300 mg of cholesterol. Weight reduction and drugs are prescribed for the management of hypertension. Counseling and educational materials are used to get the men to stop smoking.

In one clinic participating in the MRFIT program the high-density lipoprotein (HDL) cholesterol levels of 301 men were measured.[90] The mean plasma HDL cholesterol levels rose by 6% in the intervention group; these values were not significantly different from those in the control group. Plasma HDL levels were increased when plasma triglycerides and LDL cholesterol levels were reduced, cigarette smoking decreased, alcohol intake increased, weight was lost, and there was adherence to a fat-controlled diet.

FAT-CONTROLLED DIETS

The American Heart Association has published two booklets on planning fat-controlled meals either for 1200 to 1800 kcal or 2000 to 2600 kcal.[91] A programmed instruction booklet for the fat-controlled diet of 1800 kcal is also available[92] as well as a cookbook.[93]

The caloric prescription is dependent upon the patient. If the patient is overweight, then the lower caloric range is used. The calories from fat should be about 30% to 35% of the total. Saturated fats are lowered to 10% of the total. The amount of animal, dairy, and hydrogenated fat must be reduced. The polyunsaturated fats are increased to 12% to 14% of the total calories from fat. Liquid vegetable oils such as corn, safflower, soybean, and cottonseed oils are advocated. The special margarines that are high in polyunsaturated fats and low in hydrogenated fats should be used to increase the polyunsaturated/saturated fat ratio (P/S). Labels on margarine must be carefully read, for they vary in their fat content. The first item in the list of ingredients should not be a hydrogenated vegetable oil. Tub margarines have a higher P/S ratio than do the sticks of margarine. Table 8-6 shows the fat content of a margarine compared with butter. The P/S ratio of butter is much lower than that of the margarine.

To reduce fat intake, the use of beef, lamb, pork, and ham should be limited to five moderate sized portions weekly. Fish, chicken, turkey, and veal should be used more often. Lean cuts of meat must be purchased. All visible fat should be trimmed. Skimmed milk, skimmed milk cheeses, liquid vegetable oil, and margarines high in

Table 8-6. Fat composition of margarine and butter*

Component	Margarine (tub)*	Margarine (stick)†	Butter
Percent fat	80.5	80.5	80.5
Percent saturates	15	17	66
Percent polyunsaturates	67	48	1
P/S ratio	4.5	2.8	0.02

*Adapted from Peterson, D. R.: Promise margarine clinical studies, New York, 1972, Lever Brothers Co.
†Promise, Lever Brothers Co.

Table 8-7. A maximal approach to the dietary treatment of the hyperlipidemias*

Diet	Cholesterol (mg)	Percent of total calories				
		Carbohydrate	Protein	Fat	Saturated fat	Polyunsaturated fat
A	100	65	15-20	20	5.3	8.1
B	200	60	15-20	25	6.1	8.5
C	200	48	15-20	35	7.6	12.6
D	60-78	68-71	15-20	12	Not specified	Not specified

*From Subcommittee on Diet and Hyperlipidemia of the Council on Arteriosclerosis of the American Heart Association: A maximal approach to the dietary treatment of the hyperlipidemias, physician's handbook, Dallas, 1973. © American Heart Association, reprinted with permission.

polyunsaturated fat are prescribed. The cooking methods that reduce fat content, such as baking, broiling, boiling, roasting, or stewing, are advocated. The cholesterol content is restricted to 300 mg daily. Only three egg yolks a week are permitted. The use of shellfish and organ meats is limited.

A subcommittee of the American Heart Association has prepared a physicians' manual and four diets entitled *A Maximal Approach to the Dietary Treatment of the Hyperlipidemias.*[94] These diets are intended for highly motivated patients, and the objective of diet therapy is to attain a maximal lipid-lowering response. The diets are low in cholesterol, are either moderately or extremely low in fat, and are reduced in calories if the individual is over ideal weight (see Table 8-7). The diets are very restrictive and involve an alteration of food habits. A system of food exchanges is used that lists for each exchange the amounts of protein, carbohydrate, fat, monounsaturated fatty acids, polyunsaturated fatty acids, saturated fatty acids, and cholesterol.

A chart entitled Suggested Diet Prescription for Hyperlipidemias summarizes the National Heart and Lung Institute Diets, the American Heart Association Planning Fat Controlled Meals, and the American Heart Association Maximal Approach to the Dietary Treatment of the Hyperlipidemias. The chart is available from the American Heart Association.

The Prudent Diet

The Prudent Diet was developed by Jolliffee and Maslansky in 1957 for use with the New York City Anti-Coronary Club Project.[33] The distribution of fat in the typical American diet is saturated 46%, monounsaturated 40%, polyunsaturated 14%, and the P/S ratio is 0.3, whereas on the Prudent Diet the distribution of fat is 28%, 36%, and 36%, respectively, with a P/S ratio of 1.3.[95] Therefore the amount of total and saturated fat is decreased, while the polyunsaturated fat is increased. In the Prudent Diet foods are divided into six categories, and the following recommendations are made for each:

1. Fish, meats, poultry, and eggs—avoid very fat meats
   a. Fish, shellfish: at least five times a week
   b. Meats: maximum of 16 oz per week
   c. Eggs: four per week for adults
2. Milk—avoid high-fat dairy products
   a. Skim milk: 2 cups per day for adults
   b. Whole milk cheeses: not more than 4 oz per week
3. Dark green leafy and deep yellow vegetables: three to four servings per week
4. Fruits: more than one serving daily, use as desserts
5. Breads and cereals: whole grain or enriched bread or cereal at every meal
6. Vegetable oils, special shortenings, and margarines with polyunsaturated fats—avoid butter, lard, hydrogenated cooking fats, and margarines
   a. Vegetable oils: 2 tbsp per day for adults

The male participants who followed the diet were found to have lowered serum cholesterol levels, lowered blood pressure, and lost weight.[33] A lower incidence of coronary heart disease was found in the 50 to 59 year olds who followed the dietary treatment as compared to a control group. Many researchers have advocated that the general public follow the basic principles of this diet.

FOOD MODIFICATION

Within the past 70 years the fat consumption in the United States has increased. This has been paralleled by an increase in cardiovascular disease. Concern has been expressed over methods that can be developed to modify American food habits, but this will not be an easy task. One approach is to make readily available commonly used food products that contain lower amounts of fat. Many such products are currently on the market, but many more still need to be developed.

As polyunsaturated fats decrease serum cholesterol levels, attempts have been made to increase the amount of polyunsaturated fats in animals. Polyunsaturated fats can be encapsulated in a Casec-formaldehyde coating and administered to ruminants.[96] In this way the polyunsaturated fatty acids are not hydrogenated in the rumen of the animal. The linoleic acid content of milk can be increased. Antioxidants must be added to protect against oxidative rancidity. It takes 6 to 8 weeks to get meat with a P/S ratio of 1 in steers.[97]

Six persons were fed a diet containing these polyunsaturated ruminant fats.[96] The P/S ratio of the test diet was 0.89 and of the control saturated diet, 0.09. After 3 to 4 weeks of dietary treatment, five of the six subjects showed a 10% reduction of serum cholesterol. An increase in excretion of sterols by 18% was also observed. The products are acceptable, but the one disadvantage to their use is that the cholesterol content of the diet has not changed.

In another study 25 couples were randomly assigned to one of four groups: group A, saturated foods for 20 weeks; group B, polyunsaturated diet for 20 weeks; group C, saturated diet for the first 10 weeks then a polyunsaturated diet for 10 weeks; group D, the reverse order of group C.[98] The P/S ratio for the saturated diet was 0.11 to 0.14 and 0.56 to 0.62 for the polyunsaturated diet, whereas the P/S ratio for the prestudy diet was 0.43 to 0.56. The polyunsaturated meat (beef and lamb) and dairy products (milk, ice cream, butter, yogurt, sour cream, and cheese) were produced from animals fed protected lipid supplements. These products were provided to the subjects at no cost. Subjects whose initial serum cholesterol levels were elevated showed the greatest response, namely, a decrease of 10.7 mg/dl on the polyunsaturated diet and an increase of 7.8 mg/dl on the saturated diet. There was no dietary response shown by the subjects whose initial blood cholesterol levels were low.

Boys between the ages of 12 and 18 years who attended two African boarding schools participated in a dietary study consisting of three experimental periods each lasting 6 weeks.[99] The diets for the three periods consisted of the following: (1) polyunsaturated dried-filled milk, and products made from it, were substituted for the animal dairy products—P/S ratio = 1.08; (2) all meat and dairy products that were used were polyunsaturated—P/S ratio = 0.90; (3) regular diet —P/S ratio = 0.28. With the two diets that contained polyunsaturated fats there was a 14% reduction in plasma cholesterol levels. As in the previous study the greatest reduction was observed in the boys whose initial cholesterol levels were higher than 230 mg/dl. Of the 229 who were screened, 40% had serum cholesterol levels greater than 200 mg/dl, and 14% were considered to have hypercholesterolemia (> 230 mg/dl).

Brown et al. studied the effects of polyunsaturated meats and dairy products on 11 subjects, of whom eight were hyperlipidemic.[100] Six of the latter subjects were on a fat-modified diet. There was an initial adjustment period of 3 weeks and then two experimental periods of 4 weeks and a final 3-week follow-up period. During one experimental period the subjects consumed polyunsaturated beef and polyunsaturated dairy products (P/S ratio = 1.8), and during the other period they were eating saturated beef and saturated dairy products (P/S ratio = 1.4). In 10 subjects serum cholesterol levels were 6% lower on the diet with the polyunsaturated products. However, the six subjects who had been on a fat-modified diet prior to the experiment had serum cholesterol levels that were not significantly decreased by the polyunsaturated products. The five other participants who had not been on diet therapy had their serum cholesterol levels reduced by 18% with the polyunsaturated products and 11% with the saturated products. The authors concluded that polyunsaturated products along with a restriction in the amount of polyunsaturated animal fat can be used to reduce hyperlipidemia.

In Australia approximately two thirds of the fat in the diet comes from ruminant

Table 8-8. Comparison of egg and egg substitutes

Product	Manufacturer	Fat (g) per 100 g	P/S ratio	Kilocalories per serving*	Cholesterol (mg) per serving*
One large egg		10.2	0.54	80	252
Eggstra	Tillie Lewis Foods, California	13.0	0.45	44	57
Second Nature	Avoset Food Corp California	3.4	2.40	35	Trace
Egg Beaters	Standard Brands, New York	12.4	3.30	100	Trace
Egg Scramblers	Morningstar Farms, Illinois	5.8	4.25	64	0

*One serving is equivalent to one large egg.

fat, which is highly saturated.[101] It is estimated that the P/S ratio of the Australian diet is 0.2. Fat-modified foods with a high P/S ratio were produced and marketed. However, Heywood stated that the public health significance of fat-modified foods is limited.[101] The cost was approximately twice that of the conventional products. In clinical trials where there was a complete substitution of fat-modified ruminant foods, the serum cholesterol levels fell by approximately 10%. Partial substitution of these products in the diet would result in even smaller decreases in serum cholesterol levels. Therefore Heywood suggested other alternatives such as restricting the intake of butter and dairy fats, using lean cuts of meat, polyunsaturated margarines, and textured vegetable protein, using a system of meat grading in which there is a premium on lean meat, and loss of weight in the obese.

On the other hand, Hodges stated that the polyunsaturated ruminant fat foods are an important advance.[102] It is difficult for patients to stop eating products from ruminants, and as a rule dietary advice is not followed. Therefore he felt that polyunsaturated ruminant fat foods would enhance the palatability of the fat-modified diet and thus make the diet more acceptable.

Several egg substitutes are currently available that are lower in cholesterol or are cholesterol free; some have a lower caloric content (see Table 8-8). Three egg substitutes, Eggstra, Second Nature, and Egg Beaters, were evaluated by 30 home economists.[103] Initially most believed that eggs were more expensive than these three products. After being informed of the cost and cholesterol and caloric content, the women felt there was no difference in the nutritional values of these products. Fresh, whole eggs were preferred.

The fat content of many products now on the market has been reduced. Diet margarines contain half the fat content of the regular margarines. Low-fat milk with 1% to 2% fat and imitation ice cream with a low-fat content can be purchased. Polyunsaturated fats have been used in shortenings, margarines, salad oils, and salad dressings.[104]

Soybean protein has been used to fabricate meat analogues with a flavor of beef, ham, or chicken. These products contain no cholesterol, less fat, and approximately equal amounts of polyunsaturated and saturated fat and will also prove useful in alleviating the world shortage of protein.[105] Products such as Breakfast Links, Patties, and Slices and Strips are marketed by Morningstar Farms (Miles Laboratories).

CONGESTIVE HEART FAILURE

Congestive heart failure results when the heart is unable to provide sufficient blood to meet the metabolic needs of the body. A decreased blood flow to the tissues results, and congestion appears in the pulmonary and systemic circulation. Sodium and water are retained, and the volume of the extracellular fluid increases. Renal function is diminished, and sodium and water are retained. The volume of the extracellular fluid increases. Congestion in the lungs leads to pulmonary edema and dyspnea on exertion. Edema is found in the extremities, and in severe congestive heart failure ascites is present.

The common causes of congestive heart failure are hypertension, coronary atherosclerosis, and rheumatic heart disease. Treatment involves complete bed rest. Digitalis is prescribed to increase heart action, and diuretics are prescribed to increase the excretion of sodium and water. Oxygen may be needed when there is respiratory distress. Diet therapy is important. The aim is to reduce the work of the heart. Small frequent feedings are preferred; large meals should not be fed, since this distends the stomach, which elevates the diaphragm and pushes the heart upward. Obese patients must be placed on a reduction diet, since obesity also increases the work load of the heart. Caloric restriction decreases oxygen consumption, and this decreases the work of the heart. The Karell diet, prescribed first in 1866, consisted of 800 ml of milk given in four equal feedings. This is used for 3 to 4 days, and then 1000 ml of milk and some foods are gradually added back. This is prescribed for the initial stages not only of congestive heart failure but also for myocardial infarction. This dietary treatment results in diuresis, improved heart action, and a loss of symptoms.

Sodium-restricted diets are also prescribed. The degree of restriction is dependent on the severity of the heart failure and on the loss of fluid achieved through the use of diuretics. Ordinarily 500 mg sodium diets are used, although sometimes a more severe reduction of 250 mg is needed. Patients must be carefully monitored, since retention of water can develop on a low-sodium diet in which fluid intake is not restricted. Renal patients may become hyponatremic because of the inability to reabsorb sodium. When the edema has been corrected, a 1 g or a mild sodium-restricted diet is all that is necessary.

ACUTE MYOCARDIAL INFARCTION

Myocardial infarction is the result of ischemia that damages a part of the heart muscle. It is usually the result of occlusion of a coronary artery. There is severe chest pain, dyspnea, sweating, weakness, and fear of impending death. Arrhythmias, shock, and cardiac failure may develop. Many individuals die within a few minutes of the initial symptoms or before reaching medical assistance.

Electrocardiogram changes are evident but do not indicate the severity of the damage. Leukocytosis develops, and the sedimentation rate is elevated. Serum enzyme levels are elevated, and serial determinations are useful. Enzymes measured are creatine phosphokinase, glutamic oxaloacetic transaminase, lactic acid dehydrogenase, and α-hydroxybutyric dehydrogenase. See Chapter 2, Laboratory Diagnosis, for additional details.

Many hospitals have coronary care units (CCU). After an acute myocardial infarction the patient is at high risk from arrhythmias, heart failure, and cardiogenic shock. In the CCU the patient is continuously monitored by means of an electrocardiogram (ECG). When cardiac arrest occurs, a warning signal is emitted. Equipment such as defibrillators and drugs are readily available for resuscitation, which must begin immediately, for brain function is rapidly lost when oxygen is not supplied. Eight to twelve seconds after blood flow stops, the individual is unconscious, and breathing stops within 30 to 45 seconds after cardiac arrest.

The metabolic response to a myocardial infarction varies from individual to individual.[105] Abnormal glucose tolerance, delayed secretion of insulin, and hyperinsulinemia have been reported after an infarction. This all may be mediated by prior nutritional status or drug therapy, or both. Mortality caused by arrhythmias and hypotension is higher in individuals who experience metabolic acidosis after a myocardial infarction. An increase in anaerobic carbohydrate metabolism and lipid synthesis has been observed in infarcted and noninfarcted heart muscle.

Christakis and Winston suggested the following nutritional plan for a patient with a myocardial infarction.[106] For the first 2 or 3 days a liquid diet providing 500 to 800 kcal for a total volume of 1 to 1.5 L is fed. Small amounts of fruit juice, skim milk, clear soup, broth, tea, ginger ale, or water are allowed. Extremely hot or cold fluids should not be administered since this can initiate arrhythmias. Some physicians do not permit coffee or tea because of the stimulation of the heart rate. Decaffeinated beverages can be substituted. It is also important to avoid fluids that cause abdominal distention. Parenteral feeding is necessary when the patient is too ill to take fluids. A concentrated solution of dextrose (10% or 20%) has been used to provide fluids and some calories.

The sodium and potassium content of the diet must be considered. Sodium is usually restricted, especially in cases of congestive heart failure. Sodium is lost in the urine after a myocardial infarction. This coupled with a sodium restriction may precipitate shock. Therefore sodium balance must be maintained.

After the acute phase a 1000 to 1200 kcal diet is prescribed. This contains 45% carbohydrate and 30% to 35% fat and 300 mg of cholesterol. Easily digestible foods free of gastric irritants and low in roughage are allowed. The following foods are suggested: tender lean meat, fish, poultry, tender cooked vegetables, fruits, plain breads, cooked cereals, puddings, and gelatin desserts. Small amounts of coffee or tea may be permitted. Foods should not be excessively hot or cold. Small frequent feedings are best. As a patient resumes activity, a more liberal diet is allowed; however, the fat and cholesterol concentration should be controlled. Sodium restriction may be necessary for some. Reducing diets are of utmost importance for obese persons. However, the diet must not be so restrictive that it imposes an additional stress. The patients should be monitored biochemically at set intervals and the diets correlated to the results of these tests.

At one hospital the cardiac diet that is prescribed for patients who have suffered a myocardial infarction consists of six small feedings of soft food or about 1200 kcal.[107] The diet is low in cholesterol, and caffeine-containing foods and beverages are prohibited as are foods that are irritating or cause flatulence. The sodium prescription depends upon the condition of the patient.

SODIUM-RESTRICTED DIETS

Sodium-restricted diets are prescribed to prevent and eliminate edema. Since the advent of antihypertensive agents, these diets are not always prescribed for hypertension; however, in many cardiovascular, liver, and renal disorders, sodium restriction is necessary.

The American Heart Association has prepared four sodium-restricted diets. These are available in booklet or leaflet form.[108,109] Exchange lists are included to simplify menu planning (Table 8-9). These are similar to the lists used for diabetics, except that amounts of sodium for each exchange are included.

A mild restriction of 2400 to 4500 mg of sodium permits the use of light salt in cooking, but none is allowed at the table, since 5 g of salt (1 tsp) contains 1965 mg of sodium. Very salty foods cannot be eaten. A moderate sodium-restricted diet permits 1000 mg or 43 mEq of sodium. Salty foods and the use of salt in cooking and at the table are prohibited. It is necessary to use vegetables with a lower sodium content.

Table 8-9. Exchange lists for sodium-restricted diets

Exchange	Measure	Kilocalories	Carbohydrate (g)	Protein (g)	Fat (g)	Sodium (mg)
Milk, skim	0.24 L (1c)	80	12	8	—	120
Milk, low-sodium, nonfat	0.24 L	80	12	8	—	7
Vegetables	0.12 L (½c)	28	5	2	—	9
Vegetables, starchy	Varies	68	15	2	—	5
Fruit	Varies	40	10	—	—	2
Breads, cereals, low-sodium	Varies	68	15	2	—	5
Meat, lean	28 g (1 oz)	55	—	7	3	25
Fat	Varies	45	—	—	5	—

Excessive use of meat and milk should be avoided. A strict restriction allows 500 mg or 22 mEq of sodium. This diet may be prescribed for congestive heart failure, renal disease with edema, and cirrhosis with ascites. As with the previous diet, salty foods and salt at the table or in cooking are not allowed. Smaller portions of meat, milk, and eggs are permitted. Vegetables high in sodium content are excluded. If this level of restriction is ineffective, then a 250 mg or 11 mEq sodium diet may be needed. The restrictions for the 500 mg diet are followed, plus low-sodium milk and foods low in sodium are allowed. Generally the last two diets are used only with hospitalized patients.

Although most dietary sodium comes from salt or sodium chloride, there are other sodium compounds present as additives. Brine is used in processing foods to stop the growth of bacteria, for cleaning vegetables and fruits, freezing, canning, and for flavor in corned beef, pickles, and sauerkraut. Baking powder and baking soda are used as a leavening agent in breads and cakes. Baking soda is sometimes added to improve the color of vegetables as they are cooked. Disodium phosphate is found in quick-cooking cereals and processed cheese. Monosodium glutamate is used as a flavor enhancer in many foods. Sodium alginate is added to chocolate milk to keep the chocolate in suspension and to ice cream for smoother texture. Sodium benzoate is a preservative found in relishes, sauces, and salad dressings. Breads, cakes, and pasteurized cheeses contain sodium propionate to retard mold growth. Some fruit is bleached with sodium sulfite. Thus labels on food must be read carefully, and foods that contain added sodium compounds should be avoided. Difficulties are encountered with foods that come under the standards of identity. The labels on these foods do not list ingredients.

The sodium content of the water must be considered. The local heart association or health department will provide this information. Water with a sodium content higher than 5 mg per cup should not be used. This would also apply to soft drinks that are made from this water source. In areas where the water is hard, ion exchange resins may be used as water softeners. However, the water is high in sodium, because as the water passes through the resin, the calcium and magnesium ions are exchanged for sodium. Persons on sodium-restricted diets should not drink water softened by this method.

Many drugs contain sodium. Alkalizers such as bicarbonate of soda that are used for indigestion are contraindicated as are some cough medicines, laxatives, and aspirin. A physician should be consulted as to the sodium content of any unprescribed medicine that the patient may wish to take.

It is difficult to get patient acceptance of low-sodium diets. Most individuals are accustomed to ingesting large quantities of salt. When the salt is restricted, food to them is said to be tasteless, bland, and flat. Salt substitutes that contain either ammonium or potassium chloride are found by some to leave a bitter aftertaste. The ammonium salt is contraindicated in liver disease, while potassium chloride cannot be given to renal patients.

Table 8-10. Salt substitutes

Product	Manufacturer
Adolph's Salt Substitute	Adolph's, Ltd.
Co-Salt	USV Pharmaceutical Corp.
Diasal	E. Fourgera & Co.
Featherweight "K" Salt	Chicago Dietetic Supply
Neocurtasal	Winthrop Laboratories
Sweet and Low Brand	Cumberland Packing Corp.
Nu-Salt	
Featherweight Seasoned	Chicago Dietetic Supply
Salt Substitute	
Morton Salt Substitute	Morton Salt Co.

The salt substitutes listed in Table 8-10 contain between 10 and 13 mEq of potassium per gram and 0.1 mg/g or less, of sodium.[110] Another product, Lite Salt (Morton Salt Co.), contains approximately half the sodium of table salt (6.15 mEq of potassium and 8.47 mEq of sodium per gram of salt).[111] One gram of salt contains 17 mEq of sodium. Users must be cautioned that this product does indeed contain sodium and so is different from the other salt substitutes. The palatability of the sodium-restricted diet may be improved by using herbs and seasonings. Many recipes are available for use in low-sodium cooking.

The excessive use of salt substitutes can be dangerous in patients who retain potassium.[112] Two patients developed severe hyperkalemia and cardiac arrhythmias, which were corrected by a temporary pacemaker and a reduction of serum potassium. As a result of congestive heart failure, azotemia, and the taking of the drug spironolactone, the additional potassium contributed by the salt substitute could not be excreted.

REFERENCES

1. Strong, J. P., and McGill, H. D.: The pediatric aspects of atherosclerosis, Atherosclerosis 9:251, 1969.
2. Enos, W. R., Byer, J. C., and Holmes, R. H.: Pathogenesis of coronary disease in American soldiers killed in Korea, J.A.M.A. 158:912, 1955.
3. McNamara, J. J., et al.: Coronary artery disease in combat casualties in Viet Nam, J.A.M.A 216:1185, 1971.
4. Engle, H. J., Page, H. L., and Campbell, W. B.: Coronary artery disease in young women, J.A.M.A. 230:1531, 1974
5. Gotto, A. M., Jr.: Is atherosclerosis reversible? J. Am. Diet Assoc. 74:551, 1979.
6. Small, D. M.: Cellular mechanisms for lipid deposition in atherosclerosis. I, N. Engl. J. Med. 297:873, 1977.
7. Small, D. M.: Cellular mechanisms for lipid deposition in atherosclerosis. II, N. Engl. J. Med. 297:924, 1977.
8. Arteriosclerosis. A report by the National Heart and Lung Institute Task Force on Arteriosclerosis, National Institutes of Health, vol 2, June 1971, DHEW Publication No. (NIH) 72-219.
9. Kolata, G. B.: Atherosclerotic plaques: competing theories guide research, Science 194:592, 1976.
10. Platelet factor: culprit in atherosclerosis? J.A.M.A. 239:689, 1978.
11. Texon, M.: Atherosclerosis. Its hemo-

dynamic basis and implications, Med. Clin. North Am. **58**:257, 1974.

12. Gresham, G. A.: Atherosclerosis in man: natural history and effects, Proc. Nutr. Soc. **31**:303, 1972.

13. Arteriosclerosis. A report by the National Heart and Lung Institute Task Force on Arteriosclerosis, National Institutes of Health, vol 1, June 1971, DHEW Publication No (NIH) 72-137.

14. Strong, J. P.: Pathology and epidemiology of atherosclerosis, J. Am. Diet. Assoc. **62**:262, 1973.

15. Report of Inter-Society Commission for Heart Disease Resources, Circulation **42**: 1970, Revised April 1972.

16. Newer concepts of coronary heart disease, Dairy Council Digest **45**(6):31, 1974.

17. Kannel, W. B.: The role of cholesterol in coronary atherogenesis, Med. Clin. North Am. **58**:363, 1974.

18. Keys, A., and Parlin, P. W.: Serum cholesterol response to changes in dietary lipids, Am. J. Clin. Nutr. **19**:175, 1965.

19. Grande, F., Anderson, J. T., and Keys, A.: Comparison of effects of palmitic and stearic acid in the diet on serum cholesterol in man, Am. J. Clin. Nutr. **23**:1184, 1970.

20. Whyte, H. M., and Havenstein, N.: A perspective view of dieting to lower the blood cholesterol, Am. J. Clin. Nutr. **29**:784, 1976.

21. Kummerow, F. A.: Lipids in atherosclerosis, J. Food Sci. **40**:12, 1975.

22. Sturdevant, R. A. L., Pearce, M. L., and Dayton, S.: Increased gallstone prevalence in men on serum cholesterol lowering diets, N. Engl. J. Med. **288**:24, 1973.

23. Ahrens, R. A.: Sucrose, hypertension and heart disease: an historical perspective, Am. J. Clin. Nutr. **27**:403, 1974.

24. Mechanisms of carbohydrate-induced hypertriglyceridemia, Nutr. Rev. **32**:74, 1974.

25. The role of sugars in hyperlipidemia, Nutr. Rev. **32**:340, 1974.

26. Sucrose, starch and hyperlipidemia, Nutr. Rev. **33**:44, 1975.

27. Glueck, C. J., and Connor, W. E.: Diet-coronary heart disease relationships reconnoitered, Am. J. Clin. Nutr. **31**:727, 1978.

28. Truswell, A. S.: Diet and plasma lipids—a reappraisal, Am. J. Clin. Nutr. **31**:977, 1978.

29. Mann, G. V.: Current concepts diet-heart: end of an era, N. Engl. J. Med. **297**:644, 1977.

30. Reiser, R.: Oversimplification of diet: coronary heart disease relationships and exaggerated diet recommendations, Am. J. Clin. Nutr. **31**:865, 1978.

31. Castelli, W. P., et al.: HDL cholesterol and other lipids in coronary heart disease. The cooperative lipoprotein phenotyping study, Circulation **55**:767, 1977.

32. High blood lipids can be good or bad—depending on the lipid, J.A.M.A. **237**:1066, 1977.

33. Stare, F., editor: Atherosclerosis, New York, 1974, Medcom, Inc.

34. Editorial: Contrasting professional views on atherosclerosis and coronary disease, N. Engl. J. Med. **292**:105, 1975.

35. Fredrickson, D. S., Levy, R. I., and Lees, R. S.: Fat transport in lipoproteins—an integrated approach to mechanisms and disorders, N. Engl. J. Med. **276**:34, 94, 148, 215, 273, 1967.

36. Murphy, B. F.: Management of hyperlipidemias, J.A.M.A. **230**:1683, 1974.

37. The dietary management of hyperlipoproteinemia. A handbook for physicians and dietitians, Bethesda, Md., National Heart and Lung Institute, National Institutes of Health (reprinted 1974) DHEW Publication No (NIH) 75-110.

38. Margolis, S.: Treatment of hyperlipemia, J.A.M.A. **239**:2696, 1978.

39. Fleischmajer, R.: Hypolipidemic drugs, Am. Fam. Physician **17**(2):188, 1978.

40. Murphy, B. F.: Probucol (Lorelco) in treatment of hyperlipemia, J.A.M.A. **238**:2537, 1977.

41. LeLorier, J., et al.: Diet and probucol in lowering cholesterol concentrations, Arch. Intern. Med. **137**:1429, 1977.

42. Finnerty, F. A., Jr.: How to treat arterial hypertension, Am. Fam. Physician **7**(4):99, 1973.

43. Aagaard, G. N.: The management of hypertension, J.A.M.A. **224**:329, 1973.

44. Bruckheim, A. H.: Practice patterns in the management of hypertension, Am. Fam. Physician **17**(3):209, 1978.

45. Moore, M. A.: Hypertension in the ambulatory patient, Am. Fam. Physician **16**(5):188, 1977.

46. Dahl, L. K: Salt and hypertension, Am. J. Clin. Nutr. **25**:231, 1972.

47. Reisin, E., et al.: Effect of weight loss without salt restriction on the reduction of blood

pressure in overweight hypertensive patients, N. Engl. J. Med. **298:**1, 1978.

48. Meneely, G. R., and Battarbee, H. D.: Sodium and potassium, Nutr. Rev. **34:**225, 1976.

49. Kempner, W.: Treatment of kidney disease and hypertensive vascular disease with rice diet, N. C. Med. J. **5:**125, 1944.

50. Improved treatment of hypertension after physician tutorials, Nutr. Rev. **34:**334, 1976.

51. Remmers, A. R., Beathard, G. A., Lindley, J. D., and Sarles, H. E.: Diuretics, Am. Fam. Physician **8**(4):209, 1973.

52. Hutcheon, D. E.: Limitations of current diuretics, Am. Fam. Physician **8**(5):186, 1973.

53. Chrysant, S. G., and Frohlich, E. D.: Side effects of antihypertensive drugs, Am. Fam. Physician **9**(1):94, 1974.

54. Kemp, G., and Kemp, D.: Diuretics, Am. J. Nurs. **78:**1006, 1978.

55. Martinez, E. W., and Lowenthal, D. T.: Choosing a diuretic in hypertension, Am. Fam. Physician **15**(3):194, 1977.

56. Dustan, H. R., Tarazi, R. C., and Bravo, E. L.: Diuretic and diet treatment of hypertension, Arch. Intern. Med. **133:**1007, 1974.

57. Astrup, P., and Kjeldsen, K.: Carbon monoxide, smoking and atherosclerosis, Med. Clin. North Am. **58:**323, 1974.

58. Sampson, P.: Quit smoking—or suffer low blood HDL levels, J.A.M.A. **239:**690, 1978.

59. Crawford, M. D.: Hardness of drinking water and cardiovascular disease, Proc. Nutr. Soc. **31:**347, 1972.

60. Shaper, A. G.: Soft water, heart attacks and stroke, J.A.M.A. **230:**136, 1974.

61. Schroeder, H. A.: The role of trace elements in cardiovascular disease, Med. Clin. North Am. **58:**381, 1974.

62. Perry, H. M., Jr.: Minerals in cardiovascular disease, J. Am. Diet. Assoc. **62:**631, 1973.

63. Dawson, E. B. et al.: Relationship of metal metabolism to vascular disease mortality rates in Texas, Am. J. Clin. Nutr. **31:**1188, 1978.

64. Seeleg, M. S., and Heggtveit, H. A.: Magnesium interrelationship in ischemic heart disease: a review, Am. J. Clin. Nutr. **27:**59, 1974.

65. Abraham, A. S., et al.: Magnesium levels in patients with chronic ischemic heart disease, Am. J. Clin. Nutr. **31:**1400, 1978.

66. Kelvay, L. M.: Hypercholesterolemia in rats produced by an increase in the ratio of zinc to copper ingested, Am. J. Clin. Nutr. **26:**1060, 1973.

67. Kelvay, L. M.: Coronary heart disease: the zinc/copper hypothesis, Am. J. Clin. Nutr. **28:**764, 1975.

68. Cummings, J. H.: Dietary fiber, Gut **14:**69, 1973.

69. Trowell, H.: Ischemic heart disease and dietary fiber, Am. J. Clin. Nutr. **25:**926, 1972.

70. Sherman, W. C.: The case for fiber, Food Nutr. News **46**(1):1, 1974.

71. Kritchevsky, D., Tepper, S. A., and Story, J. A.: Nonnutritive fiber and lipid metabolism, J. Food Sci. **40:**8, 1975.

72. Moore, J. H.: The effect of the type of roughage in the diet on plasma cholesterol levels and aortic atheromas in rabbits, Br. J. Nutr. **21:**207, 1967.

73. Kritchevsky, D., and Story, J. A.: Binding of bile salts in vitro by nonnutritive fiber, J. Nutr. **104:**458, 1974.

74. Kritchevsky, D., et al.: Lipid metabolism and experimental atherosclerosis in baboons: influence of cholesterol-free semisynthetic diets, Am. J. Clin. Nutr. **27:**29, 1974.

75. Kay, R. M., and Truswell, A. S.: Effect of citrus pectin on blood lipids and fecal steroid excretion in man, Am. J. Clin. Nutr. **30:**171, 1977.

76. Kay, R. M., Judd, P. A., and Truswell, A. S.: The effect of pectin on serum cholesterol, Am. J. Clin. Nutr. **31:**562, 1978.

77. Palumbo, P. J., Briones, E. R., and Nelson, R. A.: High fiber diet in hyperlipemia. Comparison with cholestyramine treatment in Type IIa hyperlipoproteinemia, J.A.M.A. **240:**223, 1978.

78. Carroll, K. K.: Dietary protein in relation to plasma cholesterol levels and atherosclerosis, Nutr. Rev. **36:**1, 1978.

79. Carroll, K. K., et al.: Hypocholesterolemic effects of substituting soybean protein for animal protein in the diet of healthy young women, Am. J. Clin. Nutr. **31:**1312, 1978.

80. Rosenman, R. H., and Friedman, M.: Neurogenic factors in pathogenesis of coronary heart disease, Med. Clin. North Am. **58:**269, 1974.

81. Russek, H. I.: Behavior patterns, stress and coronary heart disease, Am. Fam. Physician **9**(4):117, 1974.

82. Diet and coronary heart disease. A joint statement of the Food and Nutrition Board, Division of Biology and Agriculture, National Academy of Sciences—National Research

Council and the Council on Foods and Nutrition, American Medical Association, Am. J. Clin. Nutr. 26:53, 1973.

83. American Heart Association, committee on nutrition, diet and coronary heart disease, New York, American Heart Association, 1965, revised 1968, 1973, 1978.

84. Gleuck, C. J., et al.: The value and safety of diet modification to control hyperlipidemia, Circulation 58:381A, 1978.

85. Diet and coronary heart disease. A report of the Advisory Panel of the British Committee on Medical Aspects of Food Policy (Nutrition) on Diet in Relation to Cardiovascular and Cerebrovascular Disease, Nutr. Today 10(1):16, 1975.

86. Reiser, R.: Saturated fat in the diet and serum cholesterol concentration: a critical examination of the literature, Am. J. Clin. Nutr. 26:524, 1973.

87. Keys, A., Grande, F., and Anderson, J. T.: Bias and misrepresentation revisited. "Perspective" on saturated fat, Am. J. Clin. Nutr. 27:188, 1974.

88. Multiple Risk Factor Intervention Trial, Nutr. Today 9(3):28, 1974.

89. The Multiple Risk Factor Intervention Trial (MRFIT). A national study of primary prevention of coronary heart disease, J.A.M.A. 235:825, 1976.

90. Hulley, S. B., Cohen, R., and Widdowson, G.: Plasma high-density lipoprotein cholesterol level. Influence of risk factor intervention, J.A.M.A. 238:2269, 1977.

91. Planning fat controlled meals for 1200 and 1800 calories and planning fat controlled meals for approximately 2000 to 2600 calories, New York, revised 1966, American Heart Association.

92. Programmed instruction for fat controlled diet 1800 calories, 1969, New York, American Heart Association.

93. Eshleman, R., and Winston, M.: The American Heart Association Cookbook, New York, 1973, David McKay Company, Inc.

94. Subcommittee on Diet and Hyperlipidemia of the Council on Arteriosclerosis of the American Heart Association: A maximal approach to the dietary treatment of the hyperlipidemias, physician's handbook, Dallas, 1973, American Heart Association.

95. Bennett, I., and Simon, M.: The prudent diet, New York, 1973, Bantam Books.

96. Nestel, P. J.: Lower plasma cholesterol after eating polyunsaturated and ruminant fats, N. Engl. J. Med. 288:379, 1973.

97. Hoover, S. R.: Decreasing the saturated fatty acid content of animal products, Food Tech. 28:22, 1974.

98. Hodges, R. E., et al.: Plasma lipid changes in young adult couples consuming polyunsaturated meats and dairy products, Am. J. Clin. Nutr. 28:1126, 1975.

99. Stein, E. A., et al.: Lowering of plasma cholesterol levels in free-living adolescent males; use of natural and synthetic polyunsaturated foods to provide balanced fat diets, Am. J. Clin. Nutr. 28:1204, 1975.

100. Brown, H. B., et al.: Polyunsaturated meat and dairy products in fat-modified food patterns for hyperlipidemia, J. Am. Diet. Assoc. 69:235, 1976.

101. Heywood, P. F.: The public health significance of fat-modulated ruminant foods, Am. J. Clin. Nutr. 30:1726, 1977.

102. Hodges, R. E.: The value of polyunsaturated ruminant fat foods, Am. J. Clin. Nutr. 30:1571, 1977.

103. Ostrander, J., et al.: Egg substitutes. Use and preference—with and without nutritional information, J. Am. Diet. Assoc. 70:267, 1977.

104. Babayan, V. K: Modification of food to control fat intake, J. Am. Oil Chem. Soc. 51:260, 1974.

105. Altschul, A. M.: Vegetable proteins in prudent diet foods, Food Tech. 28:24, 1974.

106. Christakis, G., and Winston, M.: Nutritional therapy in acute myocardial infarction, J. Am. Diet. Assoc. 63:233, 1973.

107. Hemzacek, K. I.: Dietary protocol for the patient who has suffered a myocardial infarction, J. Am. Diet. Assoc. 72:182, 1978.

108. Your mild sodium restricted diet, your 1000 milligram sodium diet, your 500 milligram sodium diet, New York, revised 1968, American Heart Association.

109. Sodium restricted diet: mild restriction, 1000 milligrams, 500 milligrams, New York, 1965, 1966, 1967, American Heart Association.

110. Sopko, J. A., and Freeman, R. M.: Salt substitutes as a source of potassium, J.A.M.A. 238:608, 1977.

111. Oexmann-Wannamaker, M. J.: Salt substitutes, Am. J. Clin. Nutr. 29:599, 1976.

112. Yap, V., Patel, A., and Thomsen, J.: Hyperkalemia with cardiac arrhythmia, J.A.M.A. 236:2775, 1976.

GLOSSARY OF TERMS USED IN CARDIOVASCULAR DISEASE

aneurysm A sac or ballooning of the wall of an artery or vein resulting from weakness of the wall.

angina pectoris A sudden severe pain in the chest and often in the left arm and shoulder. When the arteries supplying the heart muscle become narrowed, there is insufficient blood supply, and pain results. It tends to appear during stress of any kind.

angiography X-ray films taken of the heart and great blood vessels after injection of opaque substance into the circulation.

anticoagulant A substance that inhibits blood clotting such as heparin and dicumarol.

arrhythmia An irregular rhythm of the heart beat.

arteriosclerosis A thickening, hardening, and loss of elasticity of arteries.

atherogenesis The formation of atheromatous lesions in the walls of the artery.

atheroma A deposit of lipid and lipidlike substances in the intima of the artery.

atherosclerosis A deposit of lipid and lipidlike substances in the wall of the intima in the large and small arteries (atheromata), which decrease the diameter of the lumen of the arteries. This is a form of arteriosclerosis.

blood pressure The pressure of the blood on the walls of the arteries. Systolic pressure is the pressure when the heart muscle is contracted, while diastolic pressure is the pressure during the resting phase. Blood pressure is expressed as the systolic then diastolic pressure, for example 115/80.

cerebrovascular accident A decreased blood supply to the brain caused by a thrombosis, hemorrhage, embolism, or pressure on a blood vessel. It is commonly called a stroke.

congestive heart failure When the heart is unable to maintain an adequate blood flow to the tissues, blood backs up in the veins leading to the heart, as a result, fluid accumulates in various parts of the body.

coronary arteries Two arteries (left and right) that start at the aorta and branch down and carry blood into the heart.

coronary care unit (CCU) This unit in the hospital originally was designed to provide effective means of resuscitation for cardiac arrest patients. The major efforts are now directed toward prevention of complications by continuous surveillance and immediate therapy.

coronary occlusion Generally, a clot in one of the coronary arteries. Due to the lack·of blood, this part of the heart dies. This is also called a heart attack.

coronary thrombosis A clot in one of the coronary arteries. It is also called coronary occlusion.

diuretic A substance that increases the secretion of urine.

electrocardiogram (ECG or EKG) Graphic tracing of the electric current resulting from the contraction of the heart muscle.

embolism The blocking of an artery or vein by a substance that was carried to that place.

embolus A foreign substance present in the blood, such as air, a clot, fat, and cells, that circulates and finally blocks a small vessel.

essential hypertension High blood pressure for which the cause is unknown.

fatty streak A fatty lesion in the intima of a blood vessel.

heart attack See Coronary occlusion.

hypercholesterolemia Elevated blood cholesterol levels.

hyperlipemia A general term that refers to an excess of fat in the blood.

hyperlipidemia The increase of one or more blood lipid components due to environmental causes.

hyperlipoproteinemia An elevation of blood lipoproteins of genetic origin or secondary diseases.

hypertension An elevation of blood pressure. It is often called high blood pressure.

hypokalemia Low blood levels of potassium.

hyponatremia Low blood levels of sodium.

infarct Death of tissue because of an insufficient supply of blood.

intima The innermost layer of a blood vessel.

ischemia A local temporary deficiency of blood that is caused by an obstruction.

morbidity The prevalence of a disease. It is usually expressed as the number of cases of a given disease in a given population.

mortality The rate of which is expressed as the number of deaths from a given disease in a given population.

myocardial infarction The death (necrosis) of part of the myocardium because of a decrease in blood supply to that area.

myocardial insufficiency Inability of the heart to maintain normal blood flow.

myocardium The middle layer of the three layers of the heart.

plaque An elevated lesion on the intima. The base of fat is covered with a fibrous connective tissue cap.

primary hypertension Essential hypertension.

risk factor A characteristic that appears with a greater incidence in a given disease.

sclerosis Hardening caused by the growth of fibrous tissue.

secondary hypertension High blood pressure that is the result of a given disease.

stroke See Cerebrovascular accident.

thrombosis The formation of a clot.

thrombus The formation of a plug or clot in a blood vessel or the heart resulting from coagulation of the blood. It remains at the site of formation.

xanthoma A yellowish or orange growth on the skin occuring as a flat or slightly raised patch because of deposits of lipid.

9 Uncategorized clinical conditions

Although the number of critically ill hospitalized patients needing specialized diet therapy is not extensive, nevertheless diet therapy is of utmost importance to those few. Surgical and burn patients have increased nutrient requirements that may not be met by ordinary means. Other methods of feeding such as tube feeding, parenteral nutrition, or defined-formula diets may be prescribed for the critically ill patient.

PREOPERATIVE NUTRITION

Patients who undergo minor surgery lose approximately 4% to 8% of body weight postoperatively, while a weight loss of 15% to 25% may occur in complicated situations.[1] Therefore, preoperatively, the individual should have adequate body reserves. In some instances it may be desirable to postpone surgery until the nutritional status of the patient has improved. A patient in an optimal state of nutrition experiences fewer postoperative complications such as infections and has more rapid wound healing and a shorter convalescent period. Adequate glycogen stores protect the liver from the toxic effects of anesthesia. The individual of normal weight will have body stores of fat for an energy source immediately after surgery when nutritional intake is decreased. If possible, obese persons should reduce prior to surgery to avoid complications associated with excessive adipose tissue. Reserve stores of tissue and plasma protein should be as high as possible to compensate for protein blood loss and to meet the increased requirement for protein synthesis after surgery. The B complex vitamins are needed to form coenzymes for metabolic reactions. Vitamin C is necessary for wound healing and vitamin K for adequate blood clotting. Mineral deficiency must also be avoided. In particular, iron is necessary for the synthesis of hemoglobin to replace that lost during surgery.

Prior to gastrointestinal surgery, low-residue diets are prescribed. This is done to reduce the gastrointestinal contents so that the gut is clean. No food or fluids are allowed for 8 hours prior to surgery. This is to prevent vomiting and aspiration of food during anesthesia and recovery. The presence of food in the stomach leads to retention and dilatation postoperatively.

POSTOPERATIVE NUTRITION

Immediately after surgery, the patient goes into negative nitrogen balance even though he might possibly be ingesting an adequate amount of protein. Tissue

199

catabolism occurs to replace protein lost through bleeding, inflammation, or infection. To promote wound healing, large amounts of proteins, from 100 to 200 g, must be supplied daily. Sufficient calories must be provided so that protein is used for synthesis and not metabolized for energy. It is important that plasma protein be replaced to assist in avoiding shock. When plasma proteins are decreased, water flows from the circulation into the tissue spaces. Blood volume decreases, and the water in the tissues results in edema. When this occurs at the site of the wound, healing is delayed.

Calories are provided mainly from carbohydrates. Energy needs are high following surgery. The liver is protected from further damage by deposits of glycogen. It is sometimes difficult to get the patient to consume adequate calories. Special supplements may be necessary. The fluid intake should be carefully monitored to prevent dehydration. Large volumes of fluid are lost through vomiting, hemorrhaging, diuresis, and exudates. When electrolyte imbalance occurs, electrolyte mixtures may need to be administered to replace losses. Therapeutic doses of vitamins are sometimes prescribed to meet the increased needs after surgery.

During the operation and for the first day afterwards a 5% dextrose solution is administered intravenously. On the first day postoperatively about 2 to 3 L can be given. As the oral intake increases, the amount of intravenous feeding is diminished. The patient is started on a clear liquid diet when peristalsis starts, the abdomen is soft and flat, and gas is passed from the anus. The diet consists of water and clear liquids such as tea, coffee, broth, ginger ale, fruit or vegetable juice, and gelatin. This liquid diet supplies mainly fluids and electrolytes. It is nutritionally inadequate and should only be used for a short period of time. The patient progresses to a full liquid diet. This is composed of foods that are liquid or liquefy at body temperature. Milk and milk products such as puddings, ice cream, cream soups, and high-protein beverages are allowed. This is followed by a soft diet that is modified in consistency. Foods with connective tissue and indigestible carbohydrates are not allowed. After this the patient is ready for a regular diet.

Patients progress from the clear liquid to a regular diet as it is tolerated. However, when gastrointestinal surgery is performed, the progression is much slower. Water may be allowed for 2 to 4 days postoperatively followed by a liquid diet for 1 to 2 days. If this is tolerated, it is followed by a soft and then a regular diet.

In some instances, food cannot be taken orally. Then tube feeding or total parenteral feeding must be instituted.

Protein-sparing therapy

After surgery, body protein is catabolized at the rate of 75 to 150 g per day; this represents the loss of 300 to 600 g of lean body mass that is mostly muscle.[2] Blackburn et al. concluded that the administration of glucose intravenously contributed to this loss of nitrogen.[3,4] Ten surgical patients were infused with 5% dextrose (100 g glucose per day), 5% dextrose plus 3% amino acids (98 g amino acids per day), and 3% amino acids.[4] The urinary nitrogen losses were, respectively, 28.4

± 3.5 g, 15 ± 6 g, and 0.3 ± 4.8 g. The nitrogen balance was improved by the administration of an amino acid solution.

Blackburn and Flatt proposed a metabolic fuel regulatory system based on the concentration of metabolic fuels (glucose, free fatty acids, ketone bodies, and amino acids) and insulin.[5] They suggested that a 5% dextrose infusion promotes the secretion of insulin. This in turn leads to a decrease in fat mobilization and a resultant reduction in the oxidation of free fatty acids and ketone bodies. On the other hand, levels of free fatty acid and ketone bodies approached those found in starvation. Thus the infused amino acids are used for protein synthesis rather than as in the previous case for energy production.

Hoover et al. compared the effects of glucose or amino acid infusions in 20 surgical patients.[6] Although nitrogen balance was negative for both treatments it was more negative in the glucose infused patients. It was calculated that with the amino acid infusion there was approximately 50% less nitrogen lost than with the dextrose infusion. These results agree with those of Blackburn, but Hoover et al. concluded that the mechanisms for protein sparing are controversial. Insulin levels in patients on amino acid solutions are lower than in those on dextrose solutions, but there is an overlap. The roles of glucagon, catecholamines, and other metabolites are not known.

In another study 30 postoperative patients were assigned to one of four parenteral treatment groups: glucose group—150 g dextrose as 5% dextrose; protein-alone group—1 g/kg of amino acids (Travasol, 5%); protein-plus-lipid group—1 g/kg of amino acids plus 500 ml of 10% Intralipid; and protein-plus-glucose group—1 g/kg of amino acids plus 150 g of dextrose.[7] Nitrogen balance was more negative in those patients who received only dextrose infusions. However, the three groups receiving amino acids showed equivalent negative nitrogen balances. When amino acids or amino acids plus lipid were administered, higher levels of free fatty acids, ketone bodies, and glucagon and low insulin levels were observed. This is indicative of fat mobilization. The added glucose did not increase the mobilization of muscle protein even though insulin levels were high. The low insulin levels in the amino acid–plus-lipid treatment did not improve nitrogen balance; it was the same as when amino acids were administered. Therefore the authors concluded that low levels do not promote protein sparing in the hypocaloric state. They suggested that the infused amino acids are the major determinants of protein sparing in caloric deprivation, and this is not related to the degree of endogenous fat mobilization. The mechanism by which this happens is unknown, but amino acid infusions may promote protein synthesis and reduce catabolism.

Isenberg and Maxwell found that the intravenous and intraduodenal infusions of 42.5 g of amino acids gradually increased gastric acid secretion.[8] When 250 g of glucose were infused with the amino acids, the results were similar. The authors questioned whether during the constant infusion of amino acids, as is the case in total parenteral nutrition, gastric acid secretion always remains elevated. This could possibly predispose the patient to ulcer formation.

NUTRITIONAL THERAPY FOR BURN PATIENTS

Increased nutritional requirements occur after thermal injury more so than with any other kind of trauma. From the burn site there is a massive loss of fluids, electrolytes, and proteins. The accelerated rate of tissue breakdown depletes energy and protein reserves. As much as 25% to 33% of the preburn weight may be lost. Shock, wound healing, infection, and plastic surgery further increase the nutritional requirements. Adequate nutritional therapy is necessary for recovery. This becomes difficult, since the burn patients often are anorexic or incapable of consuming the large quantities of food necessary to meet their needs.

The first concern in the treatment of a burn patient is fluid replacement. An adequate nutritional intake may not be possible for several days. At first, Ringer's lactate solution is administered intravenously; this is followed by a 5% glucose solution. The blood picture and the amount of albumin lost determine whether blood, plasma, albumin, or blood substitutes such as dextran should be given.[9] A solution of glucose or Haldrane's solution (3 to 4 g salt, 1.5 to 2 g sodium bicarbonate in 1L of water flavored with lemon juice) may be given orally for fluid replacement. Generally the loss of fluid from the wound gradually decreases over 30 hours.

Caloric requirements become extensive (5000 to 6000 kcal) for severely burned patients and may not be able to be met by the oral route. Curreri and co-workers provided a 5000 kcal high-protein diet to patients with total body surface burns of from 40% to 75%.[10] The actual intakes ranged from 296 to 2279 kcal. Parenteral nutrition increased the intake to a range of 1230 to 3206 kcal. From the data collected with these patients an equation was derived to calculate the daily caloric intake, namely, sum = 25 × weight (kg) + 40 × %TBS (total body surface burn). The caloric intake calculated according to this formula should minimize weight loss during the recovery period.

The severity of a thermal injury determines the degree to which nitrogen excretion is increased. The increase in nitrogen catabolism is the result of an increased rate of basal metabolism, loss of protein from the burn site, effect of infection, breakdown of body tissue, and decreased protein synthesis by the liver and other organs.[9] The protein intake should be increased to 2 to 3 g/kg of body weight. Adequate calories must be ingested so that the protein is not used as an energy source. Amino acids may be administered intravenously. Therapeutic doses of vitamins are needed, especially vitamins A, C, and the B complex. Electrolyte levels must also be carefully monitored.[11] Sodium excretion decreases, so it may be necessary to restrict sodium intake. Therapeutic doses of iron should be given to alleviate the anemia that develops with thermal injury. Zinc plays a role in wound healing, but as yet no requirements have been established for burn patients.

Burn therapy begins with the administration of fluids and electrolytes parenterally. Some patients are anorexic or develop paralytic ileus, so other methods of feeding must be employed. Total parenteral solutions with both glucose and amino acids can meet the needs of the patient. Precautions must be taken if this method is employed to avoid infections and other metabolic complications. Tube feeding can also be used. This may be combined with oral intake, as when the patient is unable to ingest large quantities of food. In extreme cases, oral, tube, and intravenous feeding may be needed. The patient progresses to a high-protein, high-calorie diet as soon as it is feasible. High-protein liquid supplements may be prescribed for between-meal feedings.

At the Shriners Burns Institute in Cincinnati the dietary prescription for children with thermal injuries calls for one and a half times more calories and two to four times more protein than the Recommended Daily Dietary Allowance.[12] Multivitamin capsules and 250 mg of ascorbic acid are administered daily. When the total burn surface area is 15% to 20%, there is little or no decrease in appetite. Patients whose burn area is over 40% of their body cannot maintain their weight by enteral feeding alone; tube feeding then becomes necessary. An adequate nutritional intake is important for children who lose 10% of their preburn weight, for they are at risk from septic complications, which can be fatal.

Larkin and Maylan treated 15 burn patients solely by enteral nutrition.[13] The diet provided 46 kcal per kilogram, 1.6 g protein per kilogram, 1.1 g fat per kilogram, and 7.1 g carbohydrate per kilogram plus vitamin supplements. High-calorie, high-protein commercial liquid supplements were given between meals and provided 37% of the total caloric intake. Body weights ranged from a loss of 7.2% of the preburn weight to a gain of 4.6%.

A nutritional management record sheet was developed at the Bothin Burn Center in San Francisco.[14] The record sheet is placed in the patient's medical record and thus is easily accessible to all members of the health care team. The dietitian calculates the protein and energy requirement for each patient according to the following formula:

Energy
    Adult = 20 kcal × kg body weight + 70 kcal × % burn
    Child = 60 kcal × kg body weight + 35 kcal × % burn
Protein
    Adult = 1 g × kg body weight + 3 g × % burn
    Child = 3 g × kg body weight + 1 g × % burn

The physician then selects from one of the three methods of feeding, namely, tube feedings, parenteral nutrition, or the hospital diet with supplemental protein feedings. Weight is recorded twice weekly. If the patient reaches a weight loss of 10%, then the nutritional therapy must be changed.

Diet therapy is important for optimal wound healing and recovery of burn patients. For therapy to be successful the caloric and protein requirements must be adequate to maintain body weight. Enteral feeding is preferred, since parenteral feeding is associated with septicemia. However, each patient has individual needs that must be met.

Table 9-1. Blenderized tube feeding formula*

Oatmeal (strained)	10 g
Dextri-Maltose	50 g
Instant nonfat dry milk	50 g
Liver (strained)	20 g
Beef (strained)	568 g
Applesauce (strained)	402 g
Green beans (strained)	484 g
Oil	85 ml
Orange juice	200 ml
Homogenized milk	300 ml
Water	500 ml

The formula provides 1 kcal/ml in a total volume of 2500 ml.

*From Chatton, M. J., and Ullman, P. M.: Nutrition: nutritional and metabolic disorders. In Krupp, M. A., and Chatton, M. J., editors: Current medical diagnosis and treatment, Los Altos, Calif., 1975, Lange Medical Publications.

TUBE FEEDINGS

When patients cannot take food by mouth, tube feeding may be instituted. This method of feeding may be indicated after dental surgery or after surgery on the alimentary tract or respiratory system and with severe burns, paralysis, and cancer of the mouth and esophagus. Comatose, anorexic, and some mentally ill patients are also fed in this manner.

Ordinarily a pliable polyethylene tube of narrow diameter is passed through the nasal cavity into the stomach. It is important that the tube be properly placed. Diarrhea and pain result if the tube is in the duodenum. A coiled tube positioned in the wrong direction will lead to vomiting and aspiration. If the patient is unable to tolerate the tube or is to be fed for a long period of time, an incision can be made in the esophagus (esophagostomy), through the abdominal wall into the stomach (gastrostomy), or in the jejunum (jejunostomy). The tube is then inserted into the opening for feeding.

Clear fluids may be administered by means of gravity drip. More viscous solutions that have a tendency to clog the tube must be given by means of a Barron food pump.[15] This allows for delivery of a measured amount of food in regulated amounts according to the tolerance of the patient. The solutions contain approximately 1 kcal/ml, and with continuous feeding, 2000 kcal can be provided in 24 hours.

Three patients have been maintained on a milk-base convenience tube feeding for over 2 years.[16] Adequate nutrient intake is achieved when 2000 kcal are consumed in the absence of malabsorption and diarrhea. If the caloric level drops below 1500 kcal, it is difficult to meet all nutrient requirements. Two of the subjects in this study who received less than 2000 kcal showed evidence of iron deficiency anemia; in these instances it might be necessary to provide a supplement.

Table 9-2. Milk-base tube feeding formula*

Homogenized milk	800 ml
Half and half	600 ml
Powdered egg or eggnog powder	100 g
Instant nonfat dry milk	90 g
Salt	5.5 g
Vitamin preparation	5 ml to 1500 ml
Water	

The formula provides 1.4 kcal/ml in a total volume of 1500 ml.

*From Chatton, M. J., and Ullman, P. M.: Nutrition: nutritional and metabolic disorders. In Krupp, M. A., and Chatton, M. J., editors: Current medical diagnosis and treatment, Los Altos, Calif., 1975, Lange Medical Publications.

Three general types of tube feedings have been used, namely, blenderized food mixtures, milk-base formulas, and a wide variety of commercial preparations. A formula for a blenderized food mixture is given in Table 9-1. Foods are liquefied in a high-speed blender and filtered. Strained baby foods can be used. This type of feeding can be used for long periods of time. It has been accepted and well tolerated by patients with a minimum of complications. An example of a milk-base formula is given in Table 9-2. This is not tolerated as well as the blenderized food mixture, and diarrhea often develops.

Defined-formula diets

The drug industry has developed a variety of tube feedings in either liquid or powdered form (Table 9-3). Many can be used as oral supplements. In the past some of these products were referred to as chemically defined diets and elemental diets. The distinction was not very clear, but chemically defined diets contained amino acids, essential fatty acids, simple sugars, vitamins, and minerals[17]; therefore, the diets were composed of clearly defined, chemically discrete compounds.[18] These diets were low in residue and did not require digestion, and so they were useful for patients with disorders of the gastrointestinal tract. Elemental diets consisted of protein hydrolysates, simple sugars, a large portion of fat as medium chain triglycerides, vitamins, and minerals. These diets provided nutrients that were easily digested or absorbed. Since these diets are not elemental or chemically pure, the term "defined-formula diets" is now used.[19] Defined refers to the fact that the formula includes nutrients that are prepared commercially from foods or synthetic compounds. However, the precise chemical composition is not known.

Defined-formula diets require a minimum of digestion and can be used when there is impaired synthesis of digestive enzymes and bile. Residue is reduced to a minimum, and thus stool volume and the number of bowel movements decrease. Diarrhea is avoided when the diets are administered slowly and in a not too concentrated form.

Defined-formula diets can be used in many different situations.[18] They can be used with newborns and infants who have small reserves of nutrients. They are especially often used following gastrointestinal tract surgery. Prior to surgery the nutritional status of the patient may be improved by a defined-formula diet. Postoperatively, it is especially important that adequate nutrients are present to promote wound healing and resistance to infection. These low-residue diets are also useful for preoperative bowel preparation or colon x-ray film preparation. Other instances in which the defined-formula diets may be of value are chronic short bowel syndrome, diverticulitis, ulcerative colitis, malabsorption syndromes, disaccharide intolerances, fistulas, and neoplasms of the gastrointestinal tract. The low-residue diet is useful in fecal incontinence, stroke patients, and in brain-damaged individuals. Defined-formula diets may be used as supplements in the following hypermetabolic states: severe burns, long bone fractures, oral surgery or jaw fractures, multiple trauma, and severe infection.

Some of these formulations contain a high percentage of nitrogen (Codelid, Meritene, Nutrament, Precision High Nitrogen, Vivonex HN). Intact protein in the form of pureed meat, eggs, or milk and protein isolates from milk, soybean, or egg white are used in these formulas. These preparations are useful for persons in a catabolic state as a result of, for example, surgery, extensive burns, or anorexia. Patients with maldigestion, malabsorption syndromes, intestinal disorders, or biliary or pancreatic dysfunction have difficulty with intact protein. Formulations that contain protein in a predigested form, either as a protein hydrolysate (casein) or a mixture of amino acids, are useful in these instances, for example, Codelid, Flexical, Vivonex, W-T Low Residue Food, and W-T Peptide L4.

Table 9-3. Composition of commercial dietary products

| Product | Percent composition | | | Feature | Major components† |
	Carbohydrate	Protein*	Fat		
Cutter Laboratories, Inc.					
Formula 2	48	15	36	Blenderized tube feeding	Nonfat milk, beef, egg yolk, corn oil, strained vegetables, fruits, cereals
Vipep	68	10	22	Low residue	Corn syrup solids, sucrose, corn starch, tapioca flour, MCT, corn oil, fish protein hydrolysate, amino acids

*Protein or protein equivalent.
†Vitamins and minerals are also added.

Table 9-3. Composition of commercial dietary products—cont'd

Product	Percent composition			Feature	Major components
	Carbo-hydrate	Pro-tein	Fat		
Nutri-1000	40	13	47	High fat	Skim milk, soy and coco-nut oil, sucrose, corn syrup
The Doyle Pharma-ceutical Co. Compleat-B	48	16	36	Blenderized tube feeding	Pureed beef, green beans, peas, peaches, malto-dextrin, nonfat dry milk, corn oil, sucrose, orange juice
Meritene	46	24	30	High protein	Sweet skim milk, corn syrup, vegetable oil, so-dium caseinate, sucrose
Precision LR	84	8.2	0.3	Low residue	Egg white solids, maltodex-trin, sugar, vegetable oil
Precision High Nitrogen	74.9	15.1	0.2	Low residue, high nitrogen	Maltodextrin, egg white solids, sugar, vegetable oil
Precision Iso-tonic	60	12	28	Tube feeding	Glucose oligosaccharides, egg white solids, vegeta-ble oil, sucrose, sodium caseinate
Lolactene	53	26	21	Tube feeding	Nonfat dry milk, sodium caseinate, vegetable oil, monodiglycerides, corn syrup solids, sucrose, glucose, galactose
Drackett Products Co. Nutrament	54	25	21	High protein	Sweet skim milk, soy oil, sodium caseinate, sugar
Eaton Laboratories Vivonex	90.8	8.5	0.7	Low residue, elemental	Amino acids, safflower oil, glucose, and glucose oli-gosaccharides
Vivonex HN	81.34	18.26	0.4	Low residue, high nitrogen, elemental	Amino acids, safflower oil, glucose, and glucose oli-gosaccharides
Johnson & Johnson Jejunal	90	9	<1	Minimal residue, elemental	Amino acids, simple carbo-hydrates, safflower oil

Continued.

Table 9-3. Composition of commercial dietary products—cont'd

Product	Percent composition			Feature	Major components
	Carbo-hydrate	Pro-tein	Fat		
Mead Johnson					
Flexical	61	9	30	Low residue, elemental	Casein hydrolysate, essential amino acids, MCT, soy oil, corn syrup solids, sucrose
Isocal	50	13	37	Tube feeding	Corn syrup solids, soy oil, sodium and calcium caseinate, MCT oil, soy protein isolate
Portagen	46	14	40	Malabsorption, lactose intolerance	Sodium caseinate, MCT, corn oil, corn syrup solids, sugar
Sustacal	55	24	21	High protein tube feeding	Skim milk, sodium caseinate, soy, corn syrup, sugar
Sustagen	55	24	20	High protein	Whole and skim milk, calcium caseinate, maltose, dextrin
Ross Laboratories					
Ensure	54.5	14	31.5	Tube feeding	Sodium and calcium caseinate, soy protein isolate, corn oil, corn syrup solids, sucrose
Ensure Plus	53.3	14.6	31.9	Tube feeding	Sodium and calcium caseinate, soy protein isolate, corn oil, corn syrup, solids, sucrose
Ensure Osmolite	54	14	32	Low residue	Corn syrup solids, sodium and calcium caseinates, medium-chain triglycerides, corn oil, soy protein isolate, soy oil
Vital	74	16.7	9.3	Tube feeding	Hydrolyzed soy, wheat and meat, safflower oil, MCT, glucose polymers, sucrose
Schwarz-Mann					
Codelid	80.7	17.2	0	High nitrogen, chemically defined, elemental, no residue, no roughage, fat free	Amino acids, sucrose

Table 9-3. Composition of commercial dietary products—cont'd

Product	Percent composition			Feature	Major components
	Carbo-hydrate	Pro-tein	Fat		
Syntex Laboratories, Inc.					
Nutri-1000	40	13	47	High fat	Skim milk, soy and coco-nut oil, sucrose, corn syrup
Warren-Teed Pharmaceuticals Inc.					
W-T Low Residue Food	90.7	8.6	0.7	Low residue, elemental	Amino acids, safflower oil, dextrin
W-T Protein L4	89	10	1	Low residue	Sodium caseinate, nonfat dry milk, linoleic acid
W-T Peptide L4	89	10	1	Low residue	Protein hydrolysate, amino acids, linoleic acid

Fats provide a high caloric density and increase palatability but do not increase osmolality. Soy, safflower, and corn oil are used as sources of fat. One preparation contains a high percentage of fat (Nutri-1000). Steatorrhea appears in some patients; this has been alleviated by feeding medium-chain triglycerides (MCT) that are absorbed via the portal vein and easily digested soy oil. Portagen, Flexical, and Isocal contain MCT oil. The following preparations contain 1% or less fat: Jejunal, W-T Protein L4, W-T Peptide L4, W-T Low Residue Food, Vivonex, Vivonex HN, Precision LR, Precision High Nitrogen, and Codelid.

The percentage of calories supplied by carbohydrates ranges from 40% to 90% in these formulations. The sources of carbohydrate are sucrose, lactose, glucose, partially hydrolyzed starch (corn syrup solids), dextrins, and glucose oligosaccharides. Oligosaccharides are polymers containing five or more glucose molecules. The simple sugars are sweet and increase the osmolality of the solutions. Therefore they are used in small amounts.

Lactose intolerance caused by a deficiency of the enzyme lactase results in the inability to digest lactose. Therefore feeding commercial products to individuals who have this defect may not only cause symptoms but interfere with the absorption of other nutrients. Sixteen patients who were fed by nasogastric tube following surgery were fed two liquid diets that differed only in the lactose content[20]; one contained approximately 75 g of lactose per liter. Fourteen of the patients on the tube feeding with lactose exhibited an increase in stool frequency and weight and increased gastrointestinal disturbances. The unhydrolyzed lactose increases the osmotic activity, and thus fluids are pulled into the intestine. Intestinal transit increases, and there is inadequate absorption of water in the colon with diarrhea resulting. Fermentation of lactose by intestinal bacteria produces hydrogen and carbon dioxide, which leads to abdominal distention and cramps. The authors recommended that the lactose content of tube feeding diets be reduced or the sugar completely eliminated.

Commercial tube feedings low in residue are Jejunal, Precision LR, Precision High Nitrogen, Flexical, Codelid, Vivonex, Vivonex HN, W-T Low Residue Food, W-T Protein L4, W-T Peptide L4, and Ensure Osmolite. These products reduce fecal output and thus are fed for several days for presurgical bowel preparation and then postoperatively. These low-residue products are also used in gastrointestinal inflammation and digestive and absorptive disorders. Nutrition is provided while giving the lower bowel rest. Patients on low-residue diets have bowel movements every 5 to 6 days only, so this type of therapy is useful in fecal incontinence.

Shils, Block, and Chernoff have compiled the protein, fat, carbohydrate, and mineral content of a large number of nutritionally complete commercial preparations.[21] The protein, fat, carbohydrate, sodium, and potassium content of a variety of supplementary feedings is also included.

Patients may be unable to tolerate one or more nutrients in a commercial formula. Therefore at the Memorial Sloan-Kettering Cancer Center in New York three basic formulas have been prepared: a general formula for patients with normal absorption, a low-residue defined formula, and a formula with casein hydrolysate for patients with malabsorption, pancreatic insufficiency, inflammatory bowel disease, or intestinal fistulas.[21,22] These formulas are easily modified to meet the needs of the patient.

One of the complications that occurs with tube feeding is diarrhea. This might be caused by bacterial contamination, a hypertonic formula, rapid feeding, improper positioning of the feeding tube, or cold feedings.[23] Several preparations (Isocal, Ensure Osmolite, and Precision Isotonic) are isotonic and thus cause fewer complications. The other preparations are hyperosmolar and range in osmolality from 500 to 1000 milliosmoles per kilogram of water as compared to serum, which is 300 milliosmoles per kilogram of water. The term "osmolarity" is also used and refers to the number of osmotically active particles per liter of solution rather than as in osmolality, which is the number of particles per kilogram of water. As the number of particles increases, the osmolality increases. The size of the particle is inversely proportional to the osmolality; therefore, a solution of starch would have a lower osmolality than a solution of glucose.

In tube feedings the osmolarity is less than the osmolality, while in biological solutions there is only a slight difference. When osmotically active particles such as glucose, sucrose, amino acids, and electrolytes reach the intestine, water is pulled into the lumen, and diarrhea, vomiting, cramps, and nausea may result. This can be overcome by feeding slowly, diluting the formula, and then gradually increasing the concentration. As time passes, the body adapts to the hypertonic solution. If the diarrhea continues, dehydration results. High-protein intakes, dehydrated mixtures of skim milk solids, and sugars without fat have been responsible for the deaths of some patients.[23]

Supplemental fluid should also be administered not only to avoid dehydration but for excretion of urinary waste products. The nutritional state of the individual should be monitored continually especially if therapy is long term. Some tube feeding preparations may contain inadequate amounts of some vitamins or minerals or both. Individuals who are bedridden and inactive may gain excess weight if the caloric intake is too high.

Wells and Zachman compared the feeding by nasogastric and nasojejunal tubes of low-birth-weight infants.[24] On the average it took 6½ days for babies on nasojejunal feeding to regain their birth weight and 14½ days for those fed by nasogastric tube. In general, better gains were made in the first 2 weeks of nasojejunal feeding. Similar results were found by Cheek and Staub.[25] Premature (36) and full-term newborn (10) babies were fed continuously by nasojejunal tube for periods of 2 to 75 days. Such feedings provided 113.6 kcal per kilogram per day and 2.9 g protein per kilogram per day. Three of the 46 infants who did not gain weight died of hyaline membrane disease. Nasojejunal feeding meets the high nutrient requirements of the premature and ill infant. Early administration of nutrients increases the chances of survival.

Three children were maintained on Isocal, a formula diet that is primarily used in feeding adults.[26] No adverse symptoms were noted; the increase in height was normal for their state of recovery. The high caloric density and low renal solute load of Isocal make it useful for pediatric patients.

A series of defined-formula diets were fed to 15 normal male volunteers for 6 months.[27] The diets consisted of various combinations of amino acids or peptones, glucose or sucrose, ethyl linoleate, vitamins, and minerals. Physical examinations and blood and urine analyses all indicated that the men were healthy. Since the diets contained no bulk, the number of bowel movements decreased. When glucose was the carbohydrate ingested, serum cholesterol levels decreased, whereas when sucrose replaced glucose, the cholesterol levels increased. The men initially lost weight, but this was regained when they began to eat. Part of the weight loss was attributed to the lack of bulk in the gastrointestinal tract. It was concluded that the defined-formula diets could maintain normal physiological function and health of humans. Similar results were found by Copeland, Lachance, and Mohammed.[28] Sixteen male subjects were fed Jejunal for 2 weeks. All clinical and laboratory examinations were normal. Weight loss and a hypocholesterolemic effect were also noted.

The defined-formula diets have also been tested clinically and found to be beneficial.[17,29] Jejunal was administered to 30 patients.[29] The diet was most useful for patients undergoing abdominal surgery and for those with feeding difficulties. No harmful effects were observed. In another study nine patients with severe dysphagia received Flexical for 12 weeks.[17] Values for hemoglobin, serum protein, and other

Table 9-4. Supplementary feedings

Product	Manufacturer	Type
Protein (low or free)		
Cal-Power	Henkel Corporation	Carbohydrate source
Controlyte	Doyle Pharmaceutical Co.	Low electrolyte, calorie source
HYCAL	Beecham-Massengill Pharmaceuticals	Carbohydrate source
Lipomul Oral	Upjohn Company	Fat source
Lytren	Mead Johnson	Carbohydrate source
Polycose	Ross Laboratories	Carbohydrate source
Sumacal	Hospital Diet Product Corporation	Carbohydrate source
Microlipid	Hospital Diet Product Corporation	Fat emulsion
Protein supplement		
Casec	Mead Johnson	Protein source
dp High per Protein	Henkel Corporation	Protein source
EMF	Control Drug, Inc.	Liquid protein hydrolysate
Calorie supplement		
Citrotein	Doyle Pharmaceutical Co.	Calorie source
Gevral	Lederle Laboratories	Protein-calorie source

biochemical parameters were normal except for an increase in uric acid and a decrease in blood urea nitrogen. A decrease in blood urea nitrogen suggested that the formula might be of value for treating certain renal disorders. The debilitated patients gained weight on the diet.

Ten healthy subjects consumed three defined-formula diets (Vivonex, Flexical, or Precision LR) for 10 days.[30] The total stool weight was significantly lower with Vivonex than with Precision LR. There were no differences in stool frequency, fecal fat, ash, moisture, or nitrogen balance. However, all subjects were in negative nitrogen balance and lost weight when consuming the diets. It was assumed that because of the low protein-calorie ratio of the formulas, those results were in part due to insufficient consumption of the formula. Vivonex was rated the best diet by eight of the ten subjects, and all selected Precision LR as their second choice. The complaints reported by the subjects were taste, headaches, sweating, shaky weakness, diarrhea, nausea, and constipation.

However, when these three diets were tested in a patient with 120 cm of small bowel terminating in a jejunostomy, different results were obtained.[31] The best nitrogen retention was found with Vivonex HN followed by Flexical and then Precision LR. High fat retention was observed with Flexical. Thus the three diets have different effects on intestinal absorption.

Zabel et al. analyzed the selenium content of infant formulas, tube-feeding formulas, food supplements, chemically defined diets, and total parenteral nutrition solutions.[32] The content of this trace element depends on the protein source. The lowest concentrations of selenium were found in the products containing amino acid mixtures. Only two of the sixteen infant formulas tested contained more selenium than would be provided by the same amount of breast milk. Amounts of selenium equivalent to that found in the United States diet were found in three of the thirty formulas used with adults.

Much success has been attained with the defined-formula diets. Research is still needed as to the composition of these diets for various disease states to attain optimum nutrition. Patients must be observed closely to detect any biochemical or clinical signs of deficiency. The defined-formula diets should be used judiciously.

The drug companies also make a number of products that can be used for supplementary feedings. Some have high concentrations of fat and carbohydrate and can be used as calorie supplements. Some contain only protein or protein hydrolysates and are useful in rehabilitating protein-depleted patients. Other products are protein free and can be used as calorie sources for renal patients. Some of these available products are listed in Table 9-4.

PARENTERAL NUTRITION

Parenteral feeding can be used to maintain an individual who cannot be fed by mouth or by means of the digestive tract. Nutrients can be supplied by subcutaneous, intramuscular, or intravenous infusion. The method of intravenous infusion is preferred, since very limited amounts of fluid can be given via the subcutaneous and intramuscular route.

Only dilute solutions (5% or 10% glucose) can be infused into the peripheral veins without causing phlebitis or thrombosis.[33] The caloric density of the infused substances, namely, protein, carbohydrate, fat, and ethyl alcohol, limits the amount of energy that can be supplied. In addition, the adult can tolerate 35 to 50 ml of water per kilogram of body weight or a total of about 3 to 3.5 L per day. Overhydration would result if more solution were administered.

A liter of 5% to 10% glucose would provide 200 to 400 kcal respectively. Administration of 3 L a day would not provide an adequate supply of calories. Protein can be supplied by infusing a 5% amino acid mixture in a glucose solution to provide additional calories. Negative calorie and nitrogen balance lead to a breakdown of body tissue when, in fact, anabolism should be taking place. Generally patients in need of parenteral nutrition have higher nutrient requirements, and the inability to meet these needs leads to further debilitation.

In 1965 Dudrick and his co-workers fed 8-week-old beagle puppies by means of a polyvinyl catheter inserted via the external jugular vein into the mid-superior vena cava.[33] The solution fed contained glucose, fibrin hydrolysate, vitamins, and minerals. Tests performed during 1 to 2 months of feeding in this manner showed no abnormalities. The weight gains of these puppies were similar to those attained by littermates that were fed orally. Since the procedure was successful, it was adapted for use with infants and then later with adults.

The term used for this method, "hyperalimentation," refers to the administration of an excess of nutrients rather than the amount necessary for maintenance of normal body weight. The goal is to provide enough nutrients to meet the needs of the specific individual; therefore Shils suggested that the term "total parenteral nutrition" or "total parenteral alimentation" be used instead.[34]

Total parenteral nutrition is utilized only when oral or tube feeding cannot maintain the nutritional status of the patient. The criteria used by Shils are either that the edema-free body weight is 11% below the ideal body weight or that after 4 weeks of intravenous feeding there is no improvement in sight.[34] This period is shortened if the patient is in poor clinical condition.

Total parenteral nutrition has been used in a variety of situations.[35] This method has proved useful for treating malabsorptive syndromes after surgery of the gastrointestinal tract, intestinal fistulas, ulcers, incomplete bowel obstruction, short bowel syndrome, diverticulitis, ulcerative colitis, and chronic diarrhea and vomiting. Administration of mixtures of the essential l-amino acids in liver disease resulted in a decrease in blood ammonia. This amino acid mixture is also useful in reducing urea levels in acute and chronic renal failure. Malnourished patients who often exhibit malabsorption and diarrhea from enteral nutrition benefit from total parenteral nutrition. Neonates with congenital anomalies and failure-to-thrive infants also show improvement after this method of feeding, as do pediatric patients with chronic diarrhea, acute renal failure, and inflammatory bowel disease.[36] This method has been used for burn patients who may need up to 10,000 kcal per day.[35] Cancer patients who are undergoing radiation or chemotherapy and are unable to consume adequate calories can be aided by parenteral nutrition. When individuals are unable to eat because of anorexia nervosa or other psychiatric conditions, this method might prove of value.

The hypertonic solutions (1800 to 2000 milliosmoles per liter) used in total parenteral nutrition cause thrombosis in the peripheral veins, and so infusion must be into areas of high blood flow. The catheters are placed in the superior vena cava or right atrium through the subclavian or jugular vein. In infants the jugular vein is used, as the subclavian vein is too small. Aseptic and antiseptic techniques must be followed during insertion of the catheter and its maintenance to avoid the complications of bacterial and fungal infections. Arteriovenous shunts and fistulas have been used for parenteral feeding.

Solutions administered via parenteral feeding may be adjusted to meet the needs of the individual patient. Approximately 30 kcal/kg of body weight are needed by the adult and 100 to 130 kcal/kg of body weight are needed by the infant daily for weight maintenance.[34] Additional calories must be provided if the individual is underweight. Glucose is the carbohydrate used most often for a source of calories. Solutions with concentrations of 25% to 35% can be used; however, this may lead to hyperglycemia, hyperinsulinemia, and hyperosmolar syndromes. Fructose, maltose, and xylitol have also been used, but these carbohydrates have not been approved for clinical use. Alcohol has been utilized as a source of calories, but large amounts cannot be infused because of the potential for liver damage.

Parenteral fat emulsions provide for a higher caloric intake in a smaller amount of fluid. This would eliminate the need for high concentrations of glucose in large volumes. These fat emulsions had been used in the United States, but they were withdrawn from use for a period of time because of complications. A parenteral solution containing 40% to 50% of kilocalories from a 10% soya bean oil (Intralip, Pharmocia, Stockholm, Sweden) and a casein hydrolysate was tested for 31 days with 48 patients.[37] Maintenance of weight was attained with 32.5 kcal/kg of body weight per day. The lipid was rapidly cleared from the plasma, and no ill effects were noted. Positive nitrogen balance was attained. The complications associated with high concentrations of glucose were avoided.

When a fat emulsion was administered to 10 preterm infants 31 to 36 weeks old, chylomicrons appeared in the serum 40 minutes after injection and prebeta lipoprotein was seen in only one baby.[38] However, five small-for-date babies 36 to 41 weeks of age all showed prebeta lipoprotein after the lipid injection. Chylomicrons were noted 40 to 120 minutes after the lipid infusion. In a second study, 0.15 g of fat emulsion per kilogram of body weight was given hourly. The small-for-date babies had prebeta lipoprotein in the blood prior to the injection. This fraction also appeared in the plasma of the preterm babies, but in most instances it was after several lipid injections. After eight injections, the small-for-date babies had two to three times the amount of total plasma lipids as did the preterm infants. Two hours after the intravenous injection of heparin, the plasma lipid levels of the small-for-term babies were similar to those of the preterm infants. It was suggested that the heparin served to activate the enzyme lipoprotein lipase. When lipid is used in parenteral alimentation for small-for-date babies, a small dose of heparin should be administered.

The product currently being used is Intralipid (Cutter Laboratories). It contains 10% soybean oil, 1.2% egg lecithin, and 2.25% glycerol. One liter provides 1100 kcal. Since the osmolality is 280 milliosmoles per kilogram of water, it can be infused into a peripheral vein. Adverse reactions such as chills, fever, thrombocytopenia, and fatty liver are seen in some individuals. In such cases the use of the fat emulsion must be discontinued.

Three patients on total parenteral nutrition received Intralipid as a replacement for 40% of total glucose nonprotein calories.[39] The infusion time was reduced from 12 to 8 hours. Nitrogen balance remained positive, and the abnormal triene-tetraene ratio was corrected. Fasting plasma cholesterol levels were significantly higher. The use of Intralipid shortens the infusion time, and thus it would be useful for home parenteral nutrition.

Intralipid was used as the main source of kilocalories for 64 days for one patient.[40] Parenteral nutrition was stopped, but the patient refused to take food. Parenteral nutrition was administered again, but the patient died of sepsis 16 days later. An autopsy revealed free fat droplets and extreme foamy swelling of the cytoplasm of the reticuloendothelial cells in the organs that were examined. The recommended dose of Intralipid is 1 to 2 g of fat per kilogram of body weight per day, but the patient had received 2.0 to 2.5 g fat per kilogram per day for 80 days. The authors recommended that no more than 2.0 g fat per kilogram per day should be administered along with the monitoring of liver function and serum lipid levels.

Greene et al. observed that serum triglycerides were elevated in 20 normal subjects who had been infused with 500 ml of 10% Intralipid.[41] Pulmonary diffusion capacity decreased as a result of the Intralipid-induced lipemia. Therefore patients with preexisting pulmonary or vascular disease may be at risk from the lipemia produced by the infusion of Intralipid.

Essential fatty acid deficiency has been reported in infants receiving parenteral alimentation.[42,43] One infant who underwent parenteral feeding 18 days after birth showed deficiency symptoms after 6 months.[42] An enterocutaneous fistula would not heal, and scaly skin lesions, poor hair growth, and thrombocytopenia became evident. Fatty acid levels of subcutaneous fat and plasma indicated an essential fatty acid deficiency. Other researchers have suggested that the trienoic-tetraenoic fatty acid ratio is a better indicator of the degree of deficiency than is the measure of polyunsaturated fatty acids.[43] An intravenous infusion of 10% Intralipid was administered to the depleted infant for 13 days.[42] The symptoms improved, and the infant gained weight. The enterocutaneous fistula closed, and a duodenoileostomy was performed. Healing proceeded normally. Later the infant was able to take food orally. The essential fatty acid deficiency in other infants has been reversed by oral feeding.[43]

Two infants on total parenteral nutrition and four infants being fed medium-chain triglycerides developed an essential fatty acid deficiency.[44] Plasma, platelet, and red blood cell levels of linoleic and arachidonic acid were decreased, while 5, 8, 11-eicosatrienoic acid levels increased. Intravenous administration of Intralipid reversed the deficiency state.

Adults generally do not develop essential fatty acid deficiency because of large body stores. An essential fatty acid deficiency developed in four undernourished patients who were on fat-free, total parenteral nutrition for 3 weeks.[45] The deficiency was detected by measuring the triene-tetraene fatty acid ratio, as no clinical symptoms were evident. Since these patients were undernourished, their body supply of essential fatty acids most likely had been depleted. The deficiency was reversed by the oral administration of safflower oil.

However, in another study essential fatty acid deficiency developed in four patients by the second week of total parenteral nutrition.[46] At the end of the fifth week of therapy three other patients were deficient as evidenced by a triene-tetraene ratio greater than 0.4. One patient who was also deficient in zinc developed a scaly

Table 9-5. Total parenteral nutrition solutions (nitrogen source)

Solution	Company	Composition
FreAmine	McGaw Laboratories	8.5% crystalline amino acids + electrolytes
Aminosol	Abbott Laboratories	5% fibrin hydrolysate + electrolytes
Amigen	Baxter Laboratories	5% casein hydrolysate + electrolytes
Polynute	Cutter Laboratories	7% casein hydrolysate + electrolytes

eczemoid dermatitis. Plasma tocopherol levels fell during therapy and in three individuals reached a level indicative of vitamin E deficiency. There was no clinical evidence of the vitamin deficiency. The essential fatty acid deficiency was corrected by the oral administration of fat. Others have corrected the biochemical defect by topical application of 2 to 3 mg of linoleic acid per kilogram per day.[47]

Positive nitrogen balance can be achieved during total parenteral nutrition. The nitrogen is supplied either by a mixture of *l*-amino acids or protein hydrolysates (see Table 9-5). Casein and fibrin hydrolysates have been used. These are not totally hydrolyzed, and about 40% of the nitrogen is in the form of peptides. Much of this nitrogen is not used. Amino acids are added to these hydrolysates to improve the nutritive quality. The minimum daily requirements for amino acids are used to determine the concentration of amino acids in the mixtures and for supplementation of the hydrolysates; however, these requirements are based on intestinal absorption, and it is not known what effect parenteral administration has on amino acid requirements. The patients being fed in this manner are ill, and most likely their amino acid requirements are higher and similar to the requirements during growth. One or more of the essential amino acids may be needed in higher amounts, or a nonessential amino acid may now be essential. Information is needed as to the concentrations of the amino acids in the infusion mixture.

Nitrogen balance studies and blood aminograms indicated that an amino acid mixture was better than a casein hydrolysate.[48] After infusion of a casein hydrolysate the plasma levels of methionine plus cystine and phenylalanine plus tyrosine did not increase, and thus these amino acids are limiting. Plasma aminograms can be used to determine the efficiency of amino acid mixtures. This same technique was used to evaluate the effectiveness of a fibrin hydrolysate (Aminosol) and an amino acid mixture (FreAmine). Nitrogen retention was greater with the amino acid mixture.[49] The plasma amino acid ratios indicated that valine and phenylalanine are the limiting amino acids in the fibrin hydrolysate. These amino acids appear in the peptide portion of fibrin; therefore, these peptides are poorly metabolized.

Metabolic acidosis has been observed in infants after parenteral administration of amino acid mixtures and casein hydrolysates.[50-52] The pH and titratable acidity (TA) of three amino acid mixtures and eight intravenous solutions were measured.[53] The TA is a measure of the hydrogen available for buffering from the pH of the solution to the physiological pH, 7.4. The mean pH (5.3) of three amino acid mixtures, Fre-Amine, Amigen, and Hyprotigen, was similar to that of eight commonly used intravenous solutions (5.92). However, the mean TA of the latter solutions is 0.13 mEq/L, while the mean TA of the amino acid mixtures was 30.54 mEq/L. Therefore when the amino acid solutions are infused it would take 30.54 mEq of bicarbonate and non-bicarbonate buffers for neutralization, and this might result in metabolic acidosis.

Four premature infants and one 14-year-old child on total parenteral nutrition developed acidosis as a result of excessive exogenous hydrogen ion.[51] The older child was able to compensate for the acidosis in 3 to 4 days. The inability of the infants to respond to acid-base disturbances might have been caused by immature kidneys. Dilution of the amino acid mixtures resulted in a less acidogenic solution. The acidosis in the infants was corrected by infusion of sodium bicarbonate.

Eleven infants who were infused with a mixture of amino acids developed hyperchloremic metabolic acidosis.[50] There was a decrease in blood pH and in the amount of excess base and bicarbonate. Metabolic acidosis did not appear after infusion of fibrin hydrolysate. An increased loss of base through the gastrointestinal tract or kidney or excessive titratable acidity was not the cause of the acidosis in these children. The authors suggested that the metabolism of cationic amino acids causes the release of hydrogen ions, and thus acidosis results. The mixture of the amino acids contained an excess of cations, namely, lysine, histidine, and arginine. The lack of anionic amino acids would necessitate their de novo synthesis, which would result in the release of more hydrogen ions. Others suggested that the acidosis was caused by three to five times as much chloride plus sulfate as sodium plus potassium.[52] The protein hydrolysates contain higher concentrations of anions than cations.

The amino acids glutamic, aspartic, and cysteic acids have been found to be neurotoxic.[54] Subcutaneous injections of fibrin and casein hydrolysates used for parenteral nutrition were injected into mice. All the doses of the casein hydrolysate and the two highest doses of the fibrin hydrolysate produced acute degeneration of neurons in the hypothalamus. This damage has been observed previously in animals receiving amino acids via oral or parenteral administration. It was suggested that low concentrations of acidic amino acids should be used in solutions for total parenteral nutrition. Infants given protein hydrolysates parenterally do not show elevated levels of glutamic and aspartic acids.[55] Since brain damage does not occur unless the levels are elevated, others have concluded that the solutions are safe for human use.

Vitamins and minerals must be added to the parenteral solutions. The commercial vitamin mixtures for infusion do not contain all the needed vitamins.[34] These must be added to the infusion mixture or given by intramuscular injection. The requirements for parenterally administered vitamins are not known. Therefore it is possible to develop hypovitaminosis or hypervitaminosis in the case of the fat-soluble vitamins. A majority of patients on total parenteral nutrition were found initially to have serum deficiencies of vitamins A, C, and folate.[56] During alimentation, vitamins were added daily. A few patients still had below normal limits for vitamin C and folate. None of the patients were deficient in vitamin B_{12}. The authors made recommendations for parenteral vitamin requirements for vitamins A, D, C, B_{12}, and folate. Others have made recommendations for the concentrations of vitamins A, D, E, thiamine, riboflavin, niacin, B_6, pantothenic acid, folacin, ascorbic acid, B_{12}, and biotin for pediatric and adult formulations.[57] Vitamin requirements are affected by many factors; therefore, further research is indicated as to the most appropriate concentrations for parenteral solutions.

Zinc, copper, and chromium deficiencies have been reported in patients on long-term total parenteral nutrition.[58-64] Bozian and Shearer analyzed the zinc, copper, and manganese content of four amino acid and protein hydrolysates used for total parenteral nutrition.[65] All the formulas contained low levels of copper and manganese; copper should be supplemented, but it is not known whether the manganese content is adequate. The casein hydrolysates Amigen and Polynute contained adequate amounts of zinc.

Haver and Kaminski analyzed commercially prepared, total parenteral nutrition solutions of amino acids, protein hydrolysates, dextrose, lipid, and water for zinc, copper, iron, magnesium, and chromium.[66] There was a wide range of values between case lots of the same manufacturers and also with different manufacturers. The greatest differences were observed for zinc and iron content. It was recommended that the serum and urine levels of trace metals be monitored in patients on long-term total parenteral nutrition. Herlihy et al. summarized the recommendations of Dudrick and Shils for the trace elements chromium, cobalt, copper, fluorine, iodine, iron, manganese, and zinc.[57] As with vitamins, additional research is needed to determine the requirements for the trace elements.

Home total parenteral nutrition

Patients have been maintained on home parenteral nutrition for several years.[67-69] Solutions can be infused at night by means of a pump equipped with an alarm system.[67] More mobility can be provided by use of a battery pack. Jeejeebhoy et al. used a different infusion technique[68,69] in which Intralipid is infused for 2 to 3 hours by gravity drip. Then a pneumatic pressure system is used to infuse the amino acid, glucose, vitamin, and trace element mixture overnight while the patient sleeps. No alarm system is necessary.

Several patients have been able to resume normal daily routines. It is possible that small-bowel transplants will be feasible in the future, and then these patients will be able to discontinue total parenteral nutrition.

Complications

Although total parenteral nutrition is beneficial to the patient, there are many problems associated with this type of feeding.[70] Complications may arise as a result of solution preparation and catheter insertion and care. Fungal infections appear frequently, necessitating strict adherence to aseptic techniques. The following metabolic consequences can occur: dehydration, overhydration, hyperosmolar coma, hypoglycemia, metabolic acidosis, deficiencies (vitamins, trace minerals, and essential fatty acids), excesses (vitamins A and D), allergic reactions, pyrogenic reactions, and hepatic encephalopathy.

Further research is needed on dietary requirements of nutrients administered parenterally for different age groups. In disease states patients have different metabolic needs, and thus the compositions of the formulas can be varied to correct imbalances. For example, the amino acid composition for patients with liver failure would differ from that provided for renal patients.

The care of the medical and surgical patient requires the expertise of many professionals. In 1972 an Alimentation Group was formed at Boston City Hospital to provide specialized nutritional care for critically ill patients.[71] The group is composed of staff physicians, therapeutic dietitians, a nurse specializing in the care of patients receiving total parenteral nutrition, a biochemist, research assistants, and research workers. The Alimentation Group advises and supervises parenteral feeding and the use of intravenous solutions and elemental diets, conducts nutrition education for the team, and engages in clinical research. This group has been successful in managing the therapy of several high-risk patients.

The therapeutic dietitian functions as a team member and makes recommendations as to the nutritional care of the patient and participates in the education program of the house staff. The program has resulted in increased referrals and improved management of patient care.

MEDIUM-CHAIN TRIGLYCERIDES

The fat that is present in the diet is almost entirely present in the form of triglycerides. The fatty acids found in these triglycerides are palmitic, stearic, oleic, linoleic, and longer chain polyenoic acids. Only a small percentage of short-chain fatty acids appear in foods. A commercial product, MCT (medium-chain triglycerides), has been developed and is composed of esters of glycerol with saturated medium-chain fatty acids. MCT contains octanoic acid (80%), decanoic acid (17%), and 1% each of hexanoic and dodecanoic acid.[72] Coconut oil is hydrolyzed into its component fatty acids. These are then separated into fractions by molecular distillation. The fraction containing primarily octanoic and decanoic acid is then esterified with glycerol to form MCT. MCT provides 8.3 kcal per gram.

These medium-chain triglycerides are hydrolyzed more rapidly in the intestine than the longer chain fats are. Bile salts are not needed for the digestion or absorption of the fatty acids into the portal vein. The medium-chain fatty acids are carried directly to the liver. The longer chain fatty acids must be resynthesized into chylomicrons and absorbed into the lacteals and then finally into the bloodstream. The medium-chain fatty acids are oxidized into carbon dioxide, ketone bodies, and other metabolites. These fatty acids do not appear to any great extent in the lipoprotein fractions and extrahepatic tissues. A hypoglycemic effect exerted by these fatty acids is not the result of increased insulin secretion or increased peripheral uptake of glucose.

MCT has been used effectively in patients with impaired fat digestion and absorption. The treatment with MCT has reduced the steatorrhea associated with chyluria, chylothorax, pancreatitis, cystic fibrosis, tropical and nontropical sprue, biliary atresia, gastrectomy, small bowel resection, chronic liver disease, and chylomicronemia.[73] An MCT oil and a complete dietary product, Portagen, are available from the Mead Johnson Company. Portagen contains sodium caseinate, MCT oil, corn oil, corn syrup solids, sugar, vitamins, and minerals. It contains less than 0.15% lactose. Medium-chain triglycerides account for 95% of the fat content. The MCT oil can be used in food preparation in a variety of ways.[73] Recipes using MCT are available.[73-76]

REFERENCES

1. Kark, R. M.: Liquid formulas and chemically defined diets, J. Am. Diet. Assoc. **64:**476, 1974.
2. Felig, P.: Intravenous nutrition: fact and fancy, N. Engl. J. Med. **294:**1455, 1976.
3. Blackburn, G. L., et al.: Peripheral intravenous feeding with isotonic amino acid solutions, Am. J. Surg. **125:**447, 1973.
4. Blackburn, G. L., et al.: Protein sparing therapy during periods of starvation with sepsis or trauma, Ann. Surg. **177:**588, 1973.
5. Flatt, J. P., and Blackburn, G. L.: The metabolic fuel regulatory system: implications for protein-sparing therapies during caloric deprivation and disease, Am. J. Clin. Nutr. **27:**175, 1974.
6. Hoover, H. C., Jr., et al.: Nitrogen-sparing intravenous fluids in postoperative patients, N. Engl. J. Med. **293:**172, 1975.
7. Greenberg, G. R., et al.: Protein-sparing therapy in postoperative patients, N. Engl. J. Med. **294:**1411, 1976.
8. Isenberg, J. I., and Maxwell, V.: Intravenous infusion of amino acids stimulates gastric acid secretion in man, N. Engl. J. Med. **298:**27, 1978.
9. Crenshaw, C.: Nutritional support for burn patients. In Intake: perspectives in clinical nutrition, Norwich, N.Y., 1973, Eaton Laboratories.
10. Curreri, P. W., Richmond, D., Marvin, J., and Baxter, C. R.: Dietary requirements of patients with major burns, J. Am. Diet. Assoc. **65:**415, 1974.
11. Long, J. M., and Pruitt, B. A.: Ross Laboratories dietetic currents: nutritional care of the burn patient, J. Am. Diet. Assoc. **64:**309, 1974.
12. Holli, B. R., and Oakes, J. B.: Feeding the burned child, J. Am. Diet. Assoc. **67:**240, 1975.
13. Larkin, J. M., and Moylan, J. A.: Complete enteral support of thermally injured patients, Am. J. Surg. **131:**722, 1976.
14. Pennisi, V. M.: Monitoring the nutritional care of burned patients, J. Am. Diet. Assoc. **69:**531, 1976.
15. Schuman, B. M.: Tube feeding using a food pump, Am. Fam. Physician **5(3):**85, 1972.
16. Gormican, A., Liddy, E., and Thrush, L. B.: Nutritional status of patients after extended tube feeding, J. Am. Diet. Assoc. **63:**247, 1973.
17. O'Hara, J. G., Kennedy, S., and Lizewski, W.: Effects of long-term elemental nasogastric feeding on elderly debilitated patients, Can. Med. Assoc. J. **108:**977, 1973.
18. Randall, H. T.: Diet and nutrition in the care of surgical patients. In Goodhart, R. S., and Shils, M. E., editors: Modern nutrition in health and disease, ed 5, Philadelphia, 1973, Lea & Febiger.
19. Shils, M. E., editor: Defined formula diets for medical purposes, Chicago, 1977, American Medical Association.
20. Walike, B. C., and Walike, J. W.: Relative lactose intolerance. A clinical study of tube-fed patients, J.A.M.A. **238:**948, 1977.
21. Shils, M. E., Bloch, A. S., and Chernoff, R.: Liquid formulas for oral and tube feeding, Clinical Bulletin Memorial Sloan-Kettering Cancer Center **6(4):**151, 1976.
22. Chernoff, R., and Bloch, A. S.: Liquid feed-

ings: considerations and alternatives, J. Am. Diet. Assoc. **70**:389, 1977.

23. Gormican, A., and Liddy, E.: Nasogastric tube feedings, Postgrad. Med. **53**:71, 1973.

24. Wells, D., and Zachman, R.: Nasojejunal feedings in low birth weight infants, J. Pediatr. **84**:909, 1974.

25. Cheek, J. A., and Staub, G. F.: Nasojejunal alimentation for premature and full-term newborn infants, J. Pediatr. **82**:955, 1973.

26. MacLean, W. C., Jr., and Graham, G. G.: Evaluation of an isosmotic tube feeding formula in the diets of convalescent malnourished infants and children, Am. J. Clin. Nutr. **29**: 496, 1976.

27. Winitz, M., Seedman, D. A., and Graff, J.: Studies in metabolic nutrition employing chemically defined diets. I. Extended feeding of normal human adult males, Am. J. Clin. Nutr. **23**:525, 1970.

28. Copelan, H., Lachance, P., and Mohammed, K.: Short-term effects on feeding an elemental diet in healthy men, Nutr. Rep. Intern. **8**: 49, 1973.

29. Miller, J. M., and Taboado, J. C.: Clinical experience with an elemental diet, Am. J. Clin. Nutr. **28**:46, 1975.

30. McCamman, S., Beyer, P. L., and Rhodes, J. B.: A comparison of three defined formula diets in normal volunteers, Am. J. Clin. Nutr. **30**:1655, 1977.

31. Simko, V., and Linscheer, W. G.: Absorption of different elemental diets in short-bowel syndrome lasting 15 years, Am. J. Dig. Dis. **21**:419, 1976.

32. Zabel, N. L., et al.: Selenium content of commercial formula diets, Am. J. Clin. Nutr. **31**: 850, 1978.

33. Dudrick, S. J., and Rhoads, J. E.: New horizons for intravenous feeding, J.A.M.A. **215**: 939, 1971.

34. Shils, M. E.: Guidelines for total parenteral nutrition, J.A.M.A. **220**:1721, 1972.

35. Dudrick, S. J., and Ruberg, R. L.: Principles and practice of parenteral nutrition, Gastroenterology **61**:901, 1971.

36. Heird, W. C., and Winters, R. W.: Total parenteral nutrition, J. Pediatr. **86**:2, 1975.

37. Zohrab, W. J., McHattie, J. D., and Jeejeebhoy, K. N.: Total parenteral alimentation with lipid, Gastroenterology **64**:583, 1973.

38. Intravenous nutrition of newborn infants with lipid, Nutr. Rev. **32**:298, 1974.

39. Broviac, J. W., Riella, M. C., and Scribner, B. H.: The role of Intralipid in prolonged parenteral nutrition. I. As a caloric substitute for glucose, Am. J. Clin. Nutr. **29**:255, 1976.

40. Freund, V., et al.: Iatrogenic lipidosis following prolonged intravenous hyperalimentation, Am. J. Clin. Nutr. **28**:1156, 1975.

41. Greene, H. L., Hazlett, D., and Demaree, R.: Relationship between Intralipid-induced hyperlipemia and pulmonary function, Am. J. Clin. Nutr. **29**:127, 1976.

42. Caldwell, M. D., Jonsson, H. T., and Othersen, H. B.: Essential fatty acid deficiency in an infant receiving prolonged parenteral alimentation, J. Pediatr. **81**:894, 1972.

43. Fat free parenteral alimentation of infants, Nutr. Rev. **32**:134, 1974.

44. Hirono, H., et al.: Essential fatty acid deficiency induced by total parenteral nutrition and by medium-chain triglyceride feeding, Am. J. Clin. Nutr. **30**:1670, 1977.

45. Richardson, T. J., and Sgoutas, E.: Essential fatty acid deficiency in four adult patients during total parenteral nutrition, Am. J. Clin. Nutr. **28**:258, 1975.

46. Fleming, C. R., Smith, L. M., and Hodges, R. E.: Essential fatty acid deficiency in adults receiving total parenteral nutrition, Am. J. Clin. Nutr. **29**:976, 1976.

47. Press, M., Hartop, P. J., and Prottey, C.: Correction of essential fatty acid deficiency in man by the cutaneous application of sunflowerseed oil, Lancet **1**:597, 1974.

48. Evaluation of amino acid mixtures for total parenteral nutrition, Nutr. Rev. **32**:236, 1974.

49. Long, C. L., Zikria, B. A., Kinney, J. M., and Geiger, J. W.: Comparison of fibrin hydrolysates and crystalline amino acid solutions in parenteral nutrition, Am. J. Clin. Nutr. **27**: 163, 1974.

50. Heird, W. C., et al.: Metabolic acidosis after intravenous alimentation with amino acids, N. Engl. J. Med. **287**:943, 1972.

51. Chan, J. C. M., Asch, M. J., Lin, S., and Hays, D. M.: Hyperalimentation with amino acid and casein hydrolysate solutions. Mechanism of acidosis, J.A.M.A. **220**:1700, 1972.

52. Metabolic acidosis in infants infused with commercial amino acid mixtures, Nutr. Rev. **31**:173, 1973.

53. Chan, J. C. M., Malekzadeh, M., and Hurley, J.: pH and titratable acidity of amino mixtures used in hyperalimentation, J.A.M.A. **220**:1119, 1972.

54. Olney, J. W., Ho, O. L., and Rhee, V.: Brain damaging potential of protein hydrolysates, N. Engl. J. Med. **289**:391, 1973.

55. Editorial: Safety of hydrolysates in parenteral nutrition, N. Engl. J. Med. **289**:426, 1973.

56. Lowry, S. F., et al.: Parenteral vitamin requirements during intravenous feeding, Am. J. Clin. Nutr. **31**:2149, 1978.

57. Herlihy, P., Stanaszek, W. F., and Covington, T. R.: Total parenteral nutrition, J. Am. Diet. Assoc. **70**:279, 1977.

58. Vilter, R., et al.: Manifestations of copper deficiency in a patient with systemic sclerosis on intravenous hyperalimentation, N. Engl. J. Med. **291**:188, 1974.

59. Kay, R. G., et al.: A syndrome of acute zinc deficiency during total parenteral alimentation in man, Ann. Surg. **183**:331, 1976.

60. Tucker, S. B., et al.: Acquired zinc deficiency, J.A.M.A. **235**:2399, 1976.

61. Solomons, N. W., et al.: Plasma trace metals during total parenteral alimentation, Gastroenterology **70**:1022, 1976.

62. Fleming, C. R., Hodges,R. E., and Hurley, L. S.: A prospective study of serum copper and zinc levels in patients receiving total parenteral nutrition, Am. J. Clin. Nutr. **29**:70, 1976.

63. Arakawa, T., et al.: Zinc deficiency in two infants during total parenteral alimentation for diarrhea, Am. J. Clin. Nutr. **29**:197, 1976.

64. Jeejeebhoy, K. N., et al.: Chromium deficiency glucose intolerance and neuropathy reversed by chromium supplementation in a patient receiving long-term total parenteral nutrition, Am. J. Clin. Nutr. **30**:531, 1977.

65. Bozian, R. C., and Shearer, C.: Copper, zinc, and manganese content of four amino acid and protein hydrolysates, Am. J. Clin. Nutr. **29**:1331, 1976.

66. Haver, E. C., and Kaminski, M. V., Jr.: Trace metal profile of parenteral nutrition solutions, Am. J. Clin. Nutr. **31**:264, 1978.

67. Shils, M. E.: A program for total parenteral, nutrition at home, Am. J. Clin. Nutr. **28**:1429, 1975.

68. Jeejeebhoy, K. N., et al.: Total parenteral nutrition at home for 23 months without complication and with good rehabilitation, Gastroenterology **65**:811, 1973.

69. Jeejeebhoy, K. N., et al.: Total parenteral nutrition at home. Studies in patients surviving 4 months to 5 years, Gastroenterology **71**:943, 1976.

70. Law, D. H.: Current concepts in nutrition. Total parenteral nutrition, N. Engl. J. Med. **297**:1104, 1977.

71. Johnson, E. Q.: The therapeutic dietitian's role in the Alimentation Group, J. Am. Diet. Assoc. **62**:648, 1973.

72. Hashim, S. A.: Medium-chain triglycerides—chemical and metabolic aspects, J. Am. Diet. Assoc. **51**:221, 1967.

73. Schizas, A. A., Cremen, J. A., Larson, E., and O'Brien, R.: Medium-chain triglycerides—use in food preparation, J. Am. Diet. Assoc. **51**: 228, 1967.

74. Howard,B. D., and Morse, E. H.: Muffins and pastry made with medium-chain triglyceride oil, J. Am. Diet. Assoc. **62**:51, 1973.

75. Bowman, F.: MCT cookies, cakes and quick breads. Quality and acceptability, J. Am. Diet. Assoc. **62**:180, 1973.

76. Recipes using MCT oil and Portagen, Evansville, Ind., 1974, Mead Johnson & Co.

10 Inborn errors of metabolism

The term "inborn errors of metabolism" was first used by an English physician, Garrod, in 1909 to describe four diseases—albinism, alkaptonuria, cystinuria, and pentosuria. He stated that these diseases were caused by a block in a metabolic reaction. Later research proved that this was correct except in the case of cystinuria, in which the defect is the result of an error in a transport mechanism.

Inborn errors of metabolism are inherited biochemical disorders that are the result of a defect in the structure or function of a protein.[1-4] Some of these are common to all individuals. For example, many species, man included, do not have the genetic information to synthesize the enzyme that converts L-gulonolactone to ascorbic acid; thus vitamin C becomes a dietary essential. Most genetic disorders are rare. Medical advances make it possible to treat many of these disorders, and children who once died in infancy now survive to adulthood and are able to have children. There is concern that this will lead to an increase in these metabolic disorders.

The clinical expression of the metabolic disorders varies greatly. Some such as pentosuria, fructosuria, iminoglycinuria, and β-aminoisobutyric aciduria are asymptomatic. Other defects are so severe that death results in utero or early infancy. In other conditions, such as phenylketonuria, branched-chain ketoaciduria, or galactosemia, if treatment is not instituted early, severe mental retardation occurs. Symptoms of some disorders such as alkaptonuria are not expressed until adulthood.

DEFECTIVE PROTEINS

It is estimated that in the human there are approximately 600 different enzymes that control metabolic reactions and 1000 proteins that have a specific function. These proteins can be composed of several hundred amino acids or can be simple peptides made up of as few as three amino acids. When the cell undergoes the complex process of protein biosynthesis, it is possible to make a mistake and synthesize the protein incorrectly. Approximately 300 such defects or inborn errors of metabolism have been diagnosed. Of these about 200 involve the synthesis of the respiratory pigment, hemoglobin. The protein portion of hemoglobin consists of four chains and a total of 574 amino acids, yet if one amino acid, valine, is substituted for glutamic acid, the three-dimensional structure is disrupted and gives rise to an abnormal hemoglobin. As a result the shape of the erythrocytes changes, and so the disorder is called sickle cell anemia. The altered structure of the hemoglobin diminishes its capacity to carry oxygen.

Other inborn errors of metabolism are caused by loss of enzymatic activity. In the affected individual the enzyme is either completely absent or present at levels that are incompatible with normal cellular metabolism. Heterozygous individuals who carry the trait for the disease have lower levels of enzyme activity. Since enzymes are generally produced in excess of need, there are no ill effects. However, this defect can be passed on to the offspring.

Enzyme activity can be greatly decreased because of a loss of affinity for the substrate or an unstable configuration that leads to rapid destruction. Several inborn errors have been shown to be the result of the inability of the coenzyme to bind to the enzyme. Some metabolic reactions are catalyzed by two enzymes, and if one is missing, the reaction does not proceed. Disorders have been found resulting from a greatly increased activity of the enzyme. Other metabolic diseases are caused by transport membrane defects where the absence of a carrier protein results in the inability to absorb a substance or substances. These defects may be found in one site or tissue or in several sites or tissues.

RESULTS OF ENZYMATIC DEFECTS

The sequence of reactions in Fig. 10-1 illustrates the ways in which metabolism can be altered because of an enzymatic defect and thus result in an inherited disorder. Reaction 1 illustrates a membrane transport defect in which the substrate S cannot enter the cell perhaps because of the lack of a carrier protein. This is the situation that exists in glucose-galactose malabsorption. Glucose and galactose cannot be absorbed from the intestine or proximal tubule of the kidney.

An inborn error of metabolism may be caused by a lack of an enzyme to metabolize the substrate. For example, in hereditary galactokinase deficiency, galactose (S) cannot be converted to galactose-1-phosphate (A) as in reaction 2. The precursor galactose accumulates and results in cataract formation.

In other instances, when the primary reaction is blocked, alternate pathways are used. In phenylketonuria, phenylalanine (A) cannot be converted to tyrosine (B—reaction 3) but instead is converted to phenylethyl amine (E—reaction 4) and phenylpyruvic acid (F—reaction 5). Phenylpyruvic acid is converted to phenyllactic acid

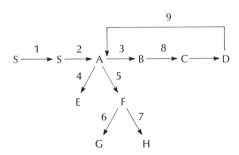

Fig. 10-1. Possible enzymatic defects in a metabolic sequence.

(reaction 6) and phenylacetic acid (reaction 7). These metabolites can be detected in the urine of phenylketonurics.

Enzyme activity can be normal, but a metabolic disorder can arise because the binding of the coenzyme to the enzyme is abnormal (reaction 8). This is the situation in vitamin B_6 dependency. It is thought that glutamic acid is not decarboxylated to γ-aminobutyric acid because the enzyme glutamic acid decarboxylase does not bind the coenzyme pyridoxal phosphate. The defect can be overcome by supplying vitamin B_6 in excessive amounts.

A block in the beginning of a metabolic sequence (reaction 3) renders the cell unable to synthesize an essential product, D, further along the normal pathway. In albinism the enzyme tyrosinase is inactive, and tyrosine cannot be metabolized through a sequence of reactions to melanin. Since this compound is responsible for pigmentation, individuals with this enzymatic defect are light skinned and have white hair.

The inability to synthesize the final product in a metabolic sequence may give rise to an inborn error of metabolism in still another way. In some reactions the final product (D) serves to inhibit a reaction (9) early in the sequence. This reaction is shut off so that the product is not made in excessive amounts. This occurs in congenital goitrous cretinism. Inadequate amounts of thyroxine do not stop the release of the thyroid stimulating hormone. Thus the gland continues to enlarge in an attempt to make more thyroxine.

DNA

The information by which the cell carries out its metabolism and transmits its characteristics to a daughter cell is found in DNA. This nucleoprotein is found only in the nucleus. It consists of hundreds of nucleotides conjugated to protein. The nucleotides are composed of nitrogen bases and the sugar deoxyribose. Each unit is hooked through a phosphate bond from the 3′ position of the deoxyribose of one nucleotide to the 5′ position of the deoxyribose of the next unit. DNA consists of two of these chains that are held together by hydrogen bonds, which results in the formation of a double helix. The variation is then in the sequence of the nitrogen bases. Four are found—two purines, adenine and guanine, and two pyrimidines, cytosine and thymine. Information is stored by means of the sequencing of these nitrogen bases.

PROTEIN BIOSYNTHESIS

The site of protein biosynthesis in the cell is the ribosome that is attached to the endoplasmic reticulum. This channel runs from the nuclear membrane to the external cellular membrane. For anabolism to proceed, all the necessary amino acids must be present. The first step involves the activation of the amino acids with ATP to form an amino acid adenylate complex. Transfer RNA (tRNA) is a polynucleotide similar to DNA. It contains the sugar ribose in place of deoxyribose and the nitrogen base uracil instead of thymine. The sequence of nitrogen bases in the tRNA forms the preliminary coding system in that each tRNA selects only one amino acid. Since there are approximately 20 structural amino acids, there are 20 tRNA. The information for the synthesis of the protein resides in the DNA in the nucleus. The double helix unwinds, and a complementary strand of messenger RNA (mRNA) is synthesized. The mRNA functions as a tape with all the information and leaves the nucleus for the ribosome. A ribosomal particle reads the information on the tape. The codon in mRNA is matched to the anticodon on tRNA. The first amino acid in the protein sequence is formylmethionine. The amino acids are brought by the tRNA to the mRNA, and the peptide bonds are formed one at a time until the last amino acid is added. The protein is released, and the amino acids in the primary structure now determine the secondary, tertiary, or quaternary structure. Several ribosomal particles can read mRNA at a time, so adequate amounts of protein are synthesized. Once the process is completed, the mRNA is destroyed. The next time the protein is synthesized, the DNA makes another mRNA.

The mRNA consists of a triplet codon. Three nitrogen bases code for each amino acid. There are four different nitrogen bases, which allows for 64 possibilities on the basis of a triplet code. Therefore there are several different codons for each amino acid. This ensures that the amino acid is brought to the mRNA more easily.

The original programming of nitrogen bases can be altered in the DNA and thus give rise to a mutant. The sequence of nitrogen bases can be changed by deletions, additions, or substitutions; this results in the synthesis of another protein with a different amino acid sequence. This may render the protein inactive. Mutations can be caused by a variety of chemicals such as acridine, lysergic acid, nitrous acid, and bromouracil. Radiation from x-rays, gamma rays, and ultraviolet light and extremes of pH and high temperatures can bring about a change in the nitrogen-base sequence of DNA.

INHERITANCE

The genetic information of the cell for inherited characteristics is passed from one generation to another. In humans the nucleus of the cell contains 46 chromosomes or 23 pairs. One pair is known as the sex chromosomes. In the female this is expressed as XX, while in the male it is XY. The other 22 pairs of chromosomes are called autosomes, and they are concerned with characteristics other than sex. The chromosomes are made up of thousands of the basic units of heredity called genes. The genes are arranged in a linear order in the chromosome. The locus refers to the site of the gene in the chromosomes. If this gene undergoes a mutation, this altered trait is then passed on to succeeding generations.

In 1959 Beadle and Tatum proposed the one gene–one enzyme concept. All metabolic processes in a cell are controlled by genes. One gene controls one enzyme. The mutation of one gene renders the cell incapable of carrying out one chemical reaction. This theory is now called the one cistron–one polypeptide concept. This would then include proteins that are not enzymes, since their synthesis is also under genic control. The cistron refers to the linear sequence of nucleotides in DNA that carry the information for the synthesis of a single polypeptide.

Most inborn errors of metabolism show an autosomal recessive mode of inheritance. This means that an affected parent has a one in four chance of producing a child with the same metabolic defect. Congenital spherocytosis and acute intermittent porphyria are two metabolic disorders that exhibit autosomal dominant inheritance. An affected parent who has a normal mate will have a one in two chance of having a child with the defect. In X-linked recessive inheritance the mutations must appear in both female X chromosomes, while the males carry the trait on the X chromosome. The defect is carried by women and expressed in their sons, while the men pass the disease through their daughters. The most well-known disease inherited in this manner is hemophilia. Familial hypophosphatemic rickets is inherited as an X-linked dominant trait. Both sexes are affected. A mother with this trait transmits the disease to half of her sons and daughters, while the father passes it to all his daughters and none of his sons.

DIAGNOSIS

Various physiological fluids can be used to detect the inborn errors of metabolism. Blood samples are used to test for phenylketonuria, galactosemia, hyperlipoproteinemias, and so forth. When a large segment of the population is screened, often blood samples are used. Such is the case for the detection of phenylketonuria. The degree of control of the disease is often followed by measuring the levels of the affected metabolite in the blood.

Urine samples have also been used for diagnosing the metabolic disorders. Alkaptonuria is easily detected, since the urine darkens on exposure to air. Abnormal urinary metabolites are found in pentosuria, cystinuria, and so on.

It is now possible to detect some disorders in utero by amniocentesis. Amniotic fluid is withdrawn from the sac surrounding the fetus. Cells from it are grown in tissue culture and then analyzed for chromosomes, enzymes, or a certain metabolite. The following inborn errors have been detected in utero: acid phosphatase deficiency, adrenogenital syndrome, branched-chain ketoaciduria, cystathioninuria, Fabry's disease, galactosemia, Gaucher's disease, homocystinuria, Hunter's syndrome, Hurler's syndrome, hypervalinemia, Krabbe's disease, Lesch-Nyhan syndrome, metachromatic leukodystrophy, methylmalonic aciduria, Niemann-Pick disease, Pompe's disease, Refsum's disease, and Tay-Sachs disease.

Tissue analysis for enzymes or various metabolites has been used to detect inborn errors. Another method involves growing human skin fibrinoblasts in tissue culture. The defect in citrullinemia and Refsum's disease was discovered by this procedure.

DETECTION OF CARRIERS

Much work has been done on devising tests for the detection of asymptomatic heterozygous carriers of these metabolic disorders. Genetic counseling services are available in some medical centers to inform parents about these metabolic diseases and the possibility of having an affected child; then amniocentesis may be performed during pregnancy if there is a possibility of one of the disorders that can be detected in this manner. If the fetus does have a metabolic defect that is fatal early in infancy, the parents may decide on an abortion.

For some inborn errors it is possible to determine the amount of the affected metabolite in a blood and urine sample of a carrier; however, in most instances heterozygous carriers show normal levels. It is then possible to perform an oral or parenteral load test, whereby a large dose of the metabolite is administered, and then blood samples are taken periodically to measure the amount that is still present. This has been done to test for carriers of galactosemia and phenylketonuria.

A tissue biopsy can be performed for the purpose of microscopic examination of the cells or the measurement of enzyme levels. The measurement of enzyme levels in skin fibroblasts grown in tissue culture has also been used for the detection of carriers.

TREATMENT

For many inborn errors of metabolism there is no treatment available at present; however, many different avenues are being investigated. One of the earliest methods of treatment involved dietary modification. This is successful only when the metabolite involved is an essential nutrient that must be ingested. Dietary treatment has no effect if the metabolite can be synthesized in vivo. Dietary treatment must be carefully monitored, for if the nutrient intake is too restrictive, growth retardation or even death may result. Several inborn errors of metabolism respond to massive doses of vitamins, such as vitamin B_6 or thiamine.

In every inborn error of metabolism a protein is either defective or missing; therefore, the aim of therapy is to supply this protein. Parenteral administration has been tried in several instances. A plasma fraction is used to treat hemophilia. Insulin is injected to treat diabetes. Fabry's disease has been treated by blood transfusions; however, this method is not very successful when dealing with enzyme defects. It is difficult to prepare sufficient quantities of enzymes for intravenous injection. In most instances the enzymes act inside the cell, and there is no evidence that the cells can take up the enzymes from the circulation. Perhaps it will be possible in the future to prepare a synthetic nonallergenic active core of an enzyme so that an immune response is not elicited from the recipient.

Some bacteria have been shown to repair their defective DNA; perhaps this can be done in human cells. One suggestion has been to inject a virus that carries the information to synthesize the correct protein into the individual with the disorder;

however, it is not known whether this would prove harmful over a long period of time.

Drugs have been administered in certain disorders to remove excessive amounts of the metabolite. Organ transplantation has also been tried. In cystinuria excessive cystine is deposited in the kidney and leads to renal failure. Kidney transplants have been tried, but eventually cystine deposits in the transplanted kidney. Liver transplants would be more useful, but at present these have not been successful.

Phillips added sperm cells to cultured mouse cells that could not divide because of a lack of the enzyme hypoxanthine-guanine phosphoribosyltransferase.[5] This corrected the defect, and the cells began to multiply, which led to the suggestion that this method might be used to treat inborn errors of metabolism. Cells from an individual with a genetic disorder and sperm from a normal individual could be grown in tissue culture. The cells would incorporate the genetic information to synthesize the missing protein from the sperm and thus overcome the defect. When enough cells were available, they could be injected into the individual who would now have the genetic information to synthesize the protein.

DISORDERS OF CARBOHYDRATE METABOLISM[2,3,4]
Disaccharidase deficiency

A deficiency of a disaccharidase such as maltase, isomaltase, sucrase, or lactase may result in diarrhea, distention, flatulence, and abdominal cramps as a result of the inability to digest the sugar. The most common disorder is lactase deficiency. When this occurs in infancy, a failure to thrive is also seen. All products that contain lactose must be omitted from the diet. The following commercial products may be used in place of milk: Meat-base formula and Lambase (Gerber Products Co.), Isomil (Ross Laboratories), Mull-Soy (Borden), Nutramigen, Prosobee, and Sobee (Mead Johnson), and Soyalac (Loma).

Low lactase levels also appear in adults. The decrease in enzyme levels has been found by some researchers in children who are 5 years old.[6] A high percentage of lactose intolerance is found in non-Caucasians. Lactose intolerance appears in some adults who have normal lactase activity. A secondary lactase deficiency may appear in celiac disease or in sprue, cystic fibrosis, colitis, enteritis, and protein calorie malnutrition.

In the standard adult a lactose tolerance test of 50 g of lactose is given, and blood samples are taken for 2 hours. Lactose malabsorption is indicated when the blood glucose level is flat (not greater than the fasting level by 20 mg/dl). The individual is considered to be lactose intolerant when diarrhea, cramps, gas, and bloating develop during or after the test.[7] Questions have been raised as to whether this is a valid test. The amount of lactose consumed is equivalent approximately to that found in a quart of milk. This amount would not normally be consumed in this short period of time. In addition, the rise in blood glucose does not always correlate with lactase activity. Therefore a more definitive diagnosis requires a biopsy of jejunal mucosa for the assay of lactase.

Another method that was found to correlate well with the standard lactose tolerance test and the lactase assay in jejunal biopsies was the 1-^{14}C lactose breath test.[8] In this test 1-^{14}C lactose was administered orally, breath was collected for 2 hours, and the $^{14}CO_2$ content was measured. Lower levels of radioactivity were found in the breath from individuals who were lactase deficient.

The measurement of respiratory hydrogen excretion has been found to be the most sensitive method for detecting lactose malabsorption in adults and children.[7] However, at the present time the methodology for the measurement of hydrogen is complex, and this limits the use of this test.

A lactose hydrolyzed milk has been prepared by heating milk with a lactase powder. Most lactose intolerant subjects are able to drink the 90% lactose hydrolyzed milk without any symptoms.[9-11] Although the milk is sweeter, it was acceptable to most individuals. This lactose hydrolyzed milk could also be used to prepare other low-lactose dairy products.

Hospital dietitians throughout the United States were surveyed as to the diets prescribed for adult lactose malabsorption.[12] Of those who responded, less than half had a lactose-free diet in their hospital manual. Six of the ninety-nine diets analyzed were galactose-free diets for galactosemia. This diet should not be prescribed for lactose malabsorption, since it is too restrictive. The remaining diets were classified as lactose-restricted, lactose-free, milk or dairy product–free, and low-lactose, and three had miscellaneous titles. The variations were primarily due to the amount of lactose allowed, and almost all the diets listed foods that were and were not permitted. Yogurt and buttermilk were allowed in some hospital diets but not in others. Some permitted goats milk, while others banned molasses, sodium monoglutamate, alcohol, and some rather improbable dietary sources of lactose. The rationale for diet therapy did not indicate that there is great variation in lactose intolerance in adults of different ethnic backgrounds or that small amounts of lactose throughout the day are better tolerated than one large feeding.

Welsh recommended that the diets be titled lactose-free. A complete diet history should be taken before any prescription is issued. If eliminating some of the lactose-containing products does not alleviate the symptoms, then a diet containing 0-3 g lactose may be necessary. A listing of the lactose content of selected milk, milk products, and substitutes was compiled by Welsh for patients on lactose-restricted diets.[12] A semiquantitative method for the determination of lactose was used to measure the lactose content of a variety of foods and drugs.[13] This data is useful as some individuals are sensitive to small amounts of lactose.

Other disaccharidase deficiencies are extremely rare. Dietary treatment involves the removal of the offending sugar.

Fructosuria

In fructosuria the enzyme fructokinase is defective, and fructose is not converted to fructose-1-phosphate. As a result, the blood levels of fructose become elevated, and fructose spills over into the urine. There are no other symptoms, and treatment is not necessary.

Fructose intolerance (fructosemia)

The enzyme aldolase, which catalyzes both of the following reactions, is defective in fructose intolerance.

Fructose-1-phosphate → Dihydroxyacetone phosphate + Glyceraldehyde
Fructose-1,6-diphosphate → Dihydroxyacetone phosphate + Glyceraldehyde-3-phosphate

If an afflicted baby is fed fructose, he begins to vomit, becomes hypoglycemic, and refuses to eat. Hepatomegaly is a result of large amounts of glycogen or fat or both in the liver. The proximal tubules of the kidney are affected, and aminoaciduria, phosphaturia, glycosuria, and renal tubular acidosis occur as a result of this. The continued administration of fructose to these babies will result in death. However, if fructose is not fed in the diet until the child is 1 year of age, the symptoms are not severe, but hypoglycemia does appear. The treatment involves the removal of both sucrose-and fructose-containing foods in the diet.

Galactokinase deficiency

Galactokinase deficiency is a rather rare variation of galactosemia. Galactose cannot be converted to galactose-1-phosphate. The high levels of galactose spill over into the urine. The only result of this metabolic defect is the formation of cataracts. This can be avoided by omitting lactose from the diet, since this is the major source of galactose.

Galactosemia[14]

Galactosemics lack the enzyme galactose-1-phosphate uridyl transferase, which catalyzes the following reaction:

Galactose-1-phosphate + UDP-glucose → UDP-galactose + Glucose-1-phosphate

As a result, galactose-1-phosphate, galactose, and the sugar alcohol galactitol accumulate in the tissues. Infants with this disorder may have anorexia, vomiting, diarrhea, hypoglycemia, hepatosplenomegaly, jaundice, and, eventually, cirrhosis, aminoaciduria, and proteinuria. The untreated babies become mentally retarded and develop cataracts.

Later in life, another metabolic pathway is available. Galactose-1-phosphate can react directly with uridine triphosphate (UTP) to form uridine diphosphate (UDP)-galactose, thus bypassing the metabolic defect. However, this pathway is not functional in infancy, so treatment must be instituted early.

The dietary treatment of this inborn error of metabolism involves the removal of galactose and lactose from the diet. Not only must milk and milk products be excluded, but labels must be read carefully as lactose or milk products are added to many foods. Since infants cannot consume milk, a proprietary formula must be used. Nutramigen (Mead Johnson), a casein hydrolysate, and two meat-containing products, Lambase and Meat Base (Gerber Products Co.), are available. Many products, contain soy protein as an ingredient, namely, Isomil (Ross Laboratories), Mull-Soy (Borden), Prosobee, Sobee (Mead Johnson), and Soyalac (Loma). The use of these soybean products has been questioned. Raffinose and stachyose are galactose-containing oligosaccharides found in soybeans. It is not known whether they are hydrolyzed to galactose by the digestive enzymes; therefore, some physicians feel they should not be used for galactosemic infants. For the same reason, beets, peas, and lima beans should not be fed. Dietary treatment is continued while the central nervous system is developing to prevent mental retardation.

A food plan, recipes, and a listing of foods that may either be included or excluded from a galactose-free diet have been compiled by Acosta and Elsas.[14]

Disorders of glycogen metabolism

Glycogen is a polymer made up of glucose units held together in α-1,4 and 1,6 linkages. This polysaccharide is stored in liver and muscle. Fig. 10-2 illustrates the reactions involved in the synthesis and hydrolysis of glycogen. Glycogen storage diseases result from a lack of one of the enzymes found in these pathways. The result is either the formation of an abnormal form of glycogen or excessive amounts from increased synthesis or decreased degradation. The polysaccharide accumulates mainly in the liver or muscle.

Eight of these disorders have been elucidated. A ninth defect results in the inability to synthesize glycogen. Only types I and IX are responsive to dietary treatment.

Type I—Gierke's disease. A lack of liver glucose-6-phosphatase leads to hepatomegaly and enlarged kidneys because of the excessive deposition of glycogen. Hypoglycemia is the result of the inability of the liver to release glucose. Lipid metabolism increases, and as a result, fat is deposited in the liver, and xanthomas are formed. Hypoglycemia also inhibits the secretion of insulin, which is needed to stimulate protein biosynthesis, and thus growth is retarded.

In some instances the symptoms are severe, and the infants die before the age of two. Others may do well, and their symptoms may improve when they attain adolescence.

A portacaval shunt and total parenteral nutrition have been used as treatments.[15,16] Clofibrate is given to lower blood lipid levels.[17]

The dietary treatment consists of small frequent feedings of glucose to minimize hypoglycemia. Normal levels of protein are prescribed. Fat intake should be reduced. Medium-chain triglycerides have been used successfully to minimize the formation of xanthomas.

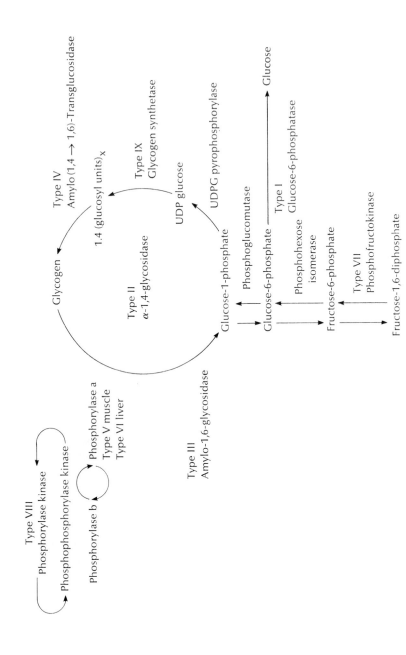

Fig. 10-2. Disorders of glycogen metabolism.

Three patients were treated with continuous intragastric feedings of Vivonex at night.[18] During the day time they received an oral feeding every 3 to 4 hours containing 60% to 70% calories as carbohydrates (high in starch), 15% calories as protein, and 13% to 25% calories as fat. The metabolic abnormalities and hepatic size were stabilized, and the patients showed an increased growth rate. It was suggested that the metabolic effects were due to the hormonal response to hypoglycemia. Thus frequent feedings to maintain normal blood glucose levels improved the metabolic and clinical effects that resulted from a deficiency of glucose-6-phosphatase.

Type II—Pompe's disease. Lysosomal acid maltase (α-1,4-glucosidase) is the enzyme missing in this disorder. Glycogen accumulates in the liver, heart, and muscle. Hepatomegaly, cardiomegaly, and muscle weakness are the most frequent symptoms. The involvement of the heart muscle most often results in early death.

Type III—Limit dextrinosis (debrancher glycogen storage disease). Since the debranching enzyme amylo-1,6-glucosidase is lacking, glycogen cannot be completely broken down. A limit dextrin is formed that still contains the branched glucose units. This short-chained glycogen is found in the liver, heart, and muscles.

Type IV—Amylopectinosis (Andersen's disease). An abnormal form of glycogen called amylopectin is synthesized in this metabolic disorder. The enzyme amylo-1,4 → 1,6-transglucosidase is defective, so a straight-chained amylopectin is synthesized instead of the highly branched normal glycogen. Hepatosplenomegaly and cirrhosis develop. Death occurs before the third year of life. This is a rare form of the glycogen storage diseases.

Type V—Muscle phosphorylase deficiency (McArdle's disease). In this disorder muscles are unable to break glycogen down, since the enzyme phosphorylase is missing. Energy is provided by glucose and fatty acids. Symptoms appear only during exercise, since the muscle cannot break down glycogen and so performs anaerobic metabolism to meet its increased energy needs. Blood lactate and pyruvate levels do not increase. Muscular pain and stiffness are observed during exercise. The treatment involves the intravenous administration of glucose.

Type VI—Liver phosphorylase deficiency (Hers' disease). Liver and muscle phosphorylase are different enzymes, so the metabolic defects occur independently of one another. When phosphorylase activity in the liver is reduced, large amounts of glycogen accumulate. Hypoglycemia and acidosis may also occur.

Type VII—Phosphofructokinase deficiency. This disorder is similar to McArdle's disease. Because of the lack of phosphofructokinase, anaerobic metabolism cannot proceed. Afflicted individuals exhibit muscular weakness and stiffness on physical exertion. Blood lactate levels do not increase.

Type VIII—Liver phosphorylase kinase deficiency. Phosphorylase cannot be converted to the active form because of a lack of the activating enzyme phosphorylase kinase. The only symptom is hepatomegaly. The heart and muscles are normal.

Type IX—Liver glycogen synthetase deficiency. A lack of the enzyme glycogen synthetase results in the inability to synthesize liver glycogen. Convulsive hypoglycemia is seen after an overnight fast. The treatment involves a high-protein diet with an additional meal at night.

Glucose-galactose malabsorption

Glucose-galactose malabsorption involves a defect in the active transport of glucose and galactose in the intestine and kidney. Fructose absorption is normal. Afflicted infants develop diarrhea, lose weight, and become dehydrated when milk is consumed; therefore, a formula that contains fructose as the carbohydrate should be fed. Older children may be able to tolerate small amounts of milk and starch.

A second case in an adult has been reported.[19] This 21-year-old male patient was fed a 2000 to 2500 kcal diet that contained 70 g of starch and 80 to 100 g of simple sugars. No lactose was fed. Extra calories were provided in the form of honey or fructose. On this regimen the patient's diarrhea improved, and he was able to gain weight.

Pentosuria

Pentosuria is a rare, harmless disorder that is found among Jews. As a result of the inactivity of the enzyme l-xylulose dehydrogenase, l-xylulose is not metabolized and instead is excreted in the urine. Normally this ketopentose is converted to xylitol and then to D-xylulose. The D-isomer then enters the pentose pathway.

DISORDERS OF LIPID METABOLISM[2-4,20,21]
Ceramide lactoside lipidosis

At present only one case of ceramide lactoside lipidosis has been described. The child was retarded and had foam cells in the bone marrow and an enlarged spleen and liver. Because of a lack of the enzyme ceramidelactoside-β-galactosidase, ceramide lactoside is not hydrolyzed to galactose and ceramide-glucose. As a result, ceramide lactoside accumulates in the tissues.

Fabry's disease

In Fabry's disease the glycolipid ceramide trihexoside accumulates in the tissues, especially the kidney glomeruli. A reddish purple skin rash appears in certain parts of the body. Corneal opacities, cardiac abnormalities, and edema may also develop. Because of a deficiency of the enzyme ceramidetrihexoside-α-galactosidase the terminal galactose is not hydrolyzed from ceramide-glucose-galactose-galactose.

The disorder is linked to the X chromosome, so that males are afflicted. Females show a mild manifestation of the disorder that is generally limited to the rash and corneal opacities.

Treatment by kidney transplantation or by intravenous infusion of human plasma has not been successful. Brady and his co-workers administered the human placental enzyme ceramidetrihexoside-α-galactosidase into two patients with Fabry's disease.[21,22] The liver took up a large portion of the enzyme. Both patients exhibited a decrease in circulating ceramide trihexoside. In 48 hours the levels had returned to preinjection levels.

Evidence suggests that the ceramide trihexoside that is deposited in the kidneys, blood vessels, and other tissues is brought to the site by the circulation.[21] Enzyme replacement then should reduce the amount of this compound.

Fucosidosis

Children with fucosidosis show cerebral degeneration, weakened and spastic muscles, emaciation, thickened skin, and cardiomegaly. The enzyme α-L-fucosidase is missing. The substrate for this enzyme is thought to be the fucoglycolipids that are found in red blood cells and in intestinal and other tissues.

Gaucher's disease

There are two forms of Gaucher's disease. The adult type is milder and characterized by hepatosplenomegaly and erosion of the cortices of the long bones and pelvis. The infantile form is more severe, and in addition the infants are mentally retarded.

A glucocerebroside (ceramide-glucose) accumulates in the reticuloendothelial cells of the liver, spleen, and bone marrow. Because of a deficiency of the enzyme glucocerebroside-β-glucosidase, glucose is not hydrolyzed from the glucocerebroside. The accumulation of this compound in the neurons is responsible for the brain damage in the infantile form.

Spleen and kidney transplantation have met with some success. When the enzyme glucocerebrosidase was injected into two patients, it was rapidly cleared from the blood.[21] The levels of liver and erythrocyte glucocerebroside decreased. This may be an effective means of therapy, since frequent injections are not necessary. The enzyme cannot cross the blood-brain barrier, so it would not be an effective method of treatment for the infantile form.

Generalized (G_{M1}) gangliosidosis

The ganglioside G_{M1} accumulates in the nervous system of individuals with generalized gangliosidosis. The clinical symptoms that occur are mental retardation, hepatomegaly, foam cells in the bone marrow, thinning of bones, and skeletal deformities, and in a majority of patients a cherry-red spot appears on the retina. The biochemical defect is because of a lack of the enzyme G_{M1}-β-galactosidase that hydrolyzes the terminal galactose from the G_{M1} ganglioside-ceramide-glucose-galactose-(N-acetylneuraminic acid)-N-acetylgalactosamine-galactose.

Globoid leukodystrophy (Krabbe's disease)

Infants with globoid leukodystrophy are severely mentally retarded. There is only a very small amount of brain myelin. Because of the deficiency of the enzyme galactocerebroside-β-galactosidase, galactocerebroside is not hydrolyzed into galactose and ceramide.

Metachromatic leukodystrophy

In the biochemical defect of metachromatic leukodystrophy, a sphingolipid, sulfatide, is not hydrolyzed by the enzyme sulfatidase into galactocerebroside and sulfuric acid. As a result, the sphingolipid accumulates in the tissues. There is a decrease in the conduction velocity of peripheral nerves. Two forms of the disorder have been identified. One type appears in infancy with severe mental retardation. In adulthood the initial symptoms are psychological changes with gradual mental deterioration. Enzyme replacement therapy has not been successful.

Niemann-Pick disease

In Niemann-Pick disease there is a deficiency of the enzyme sphingomyelinase, which hydrolyzes sphingomyelin to phosphorylcholine and ceramide. As a result, sphingomyelin accumulates in various tissues. This leads to hepatosplenomegaly, foam cells in the bone marrow, and severe mental retardation. In the infantile form of this disease, death occurs within 2 years. There is no treatment for this disease at present.

Tay-Sachs disease

Infants with Tay-Sachs disease are mentally retarded. A cherry-red spot appears on the retina of the eye and blindness develops. Death occurs by the age of 3.

The Tay-Sachs ganglioside (G_{M2}) accumulates in the neuronal cells of the brain. Normally this compound, ceramide-glucose-galactose-(N-acetylneuraminic acid)-N-acetylgalactosamine, is hydrolyzed by the enzyme G_{M2} hexosaminidase to ceramide-glucose-galactose-(N-acetylneuraminic acid) plus N-acetylgalactosamine. There are two isoenzymes—hexosaminidase A and B. In the "B-variant" of Tay-Sachs disease, the B isoenzyme exhibits normal activity, but the A enzyme activity is decreased. In the "O-variant" form (Sandhoff's disease) the activity of both enzymes is decreased.[23] In these individuals, globoside is found in other organs. A third form of the disease is the "AB variant" in which both enzymes are active, but the metabolism of the ganglioside (G_{M2}) is not normal.

Enzyme replacement therapy has been tried in this disorder.[7] However, the enzyme was removed from the circulation, but it did not pass the blood-brain barrier; the level of plasma globoside decreased. It is hoped that in the future either an alteration of the blood-brain barrier or genetic engineering may be feasible methods of therapy.

Tangier disease

Familial alpha lipoprotein deficiency is a rare disorder that is characterized by lymphadenopathy, orange tonsillar hyperplasia, hepatosplenomegaly, and the storage of cholesteryl esters, particularly in the reticuloendothelial cells. Plasma levels of cholesterol and the high-density lipoproteins are low.

Three patients with Tangier disease were found to have large, flattened, translucent particles in the plasma high-density lipoprotein fractions.[24] After 7 days of treatment with a diet containing 80% of calories from carbohydrate and less than 5 g of fat per day, it was found that there was a reduced number of these particles. This suggests that the abnormal products of chylomicron metabolism may be one of the sources of the cholesteryl esters that accumulate in the tissues.

Familial hyperlipoproteinemia

See Chapter 8, Cardiovascular Disease.

DISORDERS OF AMINO ACID METABOLISM[2-4,14,25,26]
Disorders of the urea cycle[27]

Five disorders caused by a deficiency of enzymes needed for the synthesis of urea have been described: carbamyl phosphate synthetase deficiency, ornithine trans-carbamylase deficiency, citrullinemia, argininosuccinic aciduria, and argininemia or lysine intolerance (see Fig. 10-3). Blood ammonia levels are elevated in all these inborn errors of metabolism.

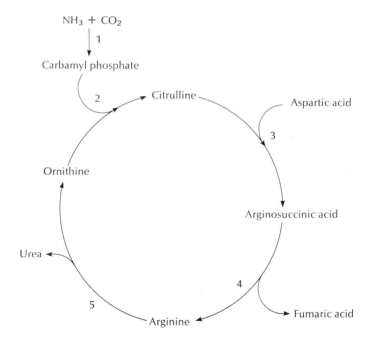

1 Carbamyl phosphate synthetase
2 Ornithine transcarbamylase
3 Argininosuccinate synthetase
4 Argininosuccinate lyase
5 Arginase

Fig. 10-3. Enzymatic defects in the urea cycle.

Carbamyl phosphate synthetase deficiency. Gelehrter and Snodgrass reported that a male infant, 6 hours after a protein feeding, became hypothermic, hypertonic, irritable, and lapsed into a coma.[28] After 4 days the infant died. Blood ammonia levels were 1480 μg/dl. Carbamyl phosphate synthetase activity was less than 16% of the lowest control value. Evidence indicated that this activity was attributed to cytoplasmic carbamyl phosphate synthetase II and that the activity of mitochondrial carbamyl phosphate synthetase I was zero. Three years earlier a male sibling with the same clinical findings survived only 4 days.

Previously, Freeman and his co-workers reported a case of an infant with hyperammonemia, vomiting, lethargy, ketoacidosis, and dehydration.[29] The carbamyl phosphate synthetase levels were decreased. The clinical symptoms improved on a low-protein diet. However, the patient died at 5 months of age.

Ornithine transcarbamylase deficiency. Ornithine transcarbamylase deficiency is inherited as an X-linked dominant trait.[30] Affected females have varying degrees of diminished enzyme activity.[31] On the other hand, affected males have no enzyme activity and die shortly after birth. The clinical symptoms are hyperammonemia, respiratory alkalosis, perspiration, and a flappy tremor of the arms. This is followed by coma and death. Several different methods have been tried to reduce the ammonia levels: complete protein restriction or only a minimum amount of essential amino acids, neomycin to decrease intestinal synthesis of ammonia, exchange transfusions, lactulase to trap ammonia, oral and intravenous hydrochloric acid to increase ammonia excretion by the kidney, and peritoneal dialysis. In all instances the blood ammonia remained elevated.

Gelehrter and Rosenberg administered N-carbamyl-L-glutamate and L-arginine to an affected infant.[32] N-Carbamyl-L-glutamate acts as an activator of carbamyl phosphate synthetase. Arginine would be metabolized to ornithine, the substrate for ornithine transcarbamylase. It was hoped that in this way, ammonia would be converted to carbamyl phosphate and then used in pyrimidine synthesis; however, these two compounds further increased the hyperammonemia, and the infant died. The authors suggested that other methods of treatment such as glucagon administration to stimulate urea cycle enzymes, administration of α-keto acids as precursors for synthesis of essential amino acids, citrulline administration, or a liver transplant might be useful.

Dietary protein restriction is necessary for females with reduced enzyme activity. Individuals with as low as 10% of normal enzyme activity can develop normally as long as the protein level of the diet is reduced.

Citrullinemia. The biochemical defect in citrullinemia is caused by a lack of the enzyme arginosuccinate synthetase. Elevated levels of citrulline appear in the plasma and urine. Hyperammonemia is evident after the ingestion of protein. The clinical symptoms that appear are vomiting, irritability, seizures, and mental retardation. Improvement was noticed when a low-protein diet was fed; however, this must be instituted early in life to prevent mental deterioration.

Argininosuccinic aciduria. Argininosuccinic aciduria is the disorder of the urea cycle that appears most frequently. Large amounts of argininosuccinic acid are excreted in the urine. Normally this substrate is not found in blood, cerebrospinal fluid, or urine. Hyperammonemia is present after the ingestion of protein; therefore dietary protein restriction is necessary.

Two forms of this disorder have been described. The condition that appears in young infants is usually fatal. The chronic disorder in older children is characterized by mental retardation or convulsions. Approximately half the children exhibit a peculiar tufted friable hair.

Argininemia. Two sisters with argininemia were mentally retarded and had seizures. Elevated levels of ammonia and arginine were found in their blood. Urinary excretion of lysine and cystine were also increased. The cystine increase was probably due to the competitive inhibition of renal tubular reabsorption of these two amino acids by the elevated load of arginine that has to be filtered. A low-protein diet reduced the blood ammonia and arginine levels. The lysinuria and cystinuria disappeared.

Homocystinuria

The occurrence of homocystinuria approaches that of phenylketonuria. The enzyme cystathionine synthase converts methionine to cystathionine (Fig. 10-4). When this enzyme is defective, plasma levels of methionine and homocystine are elevated. Excess homocystine is excreted in the urine. The clinical symptoms that appear with this metabolic defect are mental and growth retardation, light complexion, malar flush, dislocated lens, hepatomegaly, a peculiar gait, and arterial and venous thrombosis.

A dietary regimen low in protein, in particular methionine, has been successful when instituted immediately after birth. Supplements of cystine are given to provide a source of sulfur, since the metabolic block precludes the synthesis of cysteine from methionine. Three formulas are available for infants.[26] Methionaid (Ross Labora-

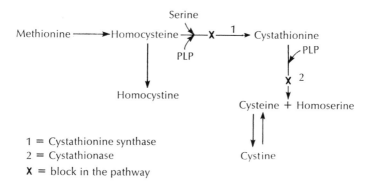

Fig. 10-4. Enzymatic defects in the metabolism of sulfur amino acids.

tories) consists of a mixture of amino acids that does not contain methionine, water-soluble vitamins, or minerals. Product 3200 K (Mead Johnson) is a soy isolate formula low in methionine containing, in addition, carbohydrate, vitamins, and minerals. Low-methionine Isomil (Ross Laboratories) is another complete infant formula that can be used. All animal sources of protein must be excluded from the diet and replaced with plant proteins low in methionine such as soybean.

Serving lists, sample prescriptions, and menus for planning methionine-restricted diets are available.[14] The diet is difficult to prepare, and it is not known whether this therapy will protect the individual from vascular complications. Diet therapy in older children and adults has not been very successful.

Pyridoxal phosphate is the coenzyme for cystathionine synthase. In some patients, administration of large doses of pyridoxine (250 to 500 mg) daily increased the activity of the enzyme and thus reversed the biochemical defect. However, not all homocystinuric children respond to the administration of vitamin B_6.

Cystathioninuria

In cystathioninuria a lack of the liver enzyme cystathionase results in the urinary excretion of cystathionine. It is suspected that this is a benign biochemical abnormality, because some individuals have been detected with no clinical symptoms. Other patients have mental deterioration. Most individuals respond to large doses of vitamin B_6 (200 to 400 mg).

Cystinosis

With cystinosis, cystine crystals deposit in tissues throughout the body. As larger amounts are deposited, the disease becomes more severe. This disorder may appear at three stages of life. In the adult form, cystine is deposited only in the cornea of the eye. The individuals suffer from headache, photophobia, and itchy eyes. The infantile and juvenile forms develop renal disease. Vitamin D–resistant rickets, chronic acidosis, polyuria, and dehydration result from the deposition of cystine in the kidney. The treatment is the same as that for chronic renal failure. Adequate fluid intake, sodium bicarbonate or citrate to correct the acidosis, and calcium and vitamin D to correct the rickets are needed. Treatment with thiol reagents to decrease the levels of cystine in the tissues has been unsuccessful. Low-cystine diets are difficult to prepare, and there is no evidence that this would be helpful. Renal transplantation has been tried in some children, but cystine crystals appear in the donor kidney after a period of time.

Pyridoxine dependency syndrome

Infants with pyridoxine dependency syndrome develop convulsions soon after birth and die within a year. There is a decrease in growth rate, and electroencephalograms show abnormal patterns. The administration of daily doses of 10 to 50 mg of pyridoxine prevents the convulsions. The enzyme responsible for this defect is not known, but some have postulated that it may be caused by the inability of glutamic acid decarboxylase to bind its coenzyme, pyridoxal phosphate. This enzyme converts glutamic acid to γ-aminobutyric acid.

Vitamin B₆ deficiency syndrome

Convulsions can be avoided in infants with vitamin B_6 deficiency syndrome by the daily administration of 2 to 10 mg of pyridoxine. Infants normally do not need more than 0.2 mg daily. No enzyme defects have been discovered. It has been suggested that the disorder is caused either by the defective synthesis of the coenzyme pyridoxal phosphate or its inability to bind to an enzyme.

Branched-chain ketoaciduria (maple syrup urine disease)

Infants with branched-chain ketoaciduria become ill shortly after birth. They are easily identified by the maple syrup odor of the body and urine. Feeding difficulties, vomiting, and convulsions are followed by death. The branched-chain amino acids— valine, isoleucine, and leucine—undergo transamination and form their corresponding keto acids (Fig. 10-5). In this inborn error of metabolism these keto acids cannot undergo oxidative decarboxylation. The blood levels of the amino acids and keto acids are elevated. Excess keto acids spill over into the urine.

Treatment must be instituted early in life to avoid mental retardation. Control is much more difficult than in the case of phenylketonuria. The plasma levels of each of the three amino acids must be regulated. The levels are not easily stabilized, particularly in times of illness. Peritoneal dialysis may be employed at first to reduce the blood levels of the branched-chain amino acids along with a synthetic formula,

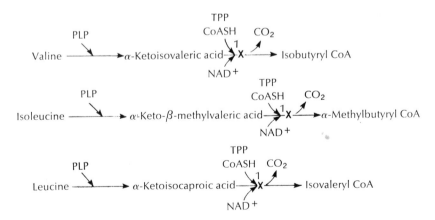

1 = branched chain α-Ketoacid decarboxylase

X = block in the pathway

Fig. 10-5. Metabolism of the branched chain amino acids.

M. S. U. D. Aid (Ross Laboratories). This product contains no leucine, isoleucine, valine, carbohydrate, and fat, so oil and dextri-maltose should be added. Another formula, MSUD Diet Powder (Mead Johnson), contains an amino acid mixture free of the branched-chain amino acids, fat, carbohydrate, vitamins, and minerals. An amino acid mix free of the branched-chain amino acids is also available (General Biochemicals). The blood levels of the branched-chain amino acids should be monitored until normal levels are reached. Then milk or a source of the branched-chain amino acids is added to the formula to meet the infant requirement.[33] Ketoacidemia and ataxia appear when the levels of leucine exceed 10 mg/dl. The urine should be checked with 2,4-dinitrophenylhydrazine to see if the child is ketoacidotic. If the test is positive, the diet must be adjusted.

As the child grows and can no longer be fed with the formula, dietary control becomes more difficult, since leucine requirements range from 300 to 800 mg depending upon age. The diet is low in protein and high in carbohydrates and fats. Noel and her co-workers have planned meals in which the main dish is a vegetable or casserole, and the high-quality protein becomes the side dish.[33] These researchers have also used protein-leucine ratios to estimate the leucine content of a variety of foods. The leucine content of foods commonly used in diets for these children and Gerber baby foods is given in tables. Acosta and Elsas have prepared serving lists giving the isoleucine, leucine, valine, protein, and kilocalorie content of a variety of foods, of Gerber baby foods, and of special low-protein products.[14]

Recently Bell, Chao, and Milne developed a new equivalency system based on the one devised by Acosta and Elsas.[34] Five categories of food are used: fruit, vegetable, cereal, free food A (little protein), and free food B (no protein). The protein, isoleucine, leucine, valine, and kilocalorie content are given for each equivalent. The parents' lists include the foods in the equivalency system along with serving sizes in gravimetric and household units. This method has been used successfully to treat patients from 4 months to 6 years of age.

Other cases of intermittent branched-chain ketonuria have been described. The biochemical defect is manifested in these individuals when they are subject to stress such as large protein intakes, infections, or surgery. Scriver and his co-workers described the correction of the biochemical defect in one patient by the administration of 10 mg of thiamine.[35]

Hypervalinemia

One case of hypervalinemia has been reported. The lack of valine transaminase resulted in elevated amounts of valine in the blood and urine. The levels of leucine and isoleucine were normal. A low-valine diet improved the clinical symptoms.

Propionyl-CoA carboxylase deficiency

In propionyl-CoA carboxylase deficiency severe ketosis and coma is followed by death early in life. The defect is the result of a lack of propionyl-CoA carboxylase, which converts propionyl-CoA to methylmalonyl-CoA. Propionic acid levels increase in the blood and spill over into the urine after a high intake of protein or isoleucine, threonine, and methionine. Leucine and valine stimulate the metabolism of isoleucine and thus can also elevate propionic acid levels.

Dietary treatment is difficult, since the levels of the aforementioned amino acids must be kept low as well as the total intake of protein. This is difficult to accomplish, and it is not known whether this therapy will prevent mental retardation. One case has been responsive to large doses of biotin (10 mg).

Methylmalonic aciduria

Because of a defect in the enzyme methylmalonyl-CoA mutase, methylmalonyl-CoA is not converted to succinyl-CoA in methylmalonic aciduria. Severe ketosis appears in a majority of the infants, and they die soon after birth. Isoleucine, threonine, valine, and methionine are metabolized to methylmalonic acid; therefore, treatment involves the restriction of these amino acids in addition to a low-protein diet.

Several cases have been described that are responsive to the administration of large doses of vitamin B_{12} (1000 μg). The vitamin-responsive patients usually exhibit a milder form of the disease.

Phenylketonuria[36]

Folling first described phenylketonuria in 1934. Two children exhibited a peculiar mousy odor because of the excretion of phenylacetic and phenylpyruvic acid in their urine. In this inborn error of metabolism a lack of the enzyme phenylalanine hydroxylase results in phenylalanine's being metabolized via other metabolic pathways rather than to tyrosine (Fig. 10-6). As a result these infants are mentally retarded, fair skinned and light haired as a result of the inability to synthesize the pigment melanin, hyperphenylalaninemic, and may have eczema. Generally if these individuals are not treated, they are institutionalized and die around the age of 30.

Many states have now passed legislation that makes screening newborn infants for phenylketonuria mandatory. The earliest screening test for this defect involved testing the urine for ketones with ferric chloride. However, this is not as sensitive as measuring the blood levels of phenylalanine either by microbiological assay, fluorometric techniques, or chromatography. Screening should be performed before 4 weeks of age so that treatment may be initiated as soon as possible.

The only mode of treatment at present is dietary. Since phenylalanine is an essential amino acid, it must be included in the diet, but the amounts must be restricted. Infants and young children tolerate about 250 to 500 mg of phenylalanine per day. Blood phenylalanine levels must be periodically monitored and the diet adjusted, so that the serum levels are between 2 to 5 mg/dl and the child shows an adequate weight gain. Hypophenylalaninemia must be avoided as it can lead to serious difficulties.

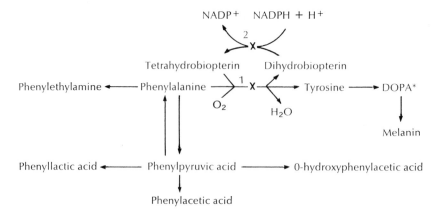

* = 3,4 Dihydroxyphenylalanine
1 = Phenylalanine hydroxylase
2 = Dihydropteridine reductase
X = Block in the pathway

Fig. 10-6. Metabolism of phenylalanine.

Since most protein foods contain approximately 5% phenylalanine, the diet must consist of low-protein foods and a milk substitute. One such product, Lofenalac (Mead Johnson), is a casein hydrolysate supplemented with methionine, tryptophan, tyrosine, corn oil, sugar, vitamins, and minerals. The powder contains approximately 0.08% phenylalanine. The product can be made into a formula to meet the nutritional needs of the infant. The phenylalanine requirement is met by adding milk. Lofenalac may also be made into a semisolid pudding or added to other recipes.

A product used in Europe called Albumaid-XP is a phenylalanine-free hydrolysate of beef serum that is supplemented with tryptophan, tyrosine, vitamins, minerals, and carbohydrate as a maize starch. In a study using Albumaid-XP and Lofenalac for phenylketonuric infants, no major differences were observed between the two formulas.[37] Lofenalac is a high-carbohydrate, fat product, whereas Albumaid-XP is high in protein. It was suggested that Albumaid-XP would be useful during adolescence when protein requirements are high, but caloric requirements are lower. More natural foods could be used as the source of phenylalanine.

For older children the product Phenyl-Free (Mead Johnson) is useful. It is a mixture of amino acids (no phenylalanine), vitamins, minerals, fat, and carbohydrate. Its protein content is higher than that of Lofenalac.

Serving lists for phenylalanine-restricted diets are useful in planning meals for older children.[14] Special commercial products that are low in phenylalanine can also be used (see Chapter 6, p. 120).

In January 1971 a collaborative study of infants treated for phenylketonuria was initiated at 18 medical centers where two treatment groups have been established:

Group I, in which serum phenylalanine levels are to be maintained at 1 to 5.4 mg/dl, and Group II, in which levels are from 5.5 to 9.9 mg/dl.[38] About 35 new babies are added to the study each year. The major protein source in the infants' diets is Lofenalac. The calculation of the nutrient intakes of 88 infants showed very few infants with low intakes. There were no differences in height and weight because of the treatments. However, it was difficult to maintain the low–serum phenylalanine levels called for in Group I.

Information has been collected on the methods used to first lower serum phenylalanine levels in newly diagnosed infants.[39] The methods used were Lofenalac, Lofenalac plus milk, Lofenalac with milk supplying 200 mg phenylalanine daily, and alternating Lofenalac and cow's milk. In a majority of the clinics the nutritionist prescribed the diet and followed up on dietary treatment. Lectures, discussions, and demonstration methods were used for dietary instruction.

Considerable controversy exists as to when the restricted phenylalanine diet should be discontinued.[40-42] Some physicians have placed children 4 to 5 years of age on regular diets, since most brain growth has been completed by that age. Although there have been no regressions, it is impossible to state whether the continuation of diet therapy would have improved mental performance; therefore, some children are maintained on the restricted diet until adolescence. For females it may be wise to continue the diet through their child-bearing years.

Prior to the cessation of the restricted phenylalanine diet, discussions should be initiated with the children and their parents.[43] In response, some parents were relieved that they no longer had to prepare special foods; a few forced their children to eat new foods. On the other hand, some children missed the attention they had received when they were on the restricted phenylalanine diet. Many children did not understand why suddenly it became permissible to eat anything.

Since diet therapy has been successful, phenylketonuric females now reach child-bearing age. As a result of the maternal hyperphenylalaninemia a majority of their infants are born mentally retarded, and a higher than normal incidence of phenylketonuria is seen. The diet of the phenylketonuric mother should meet the Recommended Daily Dietary Allowances for pregnancy. Pueschel et al. recommended a daily intake of approximately 15 mg phenylalanine per kilogram of body weight.[44]

When Lofenalac is used, natural foods are restricted, and the large volume of formula needed to meet the protein requirement also increases the caloric intake above the Recommended Daily Dietary Allowance. A new preparation, Phenyl-Free (Mead Johnson), has a higher protein content than Lofenalac. Therefore Phenyl-Free is the preferred preparation unless the mother has been accustomed to Lofenalac. Some investigators recommend that the phenylketonuric female continue a phenylalanine-restricted diet, since this would be easier than to reintroduce it again during pregnancy. Appropriate dietary management should prevent the mental retardation and congenital anomalies seen in infants born to phenylketonuric mothers in the past.

Tyrosine becomes an essential amino acid for phenylketonurics. Therefore Bessman, Williamson, and Koch have suggested that mental retardation in children of phenylketonurics can be due to a deficiency of tyrosine in utero.[45] They recommend that the maternal diet be supplemented with 3 to 4 g of tyrosine per day.

It is not feasible to treat phenylketonurics with phenylalanine hydroxylase, since the enzyme is difficult to isolate and purify. It is rapidly deactivated in the circulation. A readily available microbial enzyme, phenylalanine ammonia-lyase, metabolizes phenylalanine.[46] Since it is antigenic, the enzyme is placed on the inner wall of a multitubular enzyme reactor.

Dogs were fed high levels of phenylalanine and p-chlorophenylalanine in order to develop experimental phenylketonuria. After the reactors were inserted into an extracorporeal shunt in these dogs, blood phenylalanine levels decreased. The authors suggested that these reactors could be used temporarily in phenylketonuric individuals to reduce exceedingly high serum phenylalanine levels.

A child with a variant form of phenylketonuria was studied by Kaufman and his co-workers.[47] The activities of the enzymes phenylalanine hydroxylase, dihydropteridine reductase, and dihydrofolate reductase were normal. However, low levels of tetrahydrobiopterin were found in the liver, and the serum and urinary levels of biopterin-like compounds were low. Even though the patient had been maintained on a restricted phenylalanine diet, there was evidence of neurological damage. Hyperphenylalaninemia can result from a deficiency of the enzymes phenylalanine hydroxylase (classic phenylketonuria) and dihydropterin reductase or, as in this case, from a lack of the cofactor biopterin.

Various other forms of hyperphenylalaninemia have been described. Transient phenylketonurics develop a gradual tolerance to phenylalanine, and restriction may be harmful. Other individuals have a benign form of the defect. Although phenylalanine hydroxylase activity is decreased, serum phenylalanine levels are only elevated. Premature infants may have elevated serum levels of phenylalanine or tyrosine or both because of the inability to synthesize the enzyme. This is corrected with time.

Several publications dealing with phenylketonuria and its dietary management have been prepared to assist the parents and health professionals involved in the care of phenylketonuric infants.[48-51]

Tyrosinemia

Several disorders pertaining to the metabolism of tyrosine have been reported. Neonatal tyrosinemia often occurs in premature infants because of the immaturity of liver enzymes. Short-term dietary treatment involves the restriction of protein and the administration of vitamins.

Tyrosinemia type I results from a deficiency of the enzyme p-hydroxyphenylpyruvic acid oxidase (Fig. 10-7). The symptoms associated with this disorder are hypoglycemia, hypoprothrombinemia, jaundice, ascites, cirrhosis, a renal tubular defect that results in aminoaciduria, phosphaturia, glycosuria, and rickets. Blood

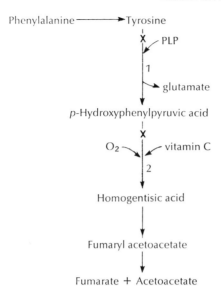

1 = Tyrosine glutamate aminotransferase
2 = p-Hydroxyphenylpyruvic acid oxidase
X = Block in the pathway

Fig. 10-7. Metabolism of tyrosine.

levels of tyrosine, phenylalanine, and methionine are elevated. The disease is often fatal if dietary treatment is not instituted at an early age.

Michals, Matalon, and Wong described the treatment of a 7-month-old girl with tyrosinemia type I.[52] At first, product 80056 (Mead Johnson), plus an amino acid mixture with no phenylalanine, tyrosine, or methionine, were fed until the blood levels of these amino acids were lowered. Then formula 3200 AB (Mead Johnson), which is low in phenylalanine and tyrosine but not in methionine, was used. Fruits, vegetables, and baby cereal were also added to the diet.

Six months later the child was hospitalized due to abnormal liver function. Since methionine blood levels were elevated, product 80056 plus an amino acid mixture free of methionine were used to reduce the levels of this amino acid. Two months later this protocol was repeated again because of liver dysfunction. Blood amino acid levels were stabilized on a diet that closely regulated methionine levels. The other symptoms improved, although the liver was still enlarged. The patient was then maintained on product 3200 AB, an amino acid mixture with phenylalanine and glucose added, and low-protein foods. The authors formulated equivalency lists of low-protein foods used in diets that are restricted in phenylalanine, tyrosine, and methionine. Additional information on the recommended phenylalanine, tyrosine, protein, and energy intake for tyrosinemic children and serving lists for phenyl-alanine-tyrosine–restricted diets have been compiled by Acosta and Elsas.[14]

Dietary treatment of an inborn error of metabolism is exceedingly complex. A severe restriction of an essential nutrient can result in a fatal outcome. Another infant with tyrosinemia type I was hospitalized because of growth failure, anorexia, vomiting, lethargy, and hypotonia.[53] The child has been maintained on formula 3200 AB (Mead Johnson) for 2 months. His symptoms were thought to be the result of a deficiency of phenylalanine and tyrosine. After administration of these amino acids there was a dramatic improvement. The liver cirrhosis was not arrested, however, and the baby died 2½ months later. These investigators also reported that this infant had hypermethioninemia, and they suggested that perhaps the dietary intake of methionine should be restricted.

Tyrosinemia type II is a less severe form of the metabolic disorder resulting from the impaired action of tyrosine-glutamate aminotransferase (Fig. 10-7). The symptoms found are mental retardation, hyperkeratosis on the palms and soles of the feet, and chronic corneal ulceration. The dietary treatment consists of a low-phenylalanine, low-tyrosine diet.

REFERENCES

1. Orten, J. M., and Orten, A. U.: DNA and inborn errors of metabolism, J. Am. Diet. Assoc. **59:**331, 1971.
2. Rosenberg, L. E.: Inborn errors of metabolism. In Bondy, P. K., and Rosenberg, L. E., editors: Duncan's diseases of metabolism, ed. 7, Philadelphia, 1974, W. B. Saunders Co.
3. Wong, P. W. K., and Hsia, D. Y-Y.: Inborn errors of metabolism. In Goodhart, R. S., and Shils, M. E., editors: Modern nutrition in health and disease, ed. 5, Philadelphia, 1973, Lea & Febiger.
4. Brady, R. O.: Inherited metabolic diseases of the nervous system, Science **193:**733, 1976.
5. Sperm seen as route to genetic therapy, Chem. Eng. News **52**(49):19, 1974.
6. Lebenthal, E., Antonowicz, I., and Shwachman, H.: Correlation of lactase activity, lactose intolerance and milk consumption in different age groups, Am. J. Clin. Nutr. **28:**595, 1975.
7. Fernandes, J., et al.: Respiratory hydrogen excretion as a parameter for lactose malabsorption in children, Am. J. Clin. Nutr. **31:**597, 1978.
8. Arvanitakis, C., et al.: Lactase deficiency—a comparative study of diagnostic methods, Am. J. Clin. Nutr. **30:**1597, 1977.
9. Paige, D. M., et al.: Lactose hydrolyzed milk, Am. J. Clin. Nutr. **28:**818, 1975.
10. Turner, S. J., et al.: Utilization of a low-lactose milk, Am. J. Clin. Nutr. **29:**739, 1976.
11. Payne-Bose, D., et al.: Milk and lactose hydrolyzed milk, Am. J. Clin. Nutr. **30:**695, 1977.
12. Welsh, J. D.: Diet therapy in adult lactose malabsorption: present practices, Am. J. Clin. Nutr. **31:**592, 1978.
13. Lee, D. E., and Lillibridge, C. B.: A method for qualitative identification of sugar and semiquantative determination of lactose content suitable for a variety of foods, Am. J. Clin. Nutr. **29:**428, 1976.
14. Acosta, P. B., and Elsas, L. J., II: Dietary management of inherited metabolic disease: phenylketonuria, galactosemia, tyrosinemia, homocystinuria, maple syrup urine disease, Atlanta, 1976, ACELMU Publishers.
15. Folkman, J., et al.: Portacaval shunt for glycogen storage disease: value of prolonged intravenous hyperalimentation before surgery, Surgery **72:**306, 1972.
16. Burr, I. M., et al.: Comparison of the effects of total parenteral nutrition, continuous intragastric feeding and portacaval shunt on a patient with type I glycogen storage disease, J. Pediatr. **85:**792, 1974.
17. Greene, H. L., et al.: Glycogen storage disease due to glucose-6-phosphatase (G6Pase) deficiency: treatment with clofibrate, Pediatr. Res. **6:**398/138, 1972.
18. Greene, H. L., et al.: Continuous nocturnal intragastric feeding for management of type I glycogen-storage disease, N. Engl. J. Med. **294:**423, 1976.
19. Glucose-galactose malabsorption, Nutr. Rev. **32:**132, 1974.
20. Brady, R. O.: The abnormal biochemistry of inherited disorders of lipid metabolism, Fed. Proc. **32:**1660, 1973.
21. Brady, R. O., Pentchev, P. G., and Gal, A. E.: Investigations in enzyme replacement therapy

in lipid storage diseases, Fed. Proc. **34**:1310, 1975.

22. Brady, R. O., et al.: Replacement therapy for inherited enzyme deficiency in Fabry's disease, N. Engl. J. Med. **289**:9, 1973.

23. Dreyfus, J., Poenaru, L., and Svennerholm, L.: Absence of hexosaminidase A and B in a normal adult, N. Engl. J. Med. **292**:61, 1975.

24. Herbert, P. N., et al.: Tangier disease, N. Engl. J. Med. **299**:519, 1978.

25. Frimpter, G.: Aminoacidurias due to inherited disorders of metabolism, Part I and II, N. Engl. J. Med. **289**:835, 895, 1973.

26. Special diets for infants with inborn errors of amino acid metabolism, Pediatrics **57**:783, 1976.

27. Hsia, Y. E.: Inherited hyperammonemic syndromes, Gastroenterology **67**:347, 1974.

28. Gelehrter, T. D., and Snodgrass, P. J.: Lethal neonatal deficiency of carbamyl phosphatase synthetase, N. Engl. J. Med. **290**:430, 1974.

29. Freeman, J. M., et al.: Ammonia intoxication due to a congenital defect in urea synthesis, J. Pediatr. **65**:1039, 1964.

30. Short, E. M., et al.: X-linked dominant inheritance of ornithine transcarbamylase deficiency, N. Engl. J. Med. **288**:7, 1973.

31. Campbell, A. G. M., et al.: Ornithine transcarbamylase deficiency: neonatal hyperammonemia in males, N. Engl. J. Med. **288**:1, 1973.

32. Gelehrter, T. D., and Rosenberg, L. E.: Ornithine transcarbamylase deficiency, N. Engl. J. Med. **292**:351, 1975.

33. Noel, M. B., et al.: Dietary treatment of maple syrup urine disease (branched chain ketoaciduria), J. Am. Diet. Assoc. **69**:62, 1976.

34. Bell, L., Chao, E., and Milne, J.: Dietary management of maple-syrup-urine disease: extension of equivalency systems, J. Am. Diet. Assoc. **74**:357, 1979.

35. Scriver, C. R., et al.: Thiamine responsive maple-syrup urine disease, Lancet **1**:310, 1971.

36. Scriver, C. R.: Inborn errors of metabolism: a new frontier of nutrition, Nutr. Today **9**(5):4, 1974.

37. Berry, H. K., et al.: Treatment of children with phenylketonuria using a phenylalanine-free protein hydrolysate (Albumaid XP), Am. J. Clin. Nutr. **29**:351, 1976.

38. Acosta, P. P., et al.: Nutrient intake of treated infants with phenylketonuria, Am. J. Clin. Nutr. **30**:198, 1977.

39. Acosta, P. B., et al.: Methods of dietary inception in infants with PKU, J. Am. Diet. Assoc. **72**:164, 1978.

40. Holtzman, N. A., et al.: Termination of restricted diet in children with phenylketonuria: a randomized controlled study, N. Engl. J. Med. **293**:1121, 1975.

41. Beckner, A. S., et al.: Effect of rapid increase of phenylalanine intake in older PKU children, J. Am. Diet. Assoc. **69**:148, 1976.

42. Diet termination for PKU. Yes or no? J.A.M.A. **240**:1471, 1978.

43. Pueschel, S. M., Yeatman, S., and Hum, C.: Discontinuing the phenylalanine restricted diet in young children with PKU: psychosocial aspects, J. Am. Diet. Assoc. **70**:506, 1977.

44. Pueschel, S. M., et al.: Nutritional management of the female with phenylketonuria during pregnancy, Am. J. Clin. Nutr. **30**:1153, 1977.

45. Bessman, S. P., Williamson, M. L., and Koch, R.: Diet, genetics, and mental retardation interaction between phenylketonuric heterozygous mother and fetus to produce nonspecific diminution of IQ: evidence in support of the justification hypothesis, Proc. Natl. Acad. Sci. U.S.A. **75**:1562, 1978.

46. Ambrus, C. M., et al.: Phenylalanine depletion for the management of phenylketonuria: use of enzyme reactors with immobilized enzymes, Science **201**:837, 1978.

47. Kaufman, S., et al.: Hyperphenylalaninemia due to a deficiency of biopterin. A variant form of phenylketonuria, N. Engl. J. Med. **299**:673, 1978.

48. Management of newborn infants with PKU, U.S. DHEW Publication-No(HSA)78-5211, 1978.

49. Acosta, P. B., Wenz, E., Schaeffler, G., and Koch, R.: PKU-a diet guide, Evansville, Ind., 1969, Mead Johnson Laboratories.

50. PKU Clinic Staff: Living with PKU, Evansville, Ind., 1972, Mead Johnson Laboratories.

51. Phenylketonuria: Evansville, Ind., 1973, Mead Johnson Laboratories.

52. Michals, K., Matalon, R., and Wong, P. W. K.: Dietary treatment of tyrosinemia type I. Importance of methionine restriction, J. Am. Diet. Assoc. **73**:507, 1978.

53. Cohn, R. M., et al.: Phenylalanine-tyrosine deficiency syndrome as a complication of the management of hereditary tyrosinemia, Am. J. Clin. Nutr. **30**:209, 1977.

11 Cancer

The second leading cause of death in the United States is cancer. It has been estimated that most human cancers are related to environmental factors. One of those factors under much investigation is nutrition. The effects of diet on cancer are difficult to study, since in many instances long-term exposure is necessary for the development of a neoplasm. Some of the dietary constituents and their relationship to cancer currently under study are caloric intake, proteins, amino acids, fats (amount and type), vitamins, minerals, fiber, cholesterol, alcohol, food additives, and food contaminants. Epidemiological studies seem to suggest that high intakes of fat are involved in breast and colon cancer. It has also been shown that the type of cancer varies from one geographic location to another; in Japan stomach cancer is prevalent, whereas in the United States the incidence of colon cancer is higher. Thus environmental factors are important in the causation of cancer. Since these can be altered, it should be possible to prevent or reduce the incidence of cancer.

THE DIET, NUTRITION AND CANCER PROGRAM

The revised National Cancer Act of 1974 states that the National Cancer Institute shall "Collect, analyze and disseminate information respecting nutrition programs for cancer patients and the relationship between nutrition and cancer, useful in prevention, diagnosis and treatment of cancer."[1] As a result, the Diet, Nutrition and Cancer Program was formed. Its objectives are "to assess the role of nutrition in the cause and prevention of disease; to define individual nutritional and dietary requirements according to somatic, behavioral and environmental parameters; to define nutrient values of food; to develop methodology for assessing individual nutritional status; to investigate the potential of diet in disease therapy; and to increase public awareness of nutrition and health maintenance."[2]

RELATIONSHIP BETWEEN NUTRITION AND CANCER

It has been estimated that 60% of cancers in women and more than 40% of cancers in men are related to nutritional factors.[2] Some of the relationships between nutrition and cancer that have been explored are carcinogens in food, nutritional deficiencies and excesses, and the incidence of cancer among certain groups of people and populations. The substances naturally present in food that have been found to cause cancer are liver cancer—mycotoxins, cycasins, and aflatoxins; gastric cancer—nitrite, nitrate, and nitrosamides; and other types of cancer—nitrosamines.[3-5] Some food additives, the sugar substitutes (cyclamates and saccharin), and contaminants such as diethylstilbestrol and DDT have been found to be carcinogenic. Yet, for example, no studies have shown an increased risk of bladder cancer in diabetics who consume greater amounts of artificial sweeteners.[3]

Several nutritional deficiencies have been implicated in the causation of cancer.[3,6,7] In areas where there is an iodine deficiency and goiter there is an increased incidence of thyroid cancer. Plummer-Vinson syndrome and iron deficiency are associated with cancer of the upper gastrointestinal tract. A deficiency of Vitamin A and a low fat intake have been related to the development of cancer of the cervix and stomach. Liver cancer is associated with low levels of vitamin B_6. Heavy alcohol consumption can lead to cancer of the upper alimentary tract. A deficiency of riboflavin enhances the susceptibility of epithelial cells to carcinogenesis.

Only two types of cancer have been shown to be related to obesity, namely, cancer of the endometrium and the kidney in the female.[3,6] A high intake of fat in the diet has been correlated to breast and colon cancer. Epidemiological data have shown a high incidence of gastric cancer in Japan, whereas in the United States there is an increased risk of colon cancer. An examination of dietary intakes has attempted to define differences in food intake to determine which foods are implicated. Studies of migrants have also been of interest; it has been shown that Japanese who have migrated to the United States have a higher incidence of colon cancer. A study of the Seventh Day Adventists have shown a reduced risk for most cancers that are unrelated to smoking or drinking.[8] The Seventh Day Adventists do not use coffee, tea, hot condiments, or spices, nor do they smoke or drink. The majority of them follow a lacto-ovo-vegetarian diet consisting of vegetables, fruits, whole grains, and nuts. Almost all of them do not eat pork. Their diet contains about 25% fat and has 50% more fiber than the average meat diet. The study is being continued to determine what dietary habits specifically contribute to the low incidence of cancer.

Alcantara and Speckmann stated that diet and nutrition do not initiate tumor growth but instead modify it.[7] Diet and nutrition affect intestinal bacteria and substrates for bacterial metabolism, the microsomal mixed function oxidase system, endocrine system, and immunological system, availability of metabolites for cell proliferation, and the rate of carcinogen transfer and duration of exposure to the carcinogen.

Some interesting relationships between nutrition and cancer have been revealed; however, much additional research is still needed. Both Gori and Wynder recommend a prudent diet for the sedentary American public.[2,6] This is the diet that has been advocated to prevent atherosclerosis: 35% or less of the total daily caloric intake of 2500 to 2800 kcal should come from fat, and the cholesterol intake should not exceed 300 mg. For further details see Chapter 8, Cardiovascular Disease.

TASTE IN CANCER PATIENTS

Cancer patients are frequently malnourished because of a poor intake of food. One of the factors thought to be involved is a change in the taste threshold. Williams and Cohen conducted taste testing in 30 normal subjects and 30 lung cancer patients to detect whether there were any differences in taste recognition for sour, bitter, sweet, or salt.[9] The cancer patients showed some differences in bitter and sweet taste and a significantly lesser sensitivity to sour tastes. There was no difference in the taste threshold for salt. It was recommended that tart items such as grapefruit, cranberry, and lemon juices might be more acceptable to these patients. However, there are taste differences between patients, and this should be taken into consideration when planning diets.

Carson and Gormican tested the taste thresholds of control subjects and patients with breast or colon cancer prior to and after chemotherapy with 5-fluorouracil.[10] In this study there were no differences observed between the bitter or sour thresholds. However, before receiving chemotherapy colon cancer patients had higher salt thresholds than did the breast cancer patients or control subjects; patients with active cancer had higher salt recognition thresholds. Sweet recognition thresholds were higher in the cancer patients than in the controls, and again the highest thresholds were found in the patients with colon cancer. After treatment there were changes in sweet, sour, and bitter taste thresholds. In those patients with extensive disease there were more taste abnormalities. A questionnaire given to patients after chemotherapy indicated that appetite and taste of food worsened. Protein items such as meat casseroles, ground beef, and eggs were negatively rated, while the ratings of cold foods such as sandwiches, ice cream, and cheese were generally unchanged. Differences existed between patients in that some craved fruit, some objected to meat, chocolate, and coffee, and some wanted sweets and others did not. Differences between cancer patients must be recognized, and each should be treated individually. On the basis of their study Carson and Gormican recommended the following to improve food acceptance: cold protein items such as salad plates of fruit, cheese, vegetables, luncheon meats, meat salads, sandwiches, and deviled eggs; cold snacks high in protein; fresh fruit in protein-containing desserts and smaller amounts of meat in casseroles; cured meats (ham, sausage, corned beef, and luncheon meats); hot chocolate and fruit juices; and seasonings, spices, and lemon juice for flavor.

DeWys also found that cancer patients with extensive disease had more taste abnormalities.[11] Patients with altered taste sensations had a significantly lower caloric intake than did the patients who were asymptomatic. Yet one patient with taste abnormalities was able to maintain a normal caloric intake. Preliminary studies have shown that when the size of the tumor was reduced, there was a tendency toward more normal taste thresholds. DeWys also stated that the physiological effects of taste stimuli are important in that the taste stimulus initiates other physiological reflexes such as the flow of saliva and increased gastric secretion. Sweetening and seasoning of food has increased the caloric intake of some patients. Patients with an aversion to beef or pork may be able to eat poultry or fish; others can eat only eggs or mild cheese.

CANCER CACHEXIA

One of the first indications of cancer in a patient may be weight loss.[12] There is a loss of weight in tissues and organs similar to that seen in starvation, except that the liver gains in weight. Anorexia appears quite frequently in cancer patients. The pathophysiology is not clearly understood; there is no way clinically to measure anorexia.[12] There are many reasons for the decreased intake of food in cancer patients. Many have an appetite, but after a few bites of food they complain of being full. Radiation and chemotherapy also contribute to oliophagia as do nausea, discomfort, and pain. It has been suggested that the tumor produces peptides and other low-molecular-weight metabolites that induce anorexia by acting on neuroendocrine cells, neuroreceptors, the hypothalamus, and other central nervous system sensor and responder cells.[13] Experiments in animals with tumors that have been force fed show that the adequate ingestion of nutrients does not prevent weight loss.[12] Malabsorption of nutrients is seen in cancer patients even when the lesion is not in the digestive tract.

The tumor acts as a parasite, and it has been proposed that perhaps as such it can more effectively obtain nutrients, and thus the host becomes malnourished.[12] Since the tumor is small in relation to the size of the host, it does not seem feasible that it could deplete the host. Cancer patients who have been force fed show an increase in weight that is due to an increase in the amount of intracellular fluid. This is lost when the therapy is discontinued.

The mechanisms dealing with the control of food intake in the cancer patient have been examined for any differences from normal individuals.[14] There is no evidence that the centers in the hypothalamus that stimulate or suppress feeding have been altered in cancer patients.[14,15] However, sensory input is altered in that changes in taste leading to a decreased food intake have been documented in cancer patients; the sense of smell is also altered, but this has not been studied.[14] It is not known whether sensors in the gastrointestinal tract that influence food intake are altered in cancer patients. Thermostatic sensors may be affected by the heat generated by the tumor and thus signal a decrease in food intake. Glucosensitive receptors in the brain and liver, liposensitive receptors, and amino acid receptors may also play a role in anorexia. The effect of hormones and anorexigenic metabolites in cancer patients needs to be further explored. There are many control mechanisms that regulate food intake. DeWys proposed that a system of rank order may be established, and if one of these cues high in the order is altered, it may predominate.[14]

Cancer cachexia is characterized by weakness, debility, anorexia, early satiety, increased basal metabolic rate, weight loss and abnormalities in carbohydrate metabolism, water, electrolyte, and hormone imbalance, anemia, and progressive decrease in vital functions.[16,17] Surgery to remove the neoplasm or remission of the cancer by radiation and chemotherapy reverses the cachexia. It is interesting that the degree of cachexia is not related to the type of tumor or its location in the body and caloric intake.[17] Body fat stores and protein are depleted as are vitamins and minerals. The condition of the patient is similar to that of a child who has a protein deficiency disease such as kwashiorkor or marasmus.

There is some evidence that suggests that cachexia in the cancer patient is severe because the normal adaptive mechanisms to starvation do not function.[18] In starvation, at first there is mobilization of amino acids from muscle, gluconeogenesis, and an increase in urinary urea nitrogen. As adaptation takes place, urinary nitrogen losses decrease, and ammonia production increases to aid in the excretion of the keto acids resulting from the metabolism of fatty acids. Glucose is produced by gluconeogenesis in limited quantities. The brain adapts to metabolizing ketone bodies for energy.

When the body suffers a major injury, a hypercatabolic state results, and lean tissue mass is lost. This is seen in patients with burns or sepsis and is similar metabolically to cancer cachexia. A major injury lasting over 30 days can lead to a loss of 30% of total body weight and is most often fatal.[18] Of the weight that is lost, 10% of the total is protein and 20% fat.

Much of the weight loss in the cancer patient is attributed to the decreased intake of food. In chronic starvation, fat is used as the major fuel, resulting in a decrease in oxygen consumption and carbon dioxide production. However, this fall in carbon dioxide production does not occur in the cancer patient. Metabolically there is an inability to decrease gluconeogenesis from protein; pyruvate and lactate are converted to glucose; increased oxidation of acetoacetate takes place in the tumor; and there is a slower rate of disappearance of glucose.[18] Force-feeding experiments with cancer patients indicate that an excessive amount of calories and nitrogen are needed to maintain positive balance. The cancer patient is unable to decrease oxidative metabolism, which in the normal person is the adaptive response to starvation. Thus lean tissue mass is broken down. The metabolic disturbances are further complicated by the decreased food intake and inefficient utilization of ingested nutrients.

TREATMENT

While cancer itself affects the nutritional status of the individual, the method of treatment that is employed (radiation, chemotherapy, surgery, and immunotherapy) may lead to many nutritional problems. Two modalities of treatment may be employed at one time. If at all possible the patient should be in good nutritional status prior to treatment so that he may better withstand the rigors of therapy.

RADIATION

The effects of radiation on nutritional status are generally dependent on the site that is being radiated. Radiation to the head, neck, abdomen, and pelvis can create nutritional problems.[19] Patients who have cancer in the area of the vocal cords, thyroid, or ear and undergo radiation therapy do not encounter eating problems. Those who are treated in the tonsillar region, palate, tongue, and nasopharynx experience severe difficulties.[20] Mucositis, stomatitis, gingivitis, dysphagia, anorexia, nausea, and vomiting lead to a decreased food intake.[21] Radiation of the salivary glands results in xerostomia.[22,23] The lack of saliva leads to dental caries and difficulties in chewing.[24] Synthetic salivas may be prescribed for the patient. Liquids and food lubricants such as gravies, sauces, butter, and milk can be helpful to the patient with a dry mouth. Lemon slices have also been used to stimulate saliva. To prevent dental caries a sodium fluoride gel is applied daily to the teeth.[20,23] The mouth is rinsed with a supersaturated solution of calcium phosphate to aid in remineralization of the teeth.[23] Solid sweets, retentive sweets, and sugar solutions must be avoided. Local anesthetics may be prescribed when it is difficult to eat and swallow as a result of pain.

Radiotherapy for oral cancer leads to hypogeusia.[23] It has been suggested that the loss of the sense of taste is caused by damage to the microvilli and outer surface of the taste cells. Zinc sulfate is administered four times a day with meals, since zinc may produce gastrointestinal toxicity. The administration of zinc prior to radiation therapy results in less severe hypogeusia.

Since radiation therapy may take several weeks, it may be difficult to maintain the patient in an optimal nutritional state because of various complications. It is important that breakfast be taken before radiotherapy. Foods should be served at room temperature. Spicy foods should be avoided, as they irritate the mouth. The diet must be individualized, and the patient must be encouraged to consume between meal nourishments. Mechanical soft, pureed, or liquid diets may be needed. If the patient cannot be maintained by oral feedings, then tube feedings may be instituted. See Chapter 9, Uncategorized Clinical Conditions, for more details.

Radiation enteritis may occur after treatment of the abdomen and pelvis. This may lead to malabsorption, diarrhea, obstruction, fistulas, stricture, ulceration or perforation, anorexia, nausea, and vomiting.[21,23] The epithelial cells lining the gastrointestinal tract are very sensitive to radiation. The low-residue diet or the exclusion of lactose may stop the diarrhea.[20] Children with radiation enteritis have been successfully treated with a diet that does not contain lactose, gluten, and cow's milk protein.[25] In some cases defined-formula diets that need a minimum of digestion are prescribed. Such diets may be provided cold, as a drink, and should be administered slowly to avoid the effects of a hyperosmolar solution.

CHEMOTHERAPY

Some of the chemotherapeutic agents used in the treatment of cancer are actinomycin D, bleomycin, cyclophosphamide, cytarabine, doxorubicin, 5-fluorouracil, hydroxyurea, melphalan, 6-mercaptopurine, methotrexate, nitrogen mustard, nitrosoureas, vinblastine, and vincristine.[21] Most of the agents affect the patient's ability to eat. Some of the symptoms that occur with the use of these drugs are anorexia, mucosal ulceration, cheilosis, glossitis, stomatitis, esophagitis, nausea, vomiting, diarrhea, constipation, and an abnormal taste in the mouth. Antiemetic agents are prescribed in cases of vomiting. Soft and mechanically soft diets may be needed in patients who have mouth ulcerations.[20] Hot and acid foods should be avoided. Defined-formula diets and tube feedings have also been used. Total parenteral nutrition may be necessary for patients who are malnourished and cannot be maintained by enteral feeding.

The dietitian must encourage the patient to eat, even though it is difficult. It is essential that the patient consume adequate amounts of calories and nutrients. Two publications are available that contain suggestions for dealing with the problems encountered by cancer patients; recipes are provided that can be used to increase the intake of calories and protein.[26,27] A publication of the Cancer Information Clearinghouse contains selected annotations of educational materials dealing with nutrition of the cancer patient.[28]

SURGERY

Nutritional problems arising as a result of surgery vary in part due to the location of the incision. Surgical procedures in the head and neck area frequently lead to difficulties in chewing and swallowing.[19,20,22,29] Liquid or pureed diets may be used. Patients who have had a supraglottic laryngectomy have difficulty swallowing liquids without aspiration. They must be retrained to swallow. It helps to feed foods of one consistency. A nasogastric tube may be inserted at the time of surgery on the head or neck.[20]

Esophagectomy with a vagotomy results in gastric stasis, gastric hypochlorhydria, diarrhea, and steatorrhea.[29] Liquid, bland, soft, mechanical semi-soft, or defined-formula diets may be used depending on the patient.[20] Small frequent feedings and MCT oil have also been administered.[29]

A gastrectomy causes rapid movement of food into the small intestine, resulting in the dumping syndrome, hypoglycemia, loss of intrinsic factor, and malabsorption.[29] On eating, the patient becomes faint, weak, and may develop abdominal pains. If the symptoms are severe, the patient restricts his intake of food. Deficiencies of iron, calcium, fat-soluble vitamins, and vitamin B_{12} may develop.[19] Frequent small meals and liquids between meals are recommended. Carbohydrate intake is decreased, and protein and fat intake is increased.[20] MCT oil may be used. Vitamin supplements may also be necessary; if the resection is extensive, vitamin B_{12} may need to be injected due to the loss of the intrinsic factor.

The degree of malabsorption resulting from intestinal resection is dependent upon the amount of bowel that is removed. Resection of the jejunum decreases the absorption of many nutrients, whereas resection of the ileum leads to vitamin B_{12} deficiency, loss of bile salts, diarrhea, steatorrhea, and hyperoxaluria.[29] Cholestyramine, a low-fat diet or MCT oil, a low-oxalate diet, and injections of vitamin B_{12} may be indicated for an ileal resection. A massive bowel resection leaves 90 cm (3 ft) or less of bowel, and this leads to severe malabsorption including water and electrolytes.[19] At first it may be necessary to use total parenteral nutrition followed by tube and oral feedings. Gastric hypersecretion can lead to diarrhea and complications of fluid and electrolyte balance. Patients may progress to a more normal diet, but this is dependent upon the degree of malabsorption. However, the patient must be carefully monitored to prevent the development of nutritional deficiencies.

Pancreatectomy leads to diabetes mellitus and malabsorption due to a loss of pancreatic digestive enzymes.[29] Diabetic diets, pancreatic enzymes, and insulin may be needed.[20] If the pancreatic tumor is inoperable, high-carbohydrate diets and frequent feedings are prescribed as treatment for hyperinsulinemia.

NUTRITIONAL THERAPY

The objective of diet therapy with the cancer patient is to maintain an optimal nutritional state. The diet must be individualized. Nutritional support is important prior to, during, and after therapy.[30] There are many ways in which the dietitian can assist the patient. The patient should be fed in a pleasant surrounding. Emotional support and encouragement are important. Frequent, small meals should be provided to those who develop early satiety.[31] Because of changes in taste sensation, patients develop aversions for certain foods, especially those high in protein. Seasoning and flavoring food might be helpful.[32] Here, again, the likes of the patient should be considered.

Medicines such as antidepressant drugs, tranquilizers, and hypnotic drugs may be prescribed.[31] Nausea may be relieved by the use of antiemetics. Analgesics are given to those who experience pain upon eating. For example, lidocaine, a local anesthetic, is given prior to meals when there is pain associated with chewing. The temperature of the food is also important, since under certain conditions food served cold or at room temperature is more acceptable than food that is hot. The consistency of food must be considered, because in cases of esophageal obstruction, liquids are better tolerated. Vitamin and mineral supplements may be necessary.[30]

The behavior modification techniques used to treat obese patients have been used to modify feeding behavior in cancer patients.[32] Since it may be difficult for the cancer patient to gain weight, a more realistic goal of weight maintenance is set. The patient is asked to keep a food diary, and at each visit he is weighed, and his food intake is discussed. Patients are encouraged to serve food family style, to eat high caloric density foods, to eat slowly in pleasant surroundings, and to consume snacks frequently.

Commercially available nutritional supplements can be used as snacks with a high nutrient content. DeWys and Herbst tested their acceptability and found that of the five products tested, Meritene ranked the highest, Precision LR and Vivonex HN were intermediate, and Vivonex standard and WT low residue were disliked.[32] In a second experiment the nutritional supplements were tested with cancer patients and control subjects. The patients preferred Ensure and rated Sustacal third, whereas the controls rated Sustacal first and Ensure third. Both groups rated Meritene and Vivonex standard the lowest. When nutritional supplements are offered to cancer patients, their taste preferences should be considered.

Tube feedings are used when oral feeding is inadequate or contraindicated as in the following conditions: obstruction, partial or total impairment of the swallowing mechanisms, ileus, fistulas, coma, symptomatic exacerbation of disease with oral intake, and severe malabsorption or diarrhea and severe vomiting.[33] Nasopharyngeal, esophagostomy, gastrostomy, or jejunostomy tubes may be used depending upon the location of the neoplasm. Aspiration of the formula may occur in a debilitated patient with a nasopharyngeal tube. The composition of the tube feeding is dependent upon the condition of the patient. A formula can be made from blenderized foods, or one of the commercially available defined-formula diets can be used. For additional details see Chapter 9, Uncategorized Clinical Conditions.

In one experiment cancer patients who were force fed gained weight and were in positive nitrogen balance.[33] The weight gain was due to the accumulation of fluid and was lost when the forced feeding was discontinued. It was questioned as to whether there was an acceleration of the cancer by this treatment; however, most patients who are nutritionally replete have not shown rapid tumor growth.

The nutritional therapy of children with cancer is very important. van Eys stated that when administering therapy for children one must take into account the different types of cancers, the child's need for continued growth and development during therapy, strong food preferences, more frequent malabsorption syndromes, and the interrelationship between nutrition, cancer, and immunity, since the immature immune system may contribute to malnutrition.[34] Since major advances have been made in cancer therapy, there is the possibility that in the absence of good nutritional support, malnutrition could be the cause of death. Much research is still needed to be able to provide optimal nutritional support for the child with cancer. It is not known when parenteral or forced hyperalimentation by other routes should be instituted. Criteria need to be established to determine when the cancer patient is malnourished and when he has attained an optimal state of nutrition. In addition, the interrelationships between treatment modality and optimal nutrition need to be studied.

Prior to 1974 total parenteral nutrition was not widely used to treat oncological patients for two reasons. It was felt that in these debilitated patients septic complications would develop more readily from the indwelling catheter that is necessary for the administration of the hyperalimentation solutions.[35] Second, there was the possibility that the infused nutrients would stimulate the growth of the tumor. A systematic clinical evaluation of total parenteral nutrition in 120 cancer patients was reported in 1974.[36] Those who were on total parenteral nutrition prior to and during chemotherapy had reduced symptoms of nausea, vomiting, and anorexia. Although some patients lost weight, a majority showed a weight gain. Patients who were hyperalimented prior to surgery rather than postoperatively showed fewer complications. Anorexia, nausea, and vomiting did not appear in patients treated with abdominal radiation and total parenteral nutrition unless they tried to eat. The patients who were hyperalimented gained strength and lean body mass, and in some there was deposition of fat; the tumors did not show excessive growth. A low rate of catheter-related sepsis was reported.

Total parenteral nutrition is now widely used for cancer patients who previously could not be treated because of their debility or cachexia.[35] The full course of chemotherapy or radiotherapy could not be continued in some patients because of their poor conditions. However, therapy can be continued in most instances if the patients are being maintained concurrently on total parenteral nutrition.[35,37-39] Surgical patients who are nutritionally rehabilitated prior to surgery by this technique and then maintained postoperatively recover more rapidly and show fewer complications.[35,37-39] Total parenteral nutrition has been used effectively to treat the malnutrition that is often associated with cancer in children.[40]

If patients cannot be maintained by enteral nutrition and are severely depleted, then they are considered candidates for total parenteral nutrition. The criteria used by Dudrick et al. are a weight loss of 4.5 kg (10 lb) or 10% of usual body weight, a serum albumin concentration of less than 3.4 g/dl, and an anergic response to a series of standard recall skin antigens.[41] The treatment can be used for patients who are well nourished but who face a major surgical procedure, prolonged radiotherapy, chemotherapy, or combinations of the above treatments. In addition to septic complications the following metabolic imbalances may occur during total parenteral nutrition: hyperglycemia, ketoacidosis, rebound hypoglycemia, hyperchloremic metabolic acidosis, serum amino acid imbalances, hyperammonemia, prerenal azotemia, essential fatty acid deficiency, hypervitaminosis A, hypovitaminosis D or hypervitaminosis D, hypovitaminosis K, hypophosphatemia, hypocalcemia or hypercalcemia, hypokalemia or hyperkalemia, hypomagnesemia or hypermagnesemia, anemia, elevated levels of serum glutamic-oxaloacetic transaminase, glutamic-pyruvic transaminase, and alkaline phosphatase, and cholestatic hepatitis.[41] In many instances total parenteral nutrition has provided the nutritional support to allow the patient to undergo treatment that results in the remission of cancer. In other instances therapy is only palliative, but total parenteral nutrition has improved the quality of the patient's life. For further details on total parenteral nutrition see Chapter 9, Uncategorized Clinical Conditions.

COLON CANCER

The second leading cause of cancer deaths is from intestinal carcinoma.[42] In 1973 it was estimated that 37,000 Americans died from colon cancer. The Colon Cancer Segment of the National Cancer Institute is investigating the role of diet as an etiological factor in the development of carcinoma of the large bowel.[43] Epidemiological data suggest that bowel cancer is caused by an environmental factor.[44] Additional studies are needed so that the factors that promote carcinogenesis or increase host vulnerability can be prevented.

Epidemiological studies have shown that the incidence is highest in urban societies.[45] As families move from rural areas to more highly developed cities, they are at greater risk. Wynder and Reddy have reviewed the demographic relationships and the incidence of colon cancer in an attempt to identify the etiological factors that are involved.[3,6,46,47] A higher incidence of colon cancer is found in the highly developed countries. There is a positive correlation between colon cancer and myocardial infarction, but there is a negative relationship to gastric cancer. Seventh Day Adventists have a low incidence rate. The incidence of gastric cancer was high in Japan, but as the diet is becoming more westernized the rate of colon cancer is increasing. Many studies have shown a relationship between colon cancer and the intake of fat and meat, especially beef.

Burkitt and his co-workers have reported that in countries with a high incidence of tumors in the bowel there are different types and amounts of fecal bacteria in the intestinal tract of such patients.[48] He also stated that there is a relationship between the fiber content of the diet and carcinoma of the colon.[49] Low-fiber diets remain in the colon for a longer period of time, thus allowing the bacteria to form carcinogens from the bile acids.[50] It was suggested that fiber acts by decreasing intestinal tract transit time, and as a result decreasing the exposure time to the carcinogens; decreasing the formation of carcinogens from bile acids; decreasing carcinogens by its bulking effect and binding water, sterols, bile acids, and fat; and decreasing bacterial degradation of bile acids and neutral sterols by altering the intestinal flora. Because of the difficulties in defining fiber, many conflicting reports appear in the literature. In addition, there have been no epidemiological studies that show a correlation between levels of dietary fiber and colon cancer.[46,51] Some researchers believe that fiber plays a complementary role.

Another hypothesis for the etiology of colon cancer is based on the relationship to the high intake of fat.[47] A high-fat diet leads to an increased excretion of bile. Bacteria in the gut metabolize bile acids and neutral sterols that are in the bile to carcinogens and cocarcinogens. It has been shown that the stools of colon cancer patients have a higher concentration of bile acids and neutral steroids than do normal individuals.[3] In animals lithocholic, taurodeoxycholic, and deoxycholic acid enhance tumor growth; however, this has not been proved in humans.[6]

The fecal enzyme 7-α-dehydroxylase that converts primary bile acids to secondary bile acids has been shown to have a higher activity in patients with colon cancer than in controls.[52] The enzyme activity of cholesterol dehydrogenase, which converts cholesterol to coprostanol and coprostanone, was also higher in those with colon cancer. However, there was no difference in the activity of β-glucuronidase. The authors suggested that measuring the activity of fecal 7-α-dehydroxylase and cholesterol dehydrogenase might be useful in identifying people at risk for developing colorectal cancer. This method is easier than identifying all the microflora and chemical constituents of the feces.

Walker reviewed other hypotheses that have been advanced as the cause of colon cancer.[53] There have been correlations between colon cancer and levels of protein intake, increased sugar intake, increased use of refined carbohydrate foods, and low fiber intake. Since the development of colon cancer takes several years, it is not possible to identify etiological factors by short-term dietary studies. As a high fat intake has been implicated as a causative agent, some researchers recommend a low-fat diet as a preventive measure.[2,6] However, additional research is needed before other dietary recommendations can be made.

REFERENCES

1. Gori, G. B.: The diet, nutrition and cancer program of the NCI National Cancer Program, Cancer Res. 35:3545, 1975.
2. Gori, G. B.: Diet and cancer, J. Am. Diet. Assoc. 71:375, 1977.
3. Wynder, E. L.: Nutrition and cancer, Fed. Proc. 35:1309, 1976.
4. Miller, J. A., and Miller, E. C.: Carcinogens occurring naturally in foods, Fed. Proc. 35: 1316, 1976.
5. Issenberg, P.: Nitrite, nitrosamines and cancer, Fed. Proc. 35:1322, 1976.
6. Wynder, E. L.: The dietary environment and cancer, J. Am. Diet. Assoc. 71:385, 1977.
7. Alcantara, E. N., and Speckmann, E. W.: Diet, nutrition and cancer, Am. J. Clin. Nutr. 29:1035, 1976.
8. Phillips, R. L.: Role of life-style and dietary habits in risk of cancer among Seventh Day Adventists, Cancer Res. 35:3513, 1975.
9. Williams, L. R., and Cohen, M. H.: Altered taste thresholds in lung cancer, Am. J. Clin. Nutr. 31:122, 1978.
10. Carson, J. S., and Gormican, A.: Taste acuity and food attitudes of selected patients with cancer, J. Am. Diet. Assoc. 70:361, 1977.
11. DeWys, W.: Taste and feeding behavior in patients with cancer. In Winick, M., editor: Nutrition and cancer, New York, 1977, John Wiley & Sons.
12. Theologides, A.: Weight loss in cancer patients, CA 27:205, 1977.
13. Theologides, A.: Anorexia producing intermediary metabolites, Am. J. Clin. Nutr. 29: 552, 1976.
14. DeWys, W. D.: Anorexia in cancer patients, Cancer Res. 37:2354, 1977.
15. Morrison, S. D.: Origins of anorexia in neoplastic disease, Am. J. Clin Nutr. 31:1104, 1978.
16. Theologides, A.: Cancer cachexia. In Winick, M., editor: Nutrition and cancer, New York, 1977, John Wiley & Sons.
17. Costa, G.: Cachexia, the metabolic component of neoplastic diseases, Cancer Res. 37:2327, 1977.

18. Brennan, M. F.: Uncomplicated starvation versus cancer cachexia, Cancer Res. 37:2359, 1977.
19. Shils, M. E.: Nutrition in disease, nutritional problems in cancer patients, Columbus, Ohio, Aug., 1976, Ross Laboratories.
20. Hegedus, S., and Pelham, M.: Dietetics in a cancer hospital, J. Am. Diet. Assoc. 67:235, 1975.
21. Donaldson, S. S.: Effect of nutrition as related to radiation and chemotherapy. In Winick, M., editor: Nutrition and cancer, New York, 1977, John Wiley & Sons.
22. Fleming, S. M., Weaver, A. W., and Brown, J. M.: The patient with cancer affecting the head and neck: problems in nutrition, J. Am. Diet. Assoc. 70:391, 1977.
23. Dreizen, S., et al.: Oral complications of cancer radiotherapy, Postgrad. Med. 61:85, 1977.
24. Rotman, M.: Supporting therapy in radiation oncology, Cancer 39:744, 1977.
25. Donaldson, S. S., et al.: Radiation enteritis in children. A retrospective review, clinicopathologic correlation and dietary management, Cancer 35:1167, 1975.
26. Nutrition for patients receiving chemotherapy and radiation treatment, 1974, American Cancer Society, Inc.
27. Rosenbaum, E. H.: Health through nutrition. A comprehensive guide for the cancer patient, San Francisco, 1978, Alchemy Books.
28. Selected annotations of education materials—nutrition for the cancer patient, PHS NIH DHEW Publication No. (NIH) 78-1511, 1977.
29. Shils, M. E.: Nutrition in the treatment of cancer. In Winick, M., editor: Nutrition and cancer, New York, 1977, John Wiley & Sons.
30. Calman, K. C.: Nutritional support in malignant disease, Proc. Nutr. Soc. 37:87, 1978.
31. Theologides, A.: Nutritional management of the patient with advanced cancer, Postgrad. Med. 61:97, 1977.
32. DeWys, W. D., and Herbst, S. H.: Oral feeding in the nutritional management of the cancer patient, Cancer Res. 37:2429, 1977.

33. Shils, M. E.: Enteral nutrition by tube, Cancer Res. **37**:2432, 1977.

34. van Eys, J.: Nutritional therapy in children with cancer, Cancer Res. **37**:2457, 1977.

35. Copeland, E. M., III, Daly, J. M., and Dudrick, S. J.: Nutrition as an adjunct to cancer treatment in the adult, Cancer Res. **37**:2451, 1977.

36. Copeland, E. M., Macfayden, B. V., and Dudrick, S. J.: Intravenous hyperalimentation in cancer patients, J. Surg. Res. **16**:241, 1974.

37. Copeland, E. M., et al.: Intravenous hyperalimentation as an adjunct to radiation therapy, Cancer **39**:609, 1977.

38. Holter, A. R., and Fischer, J. E.: The effects of perioperative hyperalimentation on complications in patients with carcinoma and weight loss, J. Surg. Res. **23**:31, 1977.

39. Dietel, M., Vasic, V., and Alexander, M. A.: Specialized nutritional support in the cancer patient: is it worthwhile, Cancer **41**:2359, 1978.

40. Filler, R., et al.: Parenteral nutritional support in children with cancer, Cancer **39**:2665, 1977.

41. Dudrick, S. J., et al.: Parenteral nutrition techniques in cancer patients, Cancer Res. **37**:2440, 1977.

42. Diet and cancer of the colon, Nutr. Rev. **31**:110, 1973.

43. Berg, J. W., Howell, M. A., and Silverman, S. J.: Dietary hypotheses and diet-related research on the etiology of colon cancer, Health Serv. Rep. **88**:915, 1973.

44. MacGregor, I. L.: Carcinoma of the colon and stomach: a review with comment on epidemiologic associations, J.A.M.A. **227**:911, 1974.

45. Malt, R. A., and Ottinger, L. W.: Current concepts: carcinoma of the colon and rectum, N. Engl. J. Med. **288**:772, 1973.

46. Wynder, E. L.: The epidemiology of large bowel cancer, Cancer Res. **35**:3388, 1975.

47. Wynder, E. L., and Reddy, B. S.: Diet and cancer of the colon. In Winick, M., editor: Nutrition and cancer, New York, 1977, John Wiley & Sons.

48. Burkitt, D. P., Walker, A. R. P., and Painter, N. S.: Dietary fiber and disease, J.A.M.A. **229**:1068, 1974.

49. Burkitt, D. P.: Epidemiology of cancer of the colon and rectum, Cancer **28**:3, 1971.

50. Huang, C. T. L., Gopalakristina, G. S., and Nichols, B. L.: Fiber, intestinal sterols and colon cancer, Am. J. Clin. Nutr. **31**:516, 1978.

51. Hill, M. J.: Metabolic epidemiology of dietary factors in large bowel cancer, Cancer Res. **35**:3398, 1975.

52. Mastromarino, A., Reddy, B. S., and Wynder, E. L.: Metabolic epidemiology of colon cancer: enzymatic activity of fecal flora, Am. J. Clin. Nutr. **29**:1455, 1976.

53. Walker, A. R. P.: Colon cancer and diet, with special reference to intakes of fat and fiber, Am. J. Clin. Nutr. **29**:1417, 1976.

12 Drugs

Drug interactions have been studied extensively for many years. Recently much interest in the relationship between drugs and nutrition has been shown. Foods may affect the absorption and metabolism of certain drugs. The long-term use of drugs may adversely affect the ingestion, digestion, absorption, and metabolism of nutrients. Drug-induced nutritional deficiencies are most often seen in long-term therapy and in individuals who are at nutritional risk as a result of their illness or improper diet. In some instances, such as with the elderly, many drugs are prescribed that could lead to several nutritional deficiencies. However, these drug-induced nutritional deficiencies can be avoided by supplementing the diet with the proper nutrients.

It is also important to give consideration to the time when the medication is taken and with what liquid it is swallowed. Food restrictions are imposed with certain types of medications.

Much of the research in the past has been carried out in animals. Further research is needed in humans to understand more fully the effects of diet on drug metabolism.

DRUG METABOLISM

The metabolism of drugs occurs for the most part in the liver and to a small extent in the blood, intestinal mucosa, and kidneys. The hepatic microsomal drug-metabolizing enzymes are bound to the membrane.[1] They are part of a multicomponent electron transport system that consists of cytochrome P-450, NADPH-cytochrome c reductase, and phosphatidylcholine. In addition to drugs, steroids, fatty acids, bile acids, carcinogens, and other foreign compounds are metabolized by this system. The drugs are detoxified by being converted to water-soluble metabolites that are excreted through the kidneys. This is accomplished either by metabolic reactions involving oxidation, reduction, and hydrolysis or by conjugation with certain endogenous compounds such as glucuronic acid, glycine, and glutamine. Chronic ingestion of alcohol leads to an increased activity of the liver microsomes, and the resulting increased metabolism of the drug decreases its activity.[2]

MECHANISMS OF DRUG ACTION

Four principal mechanisms have been proposed to explain drug action: the effect on enzymes, the effect of antimetabolites, modification of the permeability of cellular membranes, and chelation.[3] A drug may act as an enzyme inhibitor by reacting either with the apoenzyme or coenzyme. The following are examples of drugs and the enzymes that are inhibited: penicillin—transpeptidase; antidepressants—monoamine oxidase; anticholingergics—acetylcholinesterase; and some diuretics—carbonic anhydrase. An antimetabolite is structurally similar to the substrate, but it cannot substitute for it in the enzyme-catalyzed reaction. Therefore the reaction cannot take place. The anticoagulant coumarin is similar in structure to vitamin K. It exerts its action by interfering with the role of vitamin K in blood clotting. The antibacterial sulfonamides are similar to p-aminobenzoic acid, which is part of the structure of the coenzyme tetrahydrofolic acid. This coenzyme is needed for many metabolic reactions; in particular an important reaction is the synthesis of the pyrimidines and purines for the nucleic acids. Another folate antagonist, methotrexate, is used in the treatment of cancer. Other antineoplastic drugs are 6-mercaptopurine and 6-thioguanine. These are related structurally to the purines adenine and guanine, respectively. Other drugs exert their pharmacological effect by altering the integrity of the cell membrane. Digitalis glycosides (cardiac drugs) act on the sodium pump and prevent the movement of potassium ions into the cell and sodium ions out of the cell. Local anesthetics exert a similar effect on nerve cell membranes, but in this case the membrane is impermeable to sodium ions, and potassium ions cannot move out. Many antibiotics kill bacteria and fungi by altering the permeability of the cell membrane. Chelating agents act by binding to a metal ion and rendering it unavailable. Most chelating agents are used as antidotes for metal poisoning; however, penicillamine is used in Wilson's disease to chelate copper.   .

FOOD AND DRUG INTERACTIONS

There are two types of food and drug interactions. In the first type the drug may exert its effect by decreasing the absorption or utilization of nutrients, or both. In the second type of interaction certain foods in the diet may inactivate the drug (see Table 12-1).

Perhaps one of the most dangerous drug-food interactions is the one between monoamine oxidase (MAO) inhibitors and certain foods. This drug is prescribed for depression and hypertension. The enzyme monoamine oxidase regulates the level of norepinephrine, a compound found in certain nerve endings.[2,4] The MAO inhibitors interfere with the action of this enzyme, and the levels of norepinephrine increase. Normally the tyramine in foods is deactivated by the intestinal monoamine oxidase. Increased amounts of this amine are absorbed, and this causes the release of more norepinephrine. Nose bleeds, hypertension, or a cerebrovascular accident can result from elevated levels of this neurotransmitter. Therefore patients taking this drug must avoid foods with a high tyramine content.[5] Table 12-1 lists some of these foods.

Hypertension, myopathy, and myoglobinuria have been reported in individuals eating licorice.[4,5] This is due to the action of glycyrrhizic acid, a compound that exhibits mineral corticoid-like activity and promotes hypokalemia and retention of

Table 12-1. Food and drug interactions

Class of drugs	Foods to avoid

Antibiotics
  Erythromycin
  Penicillin
	Acidic foods: caffeine, citrus fruits, cola drinks, fruit juices, pickles, tomatoes, vinegar

Aspirin	Acidic foods: (see above)
Antibiotics Tetracycline	Foods high in calcium: almonds, buttermilk, cheese, cream, ice cream, milk, pizza, waffles, yogurt
Anticoagulants	Foods high in vitamin K: beef liver; oils; green, leafy vegetables—brussels sprouts, cabbage, kale, spinach
Antidepressants MAO inhibitors	Foods high in tyramine: aged cheese; anchovies; avocados; bananas; beer; broad beans; canned figs; chocolate; coffee; cola drinks; fermented meats—bologna, salami, sausage; liver—chicken, beef; mushrooms; pickled herring; raisins; yogurt; sour cream; soy sauce; tenderizers; wine—Chianti, sherry; yeast extract
Antihypertensives	Natural licorice
Diuretics	Monosodium glutamate (MSG): used in seasoned salts, meat tenderizers, frozen vegetables, Chinese foods
Thyroid preparations	Vegetables with goitrogens: brussels sprouts, cabbage, cauliflower, kale, mustard greens, rutabaga, soybeans, turnips

salt and water. Individuals on antihypertensive therapy should not eat licorice imported from other countries. A synthetic flavoring is used in licorice made in the United States; therefore, this type can be eaten.

Patients taking anticoagulants such as the coumarins should not consume vitamin K–rich foods (see Table 12-1). The vitamin K in these foods promotes blood clotting and thus diminishes the effectiveness of the drug.[4]

Some vegetables contain goitrogenic compounds that inhibit the synthesis of thyroid hormone. Patients taking thyroid preparations should not consume excessive amounts of these foods.

In Parkinson's disease, low concentrations of dopamine are found in the brain.[2] The drug treatment involves the administration of levodopa, which can cross the blood-brain barrier. Pyridoxine is needed for the decarboxylation of the drug to form the physiologically active compound dopamine. This reaction occurs in the peripheral parts of the body, so large doses of the drug must be given to ensure that enough reaches the brain. High intakes of protein and pyridoxine must be avoided so that large amounts of levodopa are not peripherally decarboxylated.

Some antibiotics such as penicillin and erythromycin are destroyed by gastric acidity.[4] Therefore these drugs should be taken 1 hour prior to meals. These drugs should not be dissolved or taken with acid foods such as fruit juices. Aspirin also should not be consumed with acid foods. Foods high in calcium content, such as dairy products, decrease the absorption of tetracycline.[2] The calcium and tetracycline form a chelate that is insoluble. Sodium bicarbonate and iron salts also impair the absorption of tetracycline.

Patients taking diuretics should be cautioned about the intake of monosodium glutamate (MSG). This compound causes transient hypernatremia. The individual develops a headache, burning sensation in the extremities, and chest pain. This has been referred to as the "Chinese restaurant syndrome," since the MSG content of Chinese foods is high.

EFFECT OF FOOD ON DRUG ABSORPTION

The absorption of drugs from the gastrointestinal tract depends on lipid solubility, rate of dissociation, pH, particle size, and physical form.[6] Drugs are absorbed by passive nonionic diffusion. Those that are weakly acidic are absorbed in the stomach, while those weakly basic are absorbed in the small intestine. Food interferes with the absorption of some drugs; therefore, the time at which the medication is taken and with what food it is taken influences the drug's effectiveness.

Drugs used to decrease gastric acid secretion and gut motility such as belladonna, propantheline, and other anticholinergic agents must be taken shortly before food is ingested.[4] Antibiotics should be administered 1 hour before or 3 hours after a meal so that the gastric acidity does not inactivate them.[2] Some drugs are irritating to the gastrointestinal tract and should be taken with meals. Table 12-2 lists some of these drugs. Foods can increase, decrease, or delay the absorption of drugs (see Table 12-3). The absorption of griseofulvin, an oral antifungal agent, is affected by the

Table 12-2. Drugs that should be ingested with meals*

Aminophylline	Isoniazid
Aminosalicylic acid	Metronidazole
Aspirin	Nitrofurantoin
Aspirin-phenacetin-caffeine	Phenformin
Chlorpromazine	Potassium salts
Chlorpropamide	Prednisolone
Cholestyramine	Reserpine
Hydrochlorothiazide	Sulfinpyrazone
Hydrocortisone	Tolbutamide
Indomethacin	Triamterene
Iron salts	Trimeprazine

*Adapted from Visconti, J. A.: Drug-food interaction, nutrition in disease, Columbus, Ohio, 1977, Ross Laboratories.

concentration of fat in the diet; high concentrations of fat increase the absorption of this drug.[2]

EFFECT OF DRUGS ON APPETITE, TASTE, AND FOOD INTAKE

The psychotropic drugs such as chlorpromazine and lithium carbonate that are taken on a long-term basis have been shown to promote weight gain.[2] Cyproheptadine increases appetite and has been used with patients who are malnourished.[7] Insulin, steroids, sulfonylureas, and some antihistamines also stimulate the appetite.[6]

For obese patients, drugs such as amphetamines have been prescribed to promote anorexia. The effect is short term, and many side effects result from using large doses. Two stimulant drugs, dextroamphetamine and methylphenidate, are used to treat hyperactive children. Lucas and Sells found that two children on these medications had anorexia and feeding problems.[8] Their caloric intake decreased when they were on the stimulants, resulting in a decrease in height and weight. It was recommended that breakfast be given before the first medication so that appetite would not be depressed. Children on stimulant medication should be observed carefully, since they are at risk for suppression of growth.

Many drugs decrease the sweet, bitter, and sour sensitivity, or they alter taste.[9] Potassium chloride liquids, chloral hydrate, paraldehyde, cholingergic agents, expectorants, and narcotic analgesics may cause nausea and decrease appetite.[4] Cancer chemotherapeutic agents cause nausea, vomiting, and irritation of the gastrointestinal tract.[4] Digitalis causes nausea, and long-term usage leads to weight loss.

Table 12-3. Effect of food on drug absorption*

Increased absorption with food	Decreased absorption with food	Delayed absorption with food
Carbamazepine	Amoxicillin	Acetaminophen
Griseofulvin	Ampicillin	Amoxicillin
Hetacillin	Aspirin	Aspirin
Hydralazine	Demethylchlortetracycline	Cephalexin
Lithium salts	Doxycycline	Digoxin
Metoprolol	Isoniazid	Furosemide
Nitrofurantoin	Levodopa	Sulfadiazine
Propanolol	Methacycline	Sulfadimethoxine
Propoxyphene	Oxytetracycline	Sulfanilamide
Spironolactone	Penicillin G and V	Sulfisoxazole
	Phenobarbital	
	Propantheline	
	Rifampicin	
	Tetracycline	

*Adapted from Roe, D. A.: Drugs, diet and nutrition, Contemp. Nutr. **3(6)**:1, 1978.

EFFECT OF DRUGS ON NUTRIENTS

The absorption of nutrients can be impaired by the following drugs: some anti-microbial agents, antimitotic agents, cathartics, antacids, hypocholesterolemics, diuretics, anticonvulsants, and oral contraceptives.[2] Drugs can induce malabsorption by exerting their effect in the intestinal lumen or by damaging the cells lining the small intestine.[10] Mineral oil is used as a laxative, but it also functions as a solvent for the fat-soluble vitamins. Cathartics may cause the food to move rapidly through the small intestine and thereby decrease the time for absorption. Excessive use of laxatives containing phenolphthalein can result in hypokalemia and protein-losing enteropathy. Neomycin and cholestyramine bind bile acids and decrease the absorption of fats, fat-soluble vitamins, and also vitamin B_{12}. Neomycin also destroys the gut mucosa and so decreases the amount of digestive enzymes and also results in malabsorption of iron, potassium, sodium, calcium, and nitrogen.[2] Pharmacological agents that damage the pancreas cause decreased synthesis of pancreatic enzymes, and as a result there is a decrease in the digestion of fat, protein, and carbohydrate.[10]

Methotrexate, 5-fluorouracil, and colchicine inhibit mitosis in the gastrointestinal tract.[2] Colchicine, an anti-inflammatory agent used in the treatment of acute gout, can cause malabsorption of lactose, fat, carotene, vitamin B_{12}, sodium, potassium, and cholesterol. Salicylazosulfapyridine, another anti-inflammatory agent, blocks the intestinal mucosal transport of folate. Para-aminosalicylic acid interferes with the absorption of fat, cholesterol, iron folate, and vitamin B_{12}. The overuse of aluminum antacids leads to a deficiency of phosphate. The anticonvulsant agents increase the catabolism of vitamin D and its metabolites and thereby reduce the intestinal absorption of calcium. Folate deficiency can also occur with the use of these agents.

Antivitamins are used as drugs to block the utilization of a specific nutrient.[7] Methotrexate that is used to treat leukemia and other cancers blocks the metabolism of folic acid. Triamterene, a diuretic, is structurally similar to folic acid. The anticoagulant coumarin is an antagonist of vitamin K. Other drugs cause vitamin deficiencies, but this is a side effect due to interference with the metabolism of the vitamin. Vitamin B_6 deficiency can result from treatment with isoniazid, hydralazine, cycloserine, or penicillamine, since these drugs form a complex with the vitamin and render it inactive.

Many studies have been concerned with the effect of oral contraceptive agents on nutritional status.[6,7,10] The pill has been reported to alter the metabolism of thiamine, riboflavin, ascorbic acid, folic acid, pyridoxine, vitamin B_{12}, vitamin A, vitamin E, calcium, phosphorus, and magnesium. Increased levels of these nutrients may be necessary. However, at present it is felt that only women with a marginal intake of nutrients may be at risk.

Table 12-4 summarizes the effects of several classes of drugs on nutrient absorption and metabolism.

March has compiled an extensive list of the interaction of selected drugs with nutritional status in man.[11] Moore and Powers have also published a booklet of food-medication interactions.[12]

Table 12-4. Effect of drugs on nutrient absorption and metabolism

Drug	Effect
Antacids	
Aluminum antacids	Decrease absorption of phosphate
Others	Alkaline destruction of thiamine; some decrease absorption of vitamin A, iron, steatorrhea
Anticonvulsants	
Phenobarbital	Decreases serum folate, vitamins B_6, B_{12}; increases catabolism of vitamin D and metabolites
Phenytoin	Decreases serum folate, vitamins B_6, B_{12}, calcium; increases catabolism of vitamin D and metabolites
Primidone	Decreases serum folate, vitamins B_6, B_{12}; decreases calcium absorption; increases catabolism of vitamin D and metabolites
Antimicrobials	
Neomycin	Binds bile acids; decreases absorption of fat, carotene, vitamins A, D, K, B_{12}, potassium, sodium, calcium, nitrogen
Salicylazosulfapyridine	Decreases absorption of folate
Para-aminosalicylic acid	Decreases absorption of folate, vitamin B_{12}, iron, cholesterol, fat
Chloramphenicol	Increases need for vitamins B_2, B_6, B_{12}
Penicillin	Hypokalemia; renal potassium wasting
Tetracycline	Decreases absorption of fat, amino acids, calcium, iron, magnesium, zinc
Cycloserine	May decrease absorption of calcium, magnesium; may decrease serum folate, vitamins B_6, B_{12}; decreases protein synthesis
Isoniazid	Vitamin B_6 deficiency
Sulfonamides	Decrease absorption of folate; decrease serum folate, iron
Nitrofurantoin	Decreases serum folate
Antimitotics	
Methotrexate	Decreases absorption of folate, vitamin B_{12};
Colchicine	Decreases absorption of vitamin B_{12}, carotene, fat, sodium, potassium, cholesterol, lactose, nitrogen
Cathartics	Malabsorption
Phenolphthalein	Hypokalemia, deficiency of vitamin D, calcium
Mineral oil	Decreases absorption of vitamins A, D, K
Diuretics	Some cause hypokalemia, hypomagnesemia; may increase urinary excretion of vitamins B_1, B_6, calcium, magnesium, potassium
Hypocholesterolemics	
Cholestyramine	Binds bile acids; decreases absorption of fat, carotene, vitamins, A, D, K, B_{12}, folate, iron
Clofibrate	Decreases absorption of carotene, vitamin B_{12}, iron, glucose
Hypotensives	
Hydralazine	Vitamin B_6 deficiency
Oral contraceptives	Vitamin B_6, folate deficiency; may increase the need for other nutrients

REFERENCES

1. Lu, A. Y. H.: Liver microsomal drug-metabolizing enzyme system: functional components and their properties, Fed. Proc. **35:**2460, 1976.
2. Visconti, J. A.: Drug-food interaction, nutrition in disease, Columbus, Ohio, 1977, Ross Laboratories.
3. Gringauz, A.: Drugs: how they act and why, St. Louis, 1978, The C. V. Mosby Co.
4. Hartshorn, E. A.: Food and drug interactions, J. Am. Diet. Assoc. **70:**15, 1977.
5. Lehmann, P.: Food and drug interactions, FDA Consumer **12:**20, 1978.
6. Diet-drug interactions, Dairy Council Dig. **48(2):**7, 1977.
7. Roe, D. A.: Drugs, diet and nutrition, Contemp. Nutr. **3(6):**1, 1978.
8. Lucas, B., and Sells, C. J.: Nutrient intake and stimulant drugs in hyperactive children, J. Am. Diet. Assoc. **70:**373, 1977.
9. Carson, J. S., and Gormican, A.: Disease-medication relationships in altered taste sensitivity, J. Am. Diet. Assoc. **68:**550, 1976.
10. Roe, D. A.: Drug-induced nutritional deficiencies, Westport, Conn., 1976, Avi Publishing Company.
11. March, D. C.: Handbook: interactions of selected drugs with nutritional status in man, Chicago, 1976, American Dietetic Association.
12. Moore, A. O., and Powers, D. E.: Food medication interactions; Paradise Valley, Ariz., 1979, Quail Run Publications, Inc.

Food and Nutrition Board, National Academy of Sciences– National Research Council recommended daily dietary allowances, revised 1980

Mean heights and weights and recommended energy intake*

Category	Age (years)	Weight kg	Weight lb	Height cm	Height in	Energy needs (with range) kcal		Energy needs (with range) MJ
Infants	0.0-0.5	6	13	60	24	kg × 115	(95-145)	kg × .48
	0.5-1.0	9	20	71	28	kg × 105	(80-135)	kg × .44
Children	1-3	13	29	90	35	1300	(900-1800)	5.5
	4-6	20	44	112	44	1700	(1300-2300)	7.1
	7-10	28	62	132	52	2400	(1650-3300)	10.1
Males	11-14	45	99	157	62	2700	(2000-3700)	11.3
	15-18	66	145	176	69	2800	(2100-3900)	11.8
	19-22	70	154	177	70	2900	(2500-3300)	12.2
	23-50	70	154	178	70	2700	(2300-3100)	11.3
	51-75	70	154	178	70	2400	(2000-2800)	10.1
	76+	70	154	178	70	2050	(1650-2450)	8.6
Females	11-14	46	101	157	62	2200	(1500-3000)	9.2
	15-18	55	120	163	64	2100	(1200-3000)	8.8
	19-22	55	120	163	64	2100	(1700-2500)	8.8
	23-50	55	120	163	64	2000	(1600-2400)	8.4
	51-75	55	120	163	64	1800	(1400-2200)	7.6
	76+	55	120	163	64	1600	(1200-2000)	6.7
Pregnancy						+300		
Lactation						+500		

*From: Recommended Dietary Allowances, Revised 1980. Food and Nutrition Board National Academy of Sciences-National Research Council, Washington, D.C.

The energy allowances for the young adults are for men and women doing light work. The allowances for the two older age groups represent mean energy needs over these age spans, allowing for a 2% decrease in basal (resting) metabolic rate per decade and a reduction in activity of 200 kcal/day for men and women between 51 and 75 years, 500 kcal for men over 75 years and 400 kcal for women over 75. . . . The customary range of daily energy output is shown for adults in parentheses, and is based on a variation in energy needs of ±400 kcal at any one age . . . emphasizing the wide range of energy intakes appropriate for any group of people.

Energy allowances for children through age 18 are based on median energy intakes of children these ages followed in longitudinal growth studies.The values in parentheses are 10th and 90th percentiles of energy intake, to indicate the range of energy consumption among children of these ages. . . .

Designed for the maintenance of good nutrition of practically all healthy people in

	Age (years)	Weight		Height		Protein (g)	Fat-soluble vitamins				Vitamin C (mg)	Thiamin (mg)
		kg	lb	cm	in		Vitamin A (μg RE)†	Vitamin D (μg)‡	Vitamin E (mg α TE)§			
Infants	0.0-0.5	6	13	60	24	kg × 2.2	420	10	3		35	0.3
	0.5-1.0	9	20	71	28	kg × 2.0	400	10	4		35	0.5
Children	1-3	13	29	90	35	23	400	10	5		45	0.7
	4-6	20	44	112	44	30	500	10	6		45	0.9
	7-10	28	62	132	52	34	700	10	7		45	1.2
Males	11-14	45	99	157	62	45	1000	10	8		50	1.4
	15-18	66	145	176	69	56	1000	10	10		60	1.4
	19-22	70	154	177	70	56	1000	7.5	10		60	1.5
	23-50	70	154	178	70	56	1000	5	10		60	1.4
	51+	70	154	178	70	56	1000	5	10		60	1.2
Females	11-14	46	101	157	62	46	800	10	8		50	1.1
	15-18	55	120	163	64	46	800	10	8		60	1.1
	19-22	55	120	163	64	44	800	7.5	8		60	1.1
	23-50	55	120	163	64	44	800	5	8		60	1.0
	51+	55	120	163	64	44	800	5	8		60	1.0
Pregnant						+30	+200	+5	+2		+20	+0.4
Lactating						+20	+400	+5	+3		+40	+0.5

*The allowances are intended to provide for individual variations among most normal persons as they live in the United States for which human requirements have been less well defined.
†Retinol equivalents. 1 Retinol equivalent = 1 μg retinol or 6 μg βcarotene.
‡As cholecalciferol. 10 μg cholecalciferol = 400 IU vitamin D.
§α tocopherol equivalents. 1 mg d-α-tocopherol = 1 α TE.
‖ 1 NE (niacin equivalent) is equal to 1 mg of niacin or 60 mg of dietary tryptophan.
¶The folacin allowances refer to dietary sources as determined by *Lactobacillus casei* assay after treatment with enzymes
**The RDA for vitamin B$_{12}$ in infants is based on average concentration of the vitamin in human milk. The allowances after factors such as intestinal absorption.
††The increased requirement during pregnancy cannot be met by the iron content of habitual American diets nor by the exist-
tion are not substantially different from those of nonpregnant women, but continued supplementation of the mother for 2-3

Estimated safe and adequate daily dietary intakes of additional selected

	Age (years)	Vitamins			Trace		
		Vitamin K (μg)	Biotin (μg)	Pantothenic acid (mg)	Copper (mg)	Manganese (mg)	Fluoride (mg)
Infants	0-0.5	12	35	2	0.5-0.7	0.5-0.7	0.1-0.5
Children and	0.5-1	10-20	50	3	0.7-1.0	0.7-1.0	0.2-1.0
adolescents	1-3	15-30	65	3	1.0-1.5	1.0-1.5	0.5-1.5
	4-6	20-40	85	3-4	1.5-2.0	1.5-2.0	1.0-2.5
	7-10	30-60	120	4-5	2.0-2.5	2.0-3.0	1.5-2.5
	11+	50-100	100-200	4-7	2.0-3.0	2.5-5.0	1.5-2.5
Adults		70-140	100-200	4-7	2.0-3.0	2.5-5.0	1.5-4.0

*Because there is less information on which to base allowances, these figures are not given in the main table of
†Since the toxic levels for many trace elements may be only several times usual intakes, the upper levels for the

the U.S.A.*

Water-soluble vitamins					Minerals					
Riboflavin (mg)	Niacin (mg NE) ‖	Vitamin B₆ (mg)	Folacin¶ (µg)	Vitamin B₁₂ (µg)	Calcium (mg)	Phosphorus (mg)	Magnesium (mg)	Iron (mg)	Zinc (mg)	Iodine (µg)
0.4	6	0.3	30	0.5**	360	240	50	10	3	40
0.6	8	0.6	45	1.5	540	360	70	15	5	50
0.8	9	0.9	100	2.0	800	800	150	15	10	70
1.0	11	1.3	200	2.5	800	800	200	10	10	90
1.4	16	1.6	300	3.0	800	800	250	10	10	120
1.6	18	1.8	400	3.0	1200	1200	350	18	15	150
1.7	18	2.0	400	3.0	1200	1200	400	18	15	150
1.7	19	2.2	400	3.0	800	800	350	10	15	150
1.6	18	2.2	400	3.0	800	800	350	10	15	150
1.4	16	2.2	400	3.0	800	800	350	10	15	150
1.3	15	1.8	400	3.0	1200	1200	300	18	15	150
1.3	14	2.0	400	3.0	1200	1200	300	18	15	150
1.3	14	2.0	400	3.0	800	800	300	18	15	150
1.2	13	2.0	400	3.0	800	800	300	18	15	150
1.2	13	2.0	400	3.0	800	800	300	10	15	150
+0.3	+2	+0.6	+400	+1.0	+400	+400	+150	††	+5	+25
+0.5	+5	+0.5	+100	+1.0	+400	+400	+150	††	+10	+50

under usual environmental stresses. Diets should be based on a variety of common foods in order to provide other nutrients

("conjugases") to make polyglutamyl forms of the vitamin available to the test organism.
weaning are based on energy intake (as recommended by the American Academy of Pediatrics) and consideration of other

ing iron stores of many women; therefore the use of 30-60 mg of supplemental iron is recommended. Iron needs during lacta-
months after parturition is advisable in order to replenish stores depleted by pregnancy.

vitamins and minerals*

elements†			Electrolytes		
Chromium (mg)	Selenium (mg)	Molybdenum (mg)	Sodium (mg)	Potassium (mg)	Chloride (mg)
0.01-0.04	0.01-0.04	0.03-0.06	115-350	350-925	275-700
0.02-0.06	0.02-0.06	0.04-0.08	250-750	425-1275	400-1200
0.02-0.08	0.02-0.08	0.05-0.1	325-975	550-1650	500-1500
0.03-0.12	0.03-0.12	0.06-0.15	450-1350	775-2325	700-2100
0.05-0.2	0.05-0.2	0.1 -0.3	600-1800	1000-3000	925-2775
0.05-0.2	0.05-0.2	0.15-0.5	900-2700	1525-4575	1400-4200
0.05-0.2	0.05-0.2	0.15-0.5	1100-3300	1875-5625	1700-5100

the RDA and are provided here in the form of ranges of recommended intakes.
trace elements given in this table should not be habitually exceeded.

Food exchange lists*

List 1—milk exchanges
Protein, 8 g; fat, 10 g; carbohydrate, 12 g.

Food	*Measure*	*Weight (g)*
Milk, whole	1 cup	240
Milk, evaporated	½ cup	120
Milk, powder, whole	¼ cup	35
Buttermilk†	1 cup	240
Milk, skim†	1 cup	240

List 2—vegetable exchanges

GROUP A VEGETABLES—negligible protein, fat, and carbohydrate; may be used as desired in amounts ordinarily used.

Asparagus	Greens:	Mushrooms
Beans, string young	beet	Okra
Broccoli	chard	Parsley
Brussels sprouts	collard	Pepper, green
Cabbage	dandelion	Radish
Cauliflower	kale	Romaine
Celery	mustard	Sauerkraut
Chicory	spinach	Squash, summer
Cucumber	turnip	Tomatoes
Eggplant	Lettuce	Watercress
Escarole		

GROUP B VEGETABLES—protein, 2 g; fat, negligible; carbohydrate, 7 g. 1 serving = ½ cup = 100 gm

Beets	Peas, small green	Squash, winter
Carrots	Pumpkin	Turnips
Onions	Rutabagas	

---

*The exchange lists are based on material in the *Exchange Lists for Meal Plannning* prepared by committees of the American Diabetes Association, Inc., and the American Dietetic Association in cooperation with the National Institute of Arthritis, Metabolism and Digestive Diseases and the National Heart and Lung Institute, National Institutes of Health, Public Health Service, U.S. Department of Health, Education, and Welfare.
†Add 2 fat exchanges if fat free.

List 3—fruit exchanges
Protein, negligible; fat, negligible; carbohydrate, 10 g.
Fruits may be used fresh, cooked, canned or frozen, unsweetened.

Food	Measure	Weight (g)
Apple	1 small, 2-inch diameter	80
Applesauce	½ cup	100
Apricots, dried	4 halves	20
Apricots, fresh	2 medium	100
Banana	½ small	50
Berries (blackberries, raspberries, strawberries)	1 cup	150
Blueberries	⅔ cup	100
Cantaloupe	¼, 6-inch diameter	200
Cherries	10 large	75
Dates	2	15
Figs, dried	1 small	15
Figs, fresh	2 large	50
Grapefruit	½ small	125
Grapefruit juice	½ cup	100
Grape juice	¼ cup	60
Grapes	12	75
Honeydew melon	⅛, 7-inch diameter	150
Mango	½ small	70
Nectarines	1 medium	80
Orange	1 small	100
Orange juice	½ cup	100
Papaya	⅓ medium	100
Peach	1 medium	100
Pear	1 small	100
Pineapple	½ cup cubed	80
Pineapple juice	⅓ cup	80
Plums	2 medium	100
Prunes, dried	2 medium	25
Raisins	2 tbsp	15
Tangerine	1 large	100
Watermelon	1 cup diced	175

List 4—bread exchanges
Protein, 2 g; fat, negligible; carbohydrate, 15 g.

Food	Measure	Weight (g)
Bread	1 slice	25
biscuit, roll (2-inch diameter)	1	30
muffin	1 medium	35
cornbread	1½-inch cube	35
Cereal, cooked	½ cup	100
Cereal, dry	¾ cup	20
Crackers, graham	2	20
oyster	20 (½ cup)	20
Saltines (2-inch square)	5	20
soda (2½-inch square)	3	20
round, thin (1½-inch diameter)	6-8	20
Grits, macaroni, noodles, rice, spaghetti, etc.	½ cup cooked	100

Food	Measure	Weight (g)
Ice cream, vanilla (omit 2 fat exchanges)	⅓ cup	70
Sponge cake, no icing	1½-inch cube	25
Vegetables		
beans and peas, dried cooked (includes kidney, lima, navy beans, blackeyed, cowpeas, split peas, etc.)	½ cup cooked	90
corn	⅓ cup or ½ small ear	80
parsnips	⅔ cup	125
potatoes, white, boiled (2-inch diameter)	1 small	100
baked (2-inch diameter)	1 small	100
mashed	½ cup	100
sweet or yam	¼ cup	50

List 5—meat exchanges
Protein, 7 g; fat, 5 g; carbohydrate, negligible.
All items are expressed in cooked weight.

Food	Measure	Weight (g)
Meat (beef, lamb, pork, veal, liver), fish, and fowl (medium fat)	1 ounce	30
cold cuts	1 slice, ⅛-inch thick 4½-inch diameter	45
frankfurter	1	50
cod, herring, etc.	1 ounce	30
crab, salmon, tuna	¼ cup	30
clams, oyster, shrimp	5 small	45
Cheese, Cheddar or American	1 ounce	30
cottage	¼ cup	45
Egg	1	50
Peanut butter*	2 tbsp	30

List 6—fat exchanges
Protein, negligible; fat, 5 g, carbohydrate, negligible.

Food	Measure	Weight (g)
Butter or margarine	1 tsp	5
Bacon, crisp	1 slice	10
Cream, light	2 tbsp	30
Cream, heavy	1 tbsp	15
Cream cheese	1 tbsp	15
French dressing	1 tbsp	15
Mayonnaise	1 tsp	5
Nuts	6 small	10
Oil or cooking fat	1 tsp	5
Olives	5 small	50
Avocado	⅛, 4-inch diameter	25

---

*Limit peanut butter to one serving per day unless adjustment is made to balance carbohydrate content.

Foods allowed as desired

Protein, fat, and carbohydrates, negligible.

Coffee	Gelatin, unsweetened	Cranberries, unsweetened
Tea	Rennet tablets	Lemon
Clear broth	Saccharin	Mustard, dry
Bouillon	Spices	Pickle, dill unsweetened
(fat free)	Vinegar	Rhubarb, unsweetened

Revised exchange list, 1976*

LIST 1: NONFAT MILK EXCHANGES

One exchange of nonfat milk contains 12 g of carbohydrate, 8 g of protein, a trace of fat, and 80 kcal.

Milk is a basic food for your Meal Plan for very good reasons. Milk is the leading source of calcium. It is a good source of phosphorus, protein, some of the B-complex vitamins including folacin and vitamin B_{12}, and vitamins A and D. Magnesium is also found in milk.

Since it is a basic ingredient in many recipes, you will not find it difficult to include milk in your Meal Plan. Milk can be used not only to drink but can be added to cereal, coffee, tea, and other foods.

This list shows the kinds and amounts of milk or milk products to use for one Milk Exchange. Those that appear in CAPS are nonfat. Low-fat and whole milk contain saturated fat.

	Weight† (g)	Amount to use
Nonfat fortified milks		
SKIM OR NONFAT MILK	240	1 cup
POWDERED (NONFAT DRY, BEFORE ADDING LIQUID)	60	⅓ cup
CANNED, EVAPORATED SKIM MILK	120	½ cup
BUTTERMILK MADE FROM SKIM MILK	240	1 cup
YOGURT MADE FROM SKIM MILK (PLAIN, UNFLAVORED)	240	1 cup
Low-fat fortified milk		
1% fat fortified milk (omit ½ Fat Exchange)	240	1 cup

	Weight (g)	Amount to use
2% fat fortified milk (omit 1 Fat Exchange)	240	1 cup
Yogurt made from 2% fortified milk (plain, unflavored) (omit 1 Fat Exchange)	240	1 cup
Whole milk (omit 2 Fat Exchanges)		
Whole milk	240	1 cup
Canned, evaporated whole milk	120	½ cup
Buttermilk made from whole milk	240	1 cup
Yogurt made from whole milk (plain, unflavored)	240	1 cup

LIST 2: VEGETABLE EXCHANGES

One exchange of vegetables contains about 5 g of carbohydrate, 2 g of protein and 25 kcal.

The generous use of many vegetables, served either alone or in other foods such as casseroles, soups, or salads, contributes to sound health and vitality.

Dark green and deep yellow vegetables are among the leading sources of vitamin A. Many of the vegetables in this group are notable sources of vitamin C—asparagus, broccoli, brussels sprouts, cabbage, cauliflower, collard greens, kale, dandelion, mustard and turnip greens, spinach, rutabagas, tomatoes, and turnips. A number are particularly good sources of potassium—broccoli, brussels sprouts, beet greens, chard, and tomato juice. High folacin values are

---

*Adapted from Meal planning with exchange lists, New York, June 1976, The American Diabetes Association Inc.

†Weights obtained from Church, F. C., and Church, H. N.: Food values, ed. 12, Philadelphia, 1975, J. B. Lippincott Co.; Adam, C. F.: Nutritive values of American foods, Handbook No. 456, U.S. Department of Agriculture, Washington, D.C., 1975, U.S. Government Printing Office.

found in asparagus, beets, broccoli, brussels sprouts, cauliflower, collards, kale, and lettuce. Moderate amounts of vitamin B_6 are supplied by broccoli, brussels sprouts, cauliflower, collards, spinach, sauerkraut, and tomatoes and tomato juice. Fiber is present in all vegetables.

Whether you serve them cooked or raw, wash all vegetables even though they look clean. If fat is added in the preparation, omit the equivalent number of Fat Exchanges. The average amount of fat contained in a Vegetable Exchange that is cooked with fat meat or other fats is one Fat Exchange.

This list shows the kinds of *vegetables* to use for one Vegetable Exchange. One exchange is ½ cup.

Asparagus	Mustard
Beans sprouts	Spinach
Beets	Turnip
Broccoli	Mushrooms
Brussels sprouts	Okra
Cabbage	Onions
Carrots	Rhubarb
Cauliflower	Rutabaga
Celery	Sauerkraut
Cucumbers	String beans, green or
Eggplant	yellow
Green pepper	Summer squash
Greens	Tomatoes
Beet	Tomato juice
Chards	Turnips
Collards	Vegetable juice cocktail
Dandelion	Zucchini
Kale	

The following *raw vegetables* may be used as desired:

Chicory	Lettuce
Chinese cab-	Parsley
bage	Radishes
Endive	Watercress
Escarole	

Starchy vegetables are found in the Bread Exchange List.

LIST 3: FRUIT EXCHANGES

One exchange of fruit contains 10 g of carbohydrate and 40 kcal.

Everyone likes to buy fresh fruits when they are in the height of their season. However, you can also buy fresh fruits and can or freeze them for off-season use. For variety, serve fruit as a salad or in combination with other foods for dessert.

Fruits are valuable for vitamins, minerals, and fiber. Vitamin C is abundant in citrus fruits and fruit juices and is found in raspberries, strawberries, mangoes, cantaloupes, honeydew melons, and papayas. The better sources of vitamin A among these fruits include fresh or dried apricots, mangoes, cantaloupes, nectarines, yellow peaches, and persimmons. Oranges, orange juice, and cantaloupe provide more folacin than most of the other fruits in this listing. Many fruits are a valuable source of potassium, especially apricots, bananas, several of the berries, grapefruit, grapefruit juice, mangoes, cantaloupes, honeydew melons, nectarines, oranges, orange juice, and peaches.

Fruit may be used fresh, dried, canned or frozen, cooked or raw, as long as no sugar is added.

This list shows the kinds and amounts of *fruits* to use for one Fruit Exchange.

	Weight (g)	Amount to use
Apple	80	1 small
Apple juice	80	⅓ cup
Applesauce (unsweetened)	100	½ cup
Apricots, fresh	80	2 medium
Apricots, dried	15	4 halves
Banana	50	½ small
Berries		
Blackberries	70	½ cup
Blueberries	70	½ cup
Raspberries	60	½ cup
Strawberries	150	¾ cup
Cherries	75	10 large
Cider	80	⅓ cup
Dates	15	2
Figs, fresh	50	1
Figs, dried	15	1
Grapefruit	125	½
Grapefruit juice	100	½ cup
Grapes	75	12
Grape juice	60	¼ cup
Mango	70	½ small
Melon		
Cantaloupe	200	¼ small
Honeydew	150	⅛ medium
Watermelon	150	1 cup
Nectarine	50	1 small
Orange	100	1 small
Orange juice	100	½ cup
Papaya	90	¾ cup
Peach	100	1 medium
Pear	75	1 small
Persimmon, native	50	1 medium
Pineapple	80	½ cup
Pineapple juice	80	⅓ cup
Plums	100	2 medium

	Weight (g)	Amount to use
Prunes	25	2 medium
Prune juice	65	¼ cup
Raisins	15	2 tbsp
Tangerine	100	1 medium

Cranberries may also be used as desired if no sugar is added.

LIST 4: BREAD EXCHANGES (Includes Breads, Cereal, and Starchy Vegetables)

One exchange of bread contains 15 g of carbohydrate, 2 g of protein, and 70 kcal.

In this list, whole-grain and enriched breads and cereals, germ and bran products, and dried beans and peas are good sources of iron and among the better sources of thiamine. The whole-grain, bran, and germ products have more fiber than products made from refined flours. Dried beans and peas are also good sources of fiber. Wheat germ, bran, dried beans, potatoes, lima beans, parsnips, pumpkin, and winter squash are particularly good sources of potassium. The better sources of folacin in this listing include whole-wheat bread, wheat germ, dried beans, corn, lima beans, parsnips, green peas, pumpkin, and sweet potato. Starchy vegetables are included in this list because they contain the same amount of carbohydrate and protein as one slice of bread.

This list shows the kinds and amounts of *breads, cereals, starchy vegetables,* and *prepared foods* to use for one Bread Exchange. Those that appear in CAPS are low fat.

	Weight (g)	Amount to use
Bread		
WHITE (INCLUDING FRENCH AND ITALIAN)	25	1 slice
WHOLE WHEAT	25	1 slice
RYE OR PUMPERNICKEL	25	1 slice
RAISIN	25	1 slice
BAGEL, SMALL	25	½
ENGLISH MUFFIN, SMALL	25	½
PLAIN ROLL, BREAD	35	1
FRANKFURTER, ROLL	20	½
HAMBURGER BUN	15	½
DRIED BREAD CRUMBS	20	3 tbsp
TORTILLAS, 6 inch	30	1
Cereal		
BRAN FLAKES	25	½ cup
OTHER READY-TO-EAT UNSWEETENED CEREAL	20	¾ cup

	Weight (g)	Amount to use
PUFFED CEREAL (UNFROSTED)	20	1 cup
CEREAL (COOKED)	20	½ cup
GRITS (COOKED)	20	½ cup
RICE OR BARLEY (COOKED)	100	½ cup
PASTA (COOKED), SPAGHETTI, NOODLES, MACARONI	100	½ cup
POPCORN (POPPED, NO FAT ADDED)	20	3 cups
CORNMEAL (DRY)	17	2 tbsp
FLOUR	20	2½ tbsp
WHEAT GERM	50	¼ cup
Crackers		
ARROWROOT	15	3
GRAHAM, 2½-inch square	15	2
MATZOTH, 4 × 6 inch	10	½
OYSTER	15	20
PRETZELS, 3⅛ inches long, ⅛-inch diameter	50	25
RYE WAFERS, 2 × 3½ inches	20	3
SALTINES	20	6
SODA, 2½-inch square	30	4
Dried beans, peas, and lentils		
BEANS, PEAS, LENTILS (DRIED AND COOKED)	90	½ cup
BAKED BEANS, NO PORK (CANNED)	50	¼ cup
Starchy vegetables		
CORN	80	⅓ cup
CORN ON COB	140	1 small
LIMA BEANS	85	½ cup
PARSNIPS	125	⅔ cup
PEAS, GREEN (CANNED OR FROZEN)	100	½ cup
POTATO, WHITE	100	1 small
POTATO (MASHED)	100	½ cup
PUMPKIN	170	¾ cup
WINTER, ACORN, OR BUTTERNUT SQUASH	100	½ cup
YAM OR SWEET POTATO	50	¼ cup
Prepared foods		
Biscuit, 2-inch diameter (omit 1 Fat Exchange)	35	1
Corn bread, 2 × 2 × 1 inch (omit 1 Fat Exchange)	35	1
Corn muffin, 2-inch diameter (omit 1 Fat Exchange)	35	1

	Weight (g)	Amount to use		Weight (g)	Amount to use
Crackers, round butter type (omit 1 Fat Exchange)	20	5	Beef: BABY BEEF (VERY LEAN), CHIPPED BEEF, CHUCK, FLANK STEAK, TENDER-	30	1 ounce
Muffin, plain small (omit 1 Fat Exchange)	35	1	LOIN, PLATE RIBS, PLATE SKIRT STEAK, ROUND		
Potatoes, french fried, 2 to 3½ inches long (omit 1 Fat Exchange)	40	8	(BOTTOM, TOP), ALL CUTS RUMP, SPARE RIBS, TRIPE		
Potato or corn chips (omit 2 Fat Exchanges)	30	15	Lamb: LEG, RIB, SIRLOIN, LOIN (ROAST AND CHOPS), SHANK, SHOULDER	30	1 ounce
Pancake, ½ × 5 inches (omit 1 Fat Exchange)	55	1	Pork: LEG (WHOLE RUMP, CENTER SHANK), HAM,	30	1 ounce
Waffle, ½ × 5 inches (omit 1 Fat Exchange)	75	1	SMOKED (CENTER SLICES)		
			Veal: LEG, LOIN, RIB, SHANK, SHOULDER, CUTLETS	30	1 ounce
			Poultry: MEAT WITHOUT SKIN OF CHICKEN, TURKEY, CORNISH HEN, GUINEA HEN, PHEASANT	30	1 ounce

LIST 5: MEAT EXCHANGES (Lean Meat)

One exchange of lean meat (1 oz) contains 7 g of protein, 3 g of fat, and 55 kcal.

- All of the foods in the Meat Exchange Lists are good sources of protein, and many are also good sources of iron, zinc, vitamin B_{12} (present only in foods of animal origin), and other vitamins of the B-complex.
- Cholesterol is of animal origin. Foods of plant origin have no cholesterol.
- Oysters are outstanding for their high content of zinc. Crab, liver, trimmed lean meats, the dark muscle meat of turkey, dried beans, peas, and peanut butter all have much less zinc than oysters but are still good sources.
- Dried beans, peas, and peanut butter are particularly good sources of magnesium and potassium.
- Your choice of meat groups through the week will depend on your blood lipid values. Consult with your diet counselor and your physician regarding your selection.
- You may use the meat, fish, or other meat exchanges that are prepared for the family when no fat or flour has been added. If meat is fried, use the fat included in the Meal Plan. Meat juices with the fat removed may be used with your meat or vegetables for added flavor. Be certain to trim off all visible fat and measure meat after it has been cooked. A 3-ounce serving of cooked meat is about equal to 4 ounces of raw meat.
- To plan a diet low in saturated fat and cholesterol, choose only those exchanges in CAPS. This list shows the kinds and amounts of *lean meat* and other *protein-rich foods* to use for one Low-Fat Meat Exchange.

	Weight (g)	Amount to use
Fish		
ANY FRESH OR FROZEN	30	1 ounce
CANNED SALMON, TUNA, MACKEREL, CRAB, AND LOBSTER		¼ cup
CLAMS, OYSTERS, SCAL- LOPS, AND SHRIMP	30	5 or 1 ounce
SARDINES, DRAINED	30	3
CHEESES CONTAINING LESS THAN 5% BUTTERFAT	30	1 ounce
COTTAGE CHEESE, DRY, AND 2% BUTTERFAT	30	¼ cup
DRIED BEANS AND PEA (omit 1 Bread Exchange)	90	½ cup

LIST 5: MEAT EXCHANGES (Medium-Fat Meat)

For each exchange of medium-fat meat omit ½ Fat Exchange (7 g protein, 5 g fat, and 75 kcal).

This list shows the kinds and amounts of *medium-fat meat* and other *protein-rich foods* to use for one Medium-Fat Meat Exchange.

	Weight (g)	Amount to use
Beef: ground (15% fat), corned beef (canned), rib eye, round (ground commercial)	30	1 ounce
Pork: loin (all cuts tenderloin), shoulder arm (picnic), shoulder blade, Boston butt, Canadian bacon, boiled ham	30	1 ounce

	Weight (g)	Amount to use
Liver, heart, kidney and sweetbreads (these are high in cholesterol)	30	1 ounce
Creamed cottage cheese	50	¼ cup
Cheese: mozzarella, ricotta, farmer's cheese, Neufchatel	30	1 ounce
Parmesan	15	3 tbsp
Egg (high in cholesterol)	50	1
PEANUT BUTTER (omit 2 additional Fat Exchanges)	30	2 tbsp

LIST 5: MEAT EXCHANGES (High-Fat Meat)

For each exchange of high-fat meat omit 1 Fat Exchange (7 g protein, 7 g fat, and 95 kcal).

This list shows the kinds and amounts of *high-fat meat* and other *protein-rich foods* to use for one High-Fat Meat Exchange.

	Weight (g)	Amount to use
Beef: brisket, corned beef (brisket), ground beef (more than 20% fat), hamburger (commercial), chuck (ground commercial), roasts (rib), steaks (club and rib)	30	1 ounce
Lamb: breast	30	1 ounce
Pork: spare ribs, loin (back ribs), pork (ground), country style ham, deviled ham	30	1 ounce
Veal: breast	30	1 ounce
Poultry: capon, duck (domestic), goose	30	1 ounce
Cheese: cheddar types	30	1 ounce
Cold cuts	45	4½ × ⅛-inch
Frankfurter	50	1

LIST 6: FAT EXCHANGES

One exchange of fat contains 5 g of fat and 45 kcal.

Fats are of both animal and vegetable origin and range from liquid oils to hard fats. Oils are fats that remain liquid at room temperature and are usually of vegetable origin. Common fats obtained from vegetables are corn oil, olive oil, and peanut oil. Some of the common animal fats are butter and bacon fat.

Since all fats are concentrated, sources of kilocalories, and foods on this list should be measured carefully to control weight. Margarine, butter, cream, and cream cheese contain vitamin A. Use the fats on this list in the amounts on the Meal Plan.

This list shows the kinds and amounts of *fat-containing foods* to use for one Fat Exchange. To plan a diet low in saturated fat select only those exchanges that appear in CAPS. They are polyunsaturated.

	Weight (g)	Amount to use
MARGARINE, SOFT, TUB OR STICK*	5	1 tsp
AVOCADO, 4-inch diameter†	25	⅛
OIL, CORN, COTTONSEED, SAFFLOWER, SOY, SUNFLOWER	5	1 tsp
OIL, OLIVE†	5	1 tsp
OIL, PEANUT†	5	1 tsp
OLIVES†	50	5 small
ALMONDS†	10	10 whole
PECANS†	5	2 large whole
PEANUTS†		
SPANISH	10	20 whole
VIRGINIA	10	10 whole
WALNUTS	15	6 small
NUTS, OTHER†	15	6 small
Margarine, regular stick	5	1 tsp
Butter	5	1 tsp
Bacon fat	5	1 tsp
Bacon, crisp	10	1 strip
Cream, light	30	2 tbsp
Cream, sour	30	2 tbsp
Cream, heavy	15	1 tbsp
Cream cheese	15	1 tbsp
French dressing‡	15	1 tbsp
Italian dressing‡	15	1 tbsp
Lard	5	1 tsp
Mayonnaise‡	5	1 tsp
Salad dressing, mayonnaise type‡	10	2 tsp
Salt pork	5	¾-inch cube

*Made with corn, cottonseed, safflower, soy, or sunflower oil only.

†Fat content is primarily monounsaturated.

‡If made with corn, cottonseed, safflower, soy, or sunflower oil, can be used on fat modified diet.

Common prefixes, suffixes, and combining forms

Prefixes		*Suffixes*	
a, an	without, as avitaminosis	algia	pain; as neuralgia
ab	away from; as abnormal	ase	enzyme; as amylase
ad	near, toward; as adrenal	cide	kill; as bactericide
ana	upward; as anabolism	clysis	drenching; as venoclysis
anti	against; as antibiotic	cule	small; as molecule
auto	self; as autodigestion	cyte	cell; as erythrocyte
bio	life; as biology	ectomy	cut off; as appendectomy
calor	heat; as calorimeter	emesis	vomiting; as hematemesis
cata	downward; as catabolism	emia	blood; as anemia
chole	bile, gall; as cholagogue	esthesia	sensation; as anesthesia
chroma	color; as chromatosis	ism	condition; as alcoholism
co	together; as coenzyme	itis	inflammation; as appendicitis
di	two, double; as diplopia	lysis	destruction; as hemolysis
dis	ill, negative; as disease	malacia	softening; as osteomalacia
dys	bad, difficult; as dyspepsia	oma	tumor, swelling; as adenoma
ec	outside; as ectopic	opsy	to view; as biopsy
encephal	brain, skull; as encephalogram	osis	condition; as tuberculosis
endo	inside; as endogenous	pathy	disease of; neuropathy
exo	outside; as exogenous	penia	poverty; as leukopenia
hemo	blood; as hemopoiesis	phagia	to eat; as polyphagia
hyper	above, excessive; as hyperacid	phil	to love; as basophil
hypo	below, little; as hypofunction	phobia	fear of; as photophobia
im	not; as immature	pnea	breath; as hyperpnea
in	not; as incurable	poiesis	to produce; as hemopoiesis
inter	between; as interstitial	ptysis	to spit; as hemoptysis
intra	within; as intravascular	rrhea	to discharge; as diarrhea
meta	change; as metaplasia	tomy	to cut; as vagotomy
necro	dead; as necrosis	trophy	growth; as hypertrophy
para	beside; as paravertebral	uria	urine; as glucosuria
peri	around; as pericardium		
post	after; as postmortem		
pre	before; as prenatal		
syn	union, together; as synthesis		

*From Lagua, R. T., Claudio, V. S., and Thiele, V. F.: Nutrition and diet therapy reference dictionary, ed. 2, St. Louis, 1974, The C. V. Mosby Co.

Combining forms

adeno	gland; as adenoma	mega	enlarged; as hepatomegaly
arthro	joint; as arthrology	micro	small; as microorganism
cephalo	head; as cephalocaudal	myo	muscle; as myoglobin
colo	colon; as colostomy	nephro	kidney; as nephrosis
costo	rib; as costochondral	neuro	nerve; as neurology
cysto	bladder; as cystogram	oligo	few, scant; as oligosaccharide
cyto	cell; as cytoblast	ophthalmo	eye; as ophthalmology
derma	skin; as dermatology	opia	sight, vision; as myopia
entero	intestines; as enterocolitis	osteo	bone; as osteoporosis
erythro	red; as erythrocyte	oto	ear; as otoscope
gastro	stomach; as gastrointestinal	pan	all, every; as pandemic
glossa	tongue; as glossitis	path	disease; as pathogenesis
hemato	blood; as hematology	phago	to eat; as phagocytosis
hepato	liver; as hepatomegaly	phlebo	vein; as phlebotomy
hetero	mixed; as heterogenous	poly	many; as polysaccharide
hydro	water; as hydrolysis	procto	anus; as proctoscopy
hystero	uterus; as hysterogram	proto	first; as protoplasm
ileo	ileum; as ileostomy	psycho	mind; as psychology
iso	equal; as isocaloric	pulmo	lung; as pulmonary
kerato	horny; as keratoderma	pyelo	kidney, pelvis; as pyelonephritis
leuko	white; as leukocyte	pyo	pus; as pyorrhea
lith	stone, calculus; as cholelith	rrhage	excessive flow; as hemorrhage
macro	large; as macrocyte	sclero	hard; as arteriosclerosis
mal	ill or bad; as malnutrition	thio	sulfur-containing; as thiochrome

Common abbreviations on patients' charts

a	ante; before	cc	cubic centimeter
a̅a̅	each; of each	CC	chief complaint
Abd	abdominal; abdomen	CCF	cephalin-cholesterol flocculation
ac	ante cibes; before meals	CCU	coronary care unit
ad lib	ad libitum; as desired; as needed	cd	cane die; daily
Adm	admission	CHF	congestive heart failure
AF	artificial	chr	chronic
A/G	albumin-globulin	ck	check
AHD	arteriosclerotic heart disease	Cl	chloride
AID	acute infectious disease	cm	centimeter
alb	albumin	CNS	central nervous system
ALK	alkaline	CO₂	carbon dioxide
amt	amount	Cpd or Comp	compound
AP	anterior-posterior	CRF	chronic renal failure
APC	anterial premature contraction	C & S	culture and sensitivity
approx	approximately	CSF	cerebrospinal fluid
Aq	aqua; water	CV	cardiovascular
ARF	acute rheumatic fever	CVA	cerebral vascular accident
ASA	aspirin; acetylsalicylic acid	CVP	central venous pressure
ASHD	arteriosclerotic heart disease	Cw	crutch walking
as tol	as tolerated	d	daily
B	born; basophils	DBW	desirable body weight
Ba	barium	D & C	dilatation and curettage
bid	bis in die; twice daily	Diag or Dx	diagnosis
bilat	bilateral	dil	dilute
BM	bowel movement	disc or D/C	discontinue
BMR	basal metabolic rate	Disch	discharge
BP	blood pressure	dl	deciliter
BPH	benign prostatic hypertrophy	DL	danger list
BR	bed rest	D₂O	deuterium or heavy water
BRP	bathroom privileges	DOA	dead on arrival
BSL	blood sugar level	DOS	day of surgery
BSP	bromosulfonphthalein	DPM	discontinue previous medication
BUN	blood urea nitrogen	DPT	diphtheria, pertussis, tetanus inoculation
c̄	cum; with		
C	centigrade	dr	dram; drachm; 3.8 g
Ca	carcinoma; cancer; calcium	DR	delivery room
cap	capsule	D/S	dextrose and saline
cath	catheterize	DSD	dry sterile dressing
cbc or CBC	complete blood count	DT	delirium tremens

*From Lagua, R. T., Claudio, V. S., and Thiele, V. F.: Nutrition and diet therapy reference dictionary, ed. 2, St. Louis, 1974, The C. V. Mosby Co.

DW	distilled water	hx	hospitalization; history
e	et; and	ibid	same as before
E or EOS	eosinophils	Ict Ind	icterus index
ECG or EKG	electrocardiogram	ICU	intensive care unit
ED	emergency department	I & D	incision and drainage
EDC	expected date of confinement	i.e.	that is
EEG	electroencephalogram	IM	intramuscularly
e.g.	for example	Imp	impression
Elix	elixir	int	internal
ENT	ear, nose, and throat	I & O	intake and output
ER	emergency room	IPPB	intermittent positive pressure
ESR	erythrocyte sedimentation rate		breathing
etc.	and so forth	irrig	irrigation
EUA	examine under anesthesia	IU	international unit
exp	expired	IV	intravenously
Expl Lap	exploratory laparotomy	IVP	intravenous pyelogram
ext	external	IVSD	intraventricular septal defect
extr	extract	K	potassium
F	father; female; Fahrenheit	kg	kilogram
FBS	fasting blood sugar	KUB	kidney, ureter, and bladder
$FeSO_4$	ferrous sulfate	L	liter
FH	family history; fetal heart	lat	lateral
Fib	fibrillation	LBBB	left bundle branch block
FLD	fluid	liq	liquid
FTT	failure to thrive	LLL	left lower lobe
FUO	fever of unknown origin	LLQ	left lower quadrant
Fx	fracture	LMP	last menstrual period
g	gram; 15.43 grains	LP	lumbar puncture
GA	gastric analysis	LR	labor room
GB	gallbladder	LUL	left upper lobe
GBD	gallbladder disease	LUQ	left upper quadrant
GBS	gallbladder series	lym	lymphocyte
GC	gonococcal count	lytes	electrolytes
GE	gastroenteritis	m	minim
GI	gastrointestinal	M	mother; monocyte; male
GIT	gastrointestinal tract	M et N	mone et nocte; day and night
gr	grain	mcg	microgram
gtt(s)	gutta; drop(s)	mec	meconium
GTT	glucose tolerance test	mEq	milliequivalent
GU	genitourinary	mg	milligram
Gyn	gynecology	MGW	magnesium sulfate, glycerine, and
h	hour		water enema
hb, Hg, or Hgb	hemoglobin	MI	mitral insufficiency; myocardial infarction
hct	hematocrit	ml	milliliter
HCVD	hypertensive cardiovascular disease	MO	mineral oil; month
		MOM	milk of magnesia
hem	blood	M & R	measure and record
HO	house officer	MS	mitral stenosis; multiple sclerosis
H_2O	water	n	nocte; night
HNV	has not voided	Na	sodium
HPN	hypertension	NaCl	sodium chloride
HR	heart rate	NDF	no diagnostic findings
hs	hora somni; at bedtime	neg	negative

N/G or NG	nasogastric	prn	pro re nata; whenever necessary
nil	nothing	prog	prognosis
no or #	number	PSP	phenolsulfonphthalein
NP	neuropsychiatry	pt	patient
NPH	isophane insulin (neutral protamine Hagedorn)	PT	physical therapy
		PTA	prior to admission
NPN	nonprotein nitrogen	PTB	pulmonary tuberculosis
NPO	nil per os; nothing by mouth	pu	peptic ulcer
NS or NSS	normal saline solution	PWB	partial weight bearing
NSR	normal sinus rhythm	PZI	protamine zinc insulin
N & T	nose and throat	q	quaque; every
NTG	nitroglycerin	qd	quaque die; every day
NWB	no weight bearing	qh	quaque hora; every hour
O	oral	qid	quater in die; four times a day
O_2	oxygen	ql	quantum libit; as much as desired
OB	obstetrics; occult blood	qn	quaque nocte; every night
od or OD	oculus dexter; right eye	qns	quantity not sufficient
oint	ointment	qod	every other day
OM	omne mone; every day	qoh	every other hour
ON	omne nocte; every night	qon	every other night
OOB	out of bed	qs	quantum sufficiat; quantity sufficient
OOR	out of room		
O & P	ova and parasites	R	respiration rate; rectal
OPD	outpatient department	RAI	radioactive isotope
ophth	ophthalmology	RBBB	right bundle branch block
OR	operating room	RBC	red blood cell
Orth(o)	orthopedics	re	concerning
os or OS	oculus sinister; left eye	RHD	rheumatic heart disease
OT	occupational therapy; old tuberculin	RLQ	right lower quadrant
		R/O	rule out
ou	both eyes	RR	recovery room; respiratory rate
oz	ounce	rt or R	right
p	post; after	RUQ	right upper quadrant
P	pulse; phosphorus	Rx	treatment; take
PA	posterior anterior (x-ray film)	$\bar{s}$	without
PAF	paroxysmal atrial fibrillation	"S"	service patient
Pap smear	Papanicoloau smear	SAH	subarachnoid hemorrhage
PAT	pregnancy at term	sbs	soft brown stool
path	pathology	sc	subcutaneous
PBI	protein-bound iodine	SCD	surgical cut down
Pc	post cibum; after meals	sed rate	sedimentation rate
PE	physical examination	sgs	soft green stool
PH	past history	sibs	brothers and sisters
PI	present illness	sig	sign; let it be labeled
PID	pelvic inflammatory disease	S & O	salpingo-oophorectomy
PKU	phenylketonuria	SOB	short of breath
PM	postmortem	Sol	solution
PMI	post myocardial infarction	spec	specimen
PMP	previous menstrual period	sp gr	specific gravity
po	per os; by mouth; orally	$\overline{ss}$	one half
Post	posterior	SSE	soapsuds enema
pp	postprandial; postpartum	Staph	staphylococcus
PPD	purified protein derivative	stat	immediately
pr	per rectum	Strep	streptococcus

SUN	serum urea nitrogen	V	ventricular
syr	syrup	vd	void
sys	soft yellow stool	VD	venereal disease
Sx	symptoms	via	by way of
Sy	syphilis	viz	namely
t or tsp	teaspoon	VNS	visiting nurse service
T	temperature	vol	volume
T or tbsp	tablespoon	VP	venous pressure
T & A	tonsils and adenoids	VPC	ventricular premature contraction
tab	tablet	VS	vital signs
TAH	total abdominal hysterectomy	WA	when awake
tbc or TBC	tuberculosis	Wass	Wassermann
TBW	total body weight	WB	weight-bearing
TCR	turn, cough, and rebreathe	WBC	white blood count; white blood cell
temp	temperature	WNL	within normal limits
tid	three times a day	wt	weight
TP	total protein	x	times
TPR	temperature, pulse, and respiration	x-match	cross match
tr or tinct	tincture	*Miscellaneous*	
Trach	tracheostomy	♂	male
TTT	thymol turbidity test	♀	female
TURP	transurethral prostatectomy	+	positive
TWE	tap water enema	−	negative
U	unit	0	nothing
ung	ointment	$\dot{\div}$	one
URI	upper respiratory infection	<	less than
USP	*United States Pharmacopoeia*	>	greater than
UTI	urinary tract infection	∴	therefore
		~	similar to

Normal constituents of blood†

Physical measurements		Hemoglobin	
Specific gravity	1.025-1.030	Adults	
Reaction	pH 7.37-7.45	Men	14-17 g/dl
Bleeding time	1-5 minutes	Women	12-15 g/dl
Coagulation time, venous blood (Lee-White method)	4-12 minutes	Children (varies with age)	10-18 g/dl
Prothrombin time, plasma (Quick method)	14-18 seconds	Volume, whole blood	70-100 ml/kg
		Total protein, serum	6-8 g/dl
Sedimentation rate (Wintrobe)		Albumin, serum	4-5.5 g/dl
		Globulin, serum	1.3-2.7 g/dl
Men	0-9 mm per hour	Albumin-globulin ratio	1.8-2.5
Women	0-20 mm per hour	Ceruloplasmin, plasma	15-30 mg/dl
Hematology		Fibrinogen, plasma	0.2-0.4 g/dl
Cell volume	39%-50%	Nitrogen constituents	
Cells, differential count		Amino acid nitrogen, blood	4-8 mg/dl
Lymphocytes	25%-35%/mm³		
Monocytes	4%-10%/mm³	Ammonia, blood	40-70 μg/dl
Neutrophils	50%-65%/mm³	Ammonia, serum	0.15-0.30 mg/dl
Eosinophils	0.5%-4%/mm³	Creatine	0.2-0.9 mg/dl
Basophils	0%-2%/mm³	Creatinine	0.8-2 mg/dl
Erythrocytes (RBCs)	4.2-5.5 million per mm³	Nonprotein nitrogen, blood	20-40 mg/dl
Leukocytes (WBCs)	5-10 thousand per mm³	Urea nitrogen, blood	10-20 mg/dl
		Urea, blood	20-35 mg/dl
Thrombocytes (platelets)	150-300 thousand per mm³	Uric acid, blood	2.5-5 mg/dl
		Amino acids	
Reticulocytes	0.5%-2% red cells	Amino acids, total	35-65 mg/dl
Hematocrit (vol % red cells)		Alanine	3.0-3.7 mg/dl
		Alpha-aminobutyric acid	0.2-0.4 mg/dl
Men	40%-54%		
Women	37%-47%	Arginine	1.2-1.9 mg/dl

*From Lagua, R. T., Claudio, V. S., and Thiele, V. F.: Nutrition and diet therapy reference dictionary, ed. 2, St. Louis, 1974, The C. V. Mosby Co.
†Compiled from the following sources: Cecil, R. L., et al.: A textbook of medicine, Philadelphia, 1955, W. B. Saunders Co.; Cooper, L. F., et al.: Nutrition in health and disease, Philadelphia, 1958, J. B. Lippincott Co.; Goldsmith, G. A.: Nutritional diagnosis, Springfield, Ill., 1959, Charles C Thomas, Publisher; Goodhart, R. S., and Wohl, M. G.: Modern nutrition in health and disease, Philadelphia, 1964, Lea & Febiger; Harper, H. A.: Review of physiological chemistry, Los Altos, Calif., 1963, Lange Medical Publications; Harrow, B., and Mazur, A.: Textbook of biochemistry, Philadelphia, 1966, W. B. Saunders Co.; Proudfit, F. T., and Robinson, C. H.: Normal and therapeutic nutrition, New York, 1961, The Macmillan Co.; White, A., Handler, P., and Smith, E. L.: Principles of biochemistry, New York, 1964, McGraw-Hill Book Co.

Asparagine	0.5-0.7 mg/dl	O_2 content	
Aspartic acid	0.01-0.07 mg/dl	Arterial blood	15-23 vol%
Cysteine and cystine	1.1-1.3 mg/dl	Venous blood	10-16 vol%
Glutamic acid	0.4-1.2 mg/dl	O_2 saturation	
Glutamine	5-12 mg/dl	Arterial blood	94%-96%
Glycine	1.3-1.7 mg/dl	Venous blood	60%-85%
Histidine	0.8-1.5 mg/dl	O_2 tension	95-100 mm Hg
Isoleucine	0.7-1.3 mg/dl	Minerals	
Leucine	1.4-2.3 mg/dl	Base, serum (total)	145-155 mEq/L
Lysine	2.5-3.0 mg/dl	Calcium, serum	9-11 mg/dl
Methionine	0.3-0.4 mg/dl		4.5-5.5 mEq/L
Ornithine	0.6-0.8 mg/dl	Chlorides, serum	355-376 mg/dl
Phenylalanine	0.7-1.0 mg/dl		100-106 mEq/L
Proline	1.8-3.3 mg/dl	Copper	130-230 μg/dl
Serine	1.1-1.2 mg/dl	Iodine	
Threonine	1.2-1.7 mg/dl	Total	8-15 mEq/L
Tryptophan	1.0-1.2 mg/dl	Protein-bound	4-8 μg/dl
Tyrosine	0.8-1.5 mg/dl	Iron, serum	80-100 μg/dl
Valine	0.4-3.7 mg/dl	Magnesium, serum	2-3 mg/dl
Carbohydrates			1.6-2.4 mEq/L
Glucose		Phosphate	1.6-2.7 mEq/L
Nelson-Somogyi	70-100 mg/dl	Phosphorus, inorganic,	3-4.5 mg/dl
Folin-Wu	80-120 mg/dl	serum	1-1.5 mEq/L
Fructose	6-8 mg/dl	Potassium, serum	16-20 mg/dl
Glycogen	5-6 mg/dl		4-5 mEq/L
Hexoses	70-105 mg/dl	Sodium, serum	310-340 mg/dl
Hexuronates (as glucu-	0.4-1.4 mg/dl		136-145 mEq/L
ronic acid)		Sulfates, inorganic, serum	2.5-5.0 mg/dl
Pentose, total	2-4 mg/dl		0.5-1.5 mEq/L
Lipid		Vitamins	
Cephalin	0-30 mg/dl	Ascorbic acid	
Cholesterol, serum		Serum	0.4-1.0 mg/dl
Total	150-240 mg/dl	White blood cells	25-40 mg/dl
Esters	100-180 mg/dl	Folic acid	3.4 μg/dl
Cholesterol, free	50-60 mg/dl	Riboflavin	20 μg/dl
Fats, neutral	150-300 mg/dl	Thiamine	3.4 μg/dl
Fatty acids, serum (total)	350-450 mg/dl	Vitamin A	40-120 IU/dl
Fatty acids, free	8-30 mg/dl	Vitamin B_6, xanthurenic	30 mg per day
Lecithin	100-200 mg/dl	acid excretion after 10 g	
Lipids, serum (total)	450-850 mg/dl	tryptophan	
Phospholipids, serum	230-300 mg/dl	Vitamin B_{12}	350-750 μg/dl
(total)		Vitamin D, alkaline phos-	5-15 Bodansky
Plasmalogen	7-8 mg/dl	phatase	units
Sphingomyelin	10-50 mg/dl	Vitamin E, serum tocoph-	
Blood gases		erol	
CO_2-combining power	50-65 vol%	Adults	1.0-1.2 mg/dl
	21-28 mEq/L	Infants	0.23-0.43 mg/dl
CO_2 content		Vitamin K, prothrombin	10-15 seconds
Serum	50-70 vol%	time	
	21-30 mEq/L	Organic acids	
Whole blood	40-60 vol%	Acetoacetic acid	0.8-2.8 mg/dl
	18-27 mEq/L	Alpha-ketoglutaric acid	0.2-1.0 mg/dl
CO_2 tension	38-40 mm Hg	Citric acid	1.4-3.0 mg/dl
O_2 capacity, whole blood	16-27 vol%	Lactic acid	8-17 mg/dl

Malic acid	0.1-0.9 mg/dl	Phosphatase, acid	
Pyruvic acid	0.4-2 mg/dl	Bodansky	0.5-2 units/dl
Succinic acid	0.1-0.6 mg/dl	Gutman	0.5-2 units/dl
Ketone bodies	0.3-2 mg/dl	King-Armstrong	1-5 units/dl
Enzymes		Shinowara	0.1-1 units/dl
Amylase, serum	80-180 Somogyi units/dl	Miscellaneous	
		Bicarbonate	24-30 mEq/L
Lipase, serum	450-850 mg/dl	Bilirubin, serum (total)	0.2-1.4 mg/dl
Phosphatase, alkaline		Direct	0.1-0.2 mg/dl
Bodanksy	1-4 units/dl	Indirect	0.1-0.6 mg/dl
Gutman	3-10 units/dl	Carotenoids	60-180 μg/dl
King-Armstrong	8-14 units/dl	Icterus index, serum	4-7 units
Shinowara	2-8 units/dl	Taurine	0.4-0.8 mg/dl

Normal constituents of urine

Specific gravity	1.008-1.030	Sugar	None (in some persons, 0.002-0.003 g per 24 hours after a heavy meal)
Reaction	pH 5.5-8.0		
Volume	1000-1500 ml per 24 hours		
Total solids	55-70 g/L	Sulfate, organic	0.06-0.2 g per 24 hours
Organic constituents			
Acetone (ketone) bodies	0.003-0.015 g per 24 hours	Urea	20-35 g per 24 hours
		Uric acid	0.5-0.8 g per 24 hours
Ammonia	0.4-1.0 g per 24 hours		
		Inorganic constituents	
Bile	None	Calcium	0.1-0.3 g per 24 hours
Creatine	None (0-0.2 g per 24 hours)		
		Chloride (as NaCl)	10-15 g per 24 hours
Creatinine	1.0-1.5 g per 24 hours	Iron	0.001-0.005 g per 24 hours
Hippuric acid	0.1-1.0 g per 24 hours	Magnesium	0.15-0.30 g per 24 hours
Indican	0.004-0.020 g per 24 hours	Phosphorus	2.0-2.5 g per 24 hours
Nitrogen, total	10-17 g per 24 hours	Potassium	1.5-2.5 g per 24 hours
Protein (albumin)	None (0-0.015 g per 24 hours)	Sodium	2.0-5.0 g per 24 hours
Purine bases	0.006-0.014 g per 24 hours	Sulfur, total	1.5-3.0 g per 24 hours

*From Lagua, R. T., Claudio, V. S., and Thiele, V. F.: Nutrition and diet therapy reference dictionary, ed. 2, St. Louis, 1974, The C. V. Mosby Co.

pH values of various body fluids

Aqueous humor of eye	7.4
Blood serum	7.35-7.45
Cerebrospinal fluid	7.35-7.45
Feces	7.0-7.5
Gallbladder bile	5.4-6.9
Gastric juice, pure	About 0.9
Hepatic duct bile	7.4-8.5
Intestinal juice	7.0-8.0
Milk	6.6-6.9
Pancreatic juice	7.5-8.0
Saliva	6.35-6.85
Skin, intracellular, various layers	6.2-7.5
Tears	7.4
Urine	4.5-7.5

---

*From Lagua, R. T., Claudio, V. S., and Thiele, V. F.: Nutrition and diet therapy reference dictionary, ed. 2, St. Louis, 1974, The C. V. Mosby Co.

Dietary management of selected disorders

Adrenocortical insufficiency. High-protein, high-calorie, and high salt diet. To avoid hypoglycemia, serve meals frequently with between-meal feedings. In ACTH therapy, mild sodium restriction is often necessary. Avoidance of salty foods and no added salt on the table is usually sufficient.

Alcoholic liver disease. Withdrawal of alcohol and a diet high in protein and vitamins, especially the B complex vitamins. Poor food intake and consequent malnutrition contribute to the fatty liver and alcoholic hepatitis. The objectives of the diet are nutritional rehabilitation, correction of deficiency states, and repair of hepatic and neural damage caused by inadequate nutrition.

Alkaptonuria. The exact dietary treatment is not yet known, although restriction of dietary protein to reduce homogentisic acid formation may be of some value.

Allergy. Avoid or exclude the offending food allergen from the diet. Take note of forms of food preparation in which the food allergen may be used. When the offending food allergen is not known, one of several test diets for allergy may be used.

Anemia, folic acid–deficiency. A diet liberal in protein of high biological value with folic acid and vitamin C supplementation. Emphasis is placed on liver, meats, fish, legumes, deep green leafy vegetables, citrus fruits, and other vitamin C–rich foods. Vitamin C is necessary for the conversion of folic acid to its metabolically active form, folinic acid.

Anemia, iron-deficiency. A diet high in iron, protein of high biological value, and vitamin C for absorption of iron. Foods high in iron include liver, egg yolk, kidney, beef, dried fruits, molasses, and whole-grain cereals.

Anemia, pernicious. Vitamin B_{12} in therapeutic doses plus a diet high in protein of good biological value with iron and vitamin supplementa-

tion. A sore mouth or gastrointestinal irritation may necessitate a soft or even liquid diet.

Anemia, protein-deficiency. The protein level in the diet should be very high (2.5 to 3.0 g/kg of body weight or approximately 120 to 150 g per day). Carbohydrate and caloric intake should be high for proper utilization of protein.

Anorexia nervosa. It is best not to press food at the beginning, since rejection of food is part of the illness. Serve attractive and palatable meals in small quantities, and gradually increase the amount until 3000 or more calories are being consumed. When the patient refuses to eat, it may be necessary to give food by tube feeding.

Arginosuccinic aciduria. The exact dietary treatment is not known. Protein restriction with arginine supplementation has been tried.

Arthritis. There is no specific dietary regimen as long as the nutritional status of the patient is satisfactory. A reduction in weight is advisable in osteoarthritis to lessen the extra weight placed on weight-bearing joints. On the other hand, patients with rheumatoid arthritis who have lost weight and are malnourished should be given a high-calorie, high-protein diet. Some sodium restriction may be necessary in ACTH therapy. Patients with a type IV plasma lipid profile may benefit from a type IV diet for hyperlipoproteinemia. See discussion of dietary management of hyperlipoproteinemia.

Ascites. Rigid sodium restriction is usually required (250 mg per day in severe cases; 500 mg per day in milder cases). Diuresis may occur within a few days or weeks. As the fluid retention subsides, the sodium restriction can be liberalized gradually up to 2000 mg per day.

Atherosclerosis. A diet aimed at lowering serum lipid concentrations. This can be achieved by decreasing caloric intake, restricting cholesterol intake to 300 mg or less per day, and substituting vegetable oils rich in polyunsaturated fats in

---

*From Lagua, R. T., Claudio, V. S., and Thiele, V. F.: Nutrition and diet therapy reference dictionary, ed. 2, St. Louis, 1974, The C. V. Mosby Co.

place of saturated fats. Weight reduction is indicated for the overweight.

Burns. A high-calorie, high-protein, high-fluid diet liberal in vitamins, especially vitamin C. Restore fluid and electrolyte balance to prevent shock. Tube feeding may be necessary if the patient is unable to eat or drink.

Calculi. Urinary calculi are seldom "pure." They are usually a mixture of several substances such as uric acid, cystine, calcium oxalate, calcium carbonate, and calcium phosphate. Once the stones are formed, no diet is effective in bringing about their dissolution. However, for the predisposed individual, dietary management may help prevent or retard the growth or recurrence of the stones. The type of diet depends on the chief component of the stones. Restrict calcium and phosphorus in calcium phosphate stones; maintain an acid urine in magnesium phosphate stones; restrict sulfur-containing amino acids and maintain an alkaline urine in cystine stones; restrict oxalate and calcium intakes in calcium oxalate stones; and maintain an alkaline urine to keep urate stones in solution. A high fluid intake is recommended in all types of stone formation.

Cancer. Appetizing food is emphasized, since anorexia is common. Cancer in the gastrointestinal tract may require a bland, low-fiber diet given in small, frequent feedings. A low-residue diet or defined-formula diet is indicated in cancer of the bowel. A mechanical soft diet consisting of smooth, semisolid foods is indicated in cancer of the esophagus. Tube feeding is often used when there is difficulty in swallowing.

Cardiac diseases. Caloric intake is adjusted to bring about weight loss and consequent lowering of blood pressure, slowing of heart rate, and reduction in the work of the heart. Rest is the primary consideration in acute heart diseases such as heart failure or coronary occlusion. Even fluids are restricted during the first few days. With improvement, soft and easily digested foods are gradually introduced in small amounts as tolerated. Sodium intake is restricted to 500 mg in edema and then maintained at 1000 to 1500 mg per day once edema disappears. In ischemic heart disease involving hypercholesterolemia and atherosclerosis the fat in the diet should be predominantly of the polyunsaturated type; cholesterol and saturated fats are restricted. In chronic heart conditions, three small meals with between-meal feedings are recommended to avoid strain on the heart. Constipa-

tion should be avoided, and maintenance of normal or slightly below normal weight is desirable. Sodium may be mildly restricted (2000 mg per day) to prevent edema.

Celiac disease. A gliadin-restricted diet high in calories and protein (6 to 8 g/kg body weight) with mineral and vitamin supplementation to correct nutritional deficiency states resulting from impaired absorption. In infants with severe diarrhea, immediate administration of fluid and electrolytes is necessary. Fat is restricted in the milk formula. Simple carbohydrates and fruits and selected starches such as corn, rice, arrowroot, cassava, and potato supply the remaining calories. The restriction in gliadin intake should be regarded as permanent in this condition.

Cerebral palsy. A high-calorie diet (up to 4000 kcal) for the athetoid type or for those who are constantly in motion and are often underweight, and a low-calorie diet for the spastic type or those who are prone to obesity because of limited activity. Vitamins, especially the B complex, and mineral supplements are usually needed. Tube feeding may be indicated when there is difficulty in swallowing.

Cholecystectomy. After surgery, a low-fat diet for a month or longer, then a gradual increase of fat intake as tolerated. The amount of fat tolerated varies with individual patients. Avoid excessive intake of bulky, rich, and fatty foods in one meal.

Cholecystitis. A low-fat, bland diet is indicated. Restriction in fat intake will prevent stimulation of gallbladder contraction. In acute cases, nothing is given orally for 24 hours or more. Then a clear liquid diet is given for 2 to 3 days, and the diet is progressed to one low in fat (20 to 30 g per day) and restricted in coarse fiber. In chronic cholecystitis a moderate intake of fat (40 to 50 g per day) is indicated to promote the flow of bile and induce drainage of the biliary tract. Weight reduction is desirable for the overweight.

Cholelithiasis. When stones form an obstruction or the gallbladder is inflamed, give a low-fat diet to decrease gallbladder contraction and to lessen the pain. A moderate fat intake is desirable if the gallbladder is sluggish or "lazy" to stimulate its contraction and prevent stagnation of bile. It is unlikely that restriction of cholesterol in the diet has any appreciable effect on reducing cholesterol stones. Weight reduction is indicated for the overweight.

Cirrhosis. A high-calorie, high-protein, high-carbohydrate diet with a moderate amount of fat and plenty of vitamins, especially B complex vitamins. The objectives of dietary treatment are to promote healing and regeneration of liver tissue and to prevent fat stasis and formation of fibrous tissues. Allow 2 g protein per kilogram of desirable body weight and 300 to 350 g carbohydrate to spare protein. Protein should be immediately curtailed in impending coma. Restrict sodium to 500 mg or less if ascites and peripheral edema are present, and avoid fibrous and coarse foods if esophageal varices are present. Alcohol is not allowed.

Citrullinemia. The exact dietary treatment is not known. Protein restriction is recommended to control blood ammonia.

Cleft palate. Inability to suck adequately presents a problem. In the newborn a medicine dropper or a plastic bottle and a soft nipple with an enlarged hole may be used. Milk can be squeezed a little at a time in coordination with the infant's chewing motions. When starting solid foods, pureed baby foods may be mixed with milk in the bottle or diluted with milk and spoon-fed.

Colostomy. Start with a clear liquid diet and progress gradually to one low in residue. Then give soft and short-fibered foods as tolerated. A high calorie, high protein intake will speed up recovery and prevent weight loss.

Constipation. Diet is not a cure but provides relief or comfort to the patient. In atonic constipation a high-fiber diet will stimulate peristalsis, provide bulk to the intestinal contents, and help retain water in the feces to facilitate bowel movement. Emphasis is placed on liberal intakes of whole-grain cereals, raw fruits, and vegetables. In spastic constipation a low-fiber diet will prevent undue distention and stimulation of the bowel.

Coronary heart disease. Weight reduction or maintenance of desirable weight by an appropriate combination of physical activity and caloric intake is desirable. Specific dietary advice varies with the nature of the blood lipid profile. For details, see discussion of the dietary management of hyperlipoproteinemia.

Cystathioninuria. Large intakes of pyridoxine (vitamin B_6) seem beneficial. A commercial powder preparation low in methionine and cystine has been used.

Cystic fibrosis. A high-calorie, high-protein, low-fat diet supplemented with fat-soluble vitamins. A pancreatic enzyme preparation (e.g., pancreatin and Cotazym) should be taken at each meal and even with snacks to compensate for the pancreatic deficiency. For infants a halved skim milk formula is suggested. Several formulated milk preparations high in protein and low in fat are available commercially. As much fat as can be tolerated should be given as determined by the number and bulk of stools and the presence of abdominal discomfort. If fat has to be severely restricted, MCT oil may be used to increase fat intake. During the acute stage, starch is often not well tolerated. Give only simple carbohydrates. Generous salt intake may be necessary to replace sodium losses in sweat. As the condition improves, fat and starchy carbohydrates are gradually introduced and adjusted to the individual's tolerance.

Cystinuria. A high fluid intake is desirable to dilute the urine. An alkaline-ash diet is sometimes prescribed.

Diabetes mellitus. The most important dietary consideration is control of total caloric intake to attain or maintain desirable weight. This means weight reduction for the overweight and weight increase to achieve desirable weight for the underweight, especially the young diabetics who are insulin dependent. Individualizing the diet to specific needs of the patient is essential. A more liberal intake of carbohydrate (up to 60% of kilocalories) in the form of polysaccharides may be allowed. However, ingestion of concentrated simple sugars should be minimized to avoid hyperglycemic peaks. Limitation in intake of saturated fat and cholesterol is recommended to reduce the predisposition to the development of atherosclerotic disease. Also important is regular spacing of meals to avoid intermittent hypoglycemia, particularly among those receiving insulin therapy.

Diabetic coma. Immediate treatment consisting of insulin, electrolytes, and fluids is essential. In severe ketoacidosis, fluid and electrolyte administration must usually be intravenous. A 5% glucose solution is given as hyperglycemia and glycosuria subside. If there is no vomiting, salty broth and tea may be given, followed by fruit juices and other liquids.

Diarrhea. Food is withheld for 12 to 24 hours, and fluids and electrolytes are given to prevent dehydration. As the stools are formed, small amounts of food may be gradually introduced. In infants, give a half-strength formula low in carbohydrate and fat, or use a special proprietary milk preparation such as Probana or Nutramigen. The addition of 5% to 10% apple powder, banana flakes, or pectin-agar mixture may hasten the development of formed stools. In adults, start with simple foods such as broth, tea, and toast. Gradually introduce foods low in residue, and build up to a normal diet as the condition improves.

Disaccharide intolerance. Exclude the poorly tolerated disaccharide from the diet and replace with utilizable carbohydrate. Supplementation with the deficient enzyme is beneficial in the initial stage. The enzyme deficiency is apparently compensated for in later years.

Diverticular disease. The main therapeutic goal is to increase the caliber of the stools and distend the bowel wall. Thus the low-residue diet is not recommended except during acute phases of diverticulitis, ulcerative colitis, or infectious enterocolitis when the bowel is markedly inflamed. Initially, clear liquids or a defined-formula diet may be given. The diet may gradually progress to a regular diet. However, it is still advisable to avoid excessive intake of raw fruits and vegetables because of their mild laxative effect. Excessive intake of spices such as pepper and chili pepper should also be avoided. A bulk-forming agent such as methylcellulose is beneficial in initiating normal colonic function and regular bowel action.

Dumping syndrome. Dietary management consists of small, dry meals given at frequent intervals with liquids taken between meals (usually 30 to 45 minutes after meals). The diet should be high in protein, moderate in fat, and low in carbohydrate. Foods that have a strong osmolar effect such as sugars, sweets, and jellies are omitted. Artificial sweeteners may be used. Milk and dishes containing milk frequently precipitate symptoms and hence should also be omitted or limited. It is important to rest before meals, eat slowly, chew well, and relax after meals.

Dysentery. During the acute stage give only clear liquids in the form of broth, tea, and thin gruel. Gradually add strained fruit juices and boiled milk as tolerated. When the condition improves, nonirritating foods low in fiber may be gradually added to the diet.

Dyspepsia. No simple dietary rule can be set. Food should be adequate, well cooked, not too spicy, and served in a relaxed atmosphere. It is best to eat small meals. In the majority of cases, dyspepsia is of nervous origin and disappears once the psychoneurotic cause is removed. If due to organic causes, a soft diet low in fat may be beneficial.

Emphysema. A soft, high-calorie diet is usually indicated. Patients experience difficulty in eating breakfast and are short of breath after a night's sleep. Give concentrated foods in small, frequent feedings. Avoid fibrous fruits and vegetables and tough meats that will require much chewing.

Enteritis. A high-calorie, liberal-protein, low-fiber diet with vitamin and mineral supplementation. Moderately restrict fats (25% of kilocalories) in regional enteritis with malabsorption steatorrhea. In severe cases strict fat restriction (as low as 10% of kilocalories) may be necessary. The use of MCT oil is desirable in such cases.

Epilepsy. As a rule, a normal diet for the individual's age and activity is prescribed when drug therapy is used. However, the ketogenic diet is still valuable in the control of some specific types of seizures that do not respond to drug therapy alone. To produce a state of ketosis, a ketogenic-antiketogenic ratio of 3-1 or 4-1 is maintained. To obtain this, carbohydrate is drastically reduced and the bulk of calories is taken from fat. Protein is maintained at normal levels. A typical 1800 kcal ketogenic diet would have a nutrient distribution of 50 g protein, 30 g carbohydrate, and 170 g fat. The regimen is instituted with a starvation period of 3 to 5 days. Nothing is given orally except for small amounts of water until the patient has lost about 10% of his weight and/or his urine reveals marked acidosis. The use of medium-chain triglycerides (MCT oil) is found to be more effective than dietary fats in inducing ketosis. It also allows more carbohydrate, making the diet more palatable. A typical MCT-ketogenic diet has a kilocalorie distribution of 60% MCT oil, 10% dietary fat, 10% protein, and 20% carbohydrate.

Fever and febrile conditions. The diet should be high in calories, protein, carbohydrate, salt, and fluid. Recommended intakes are 3000 to 3500 kcal to meet increased energy needs due to higher basal metabolic rate; 100 to 120 g protein to replace nitrogen losses and tissue destruction characteristic of febrile conditions; 300 to 350 g carbohydrate to replenish depleted glycogen stores and spare protein; and 2.4 to 3.6 L (10 to 15 c) of liquid per day, preferably as salty broths, fruit juices, and milk, to replace fluid lost through perspiration and to facilitate elimination of toxins through increased urination. The consistency of the diet varies with the condition. In acute fever it may be necessary to give a full liquid diet. With recovery, progress the diet to soft and then to regular consistency. Frequent small feedings are better tolerated than large meals.

Fracture. A high-calorie, liberal-protein diet with mineral and vitamin supplementation. Important nutrients to consider are protein for bone matrix formation; calcium and phosphorus for deposition in bone; vitamin D for efficient utilization of calcium; and vitamin C for intercellular cementing substance.

Galactosemia. Give a galactose-free diet. Milk and milk products are not allowed. Nonmilk formulas are available commercially for infants.

Gastrectomy. Small but frequent feeding of easily digested foods. The progression of the diet varies with the extent of gastric resection and tolerance of the patient for food. The usual progression consists of hourly feedings, of 60 to 90 ml water on the first day, clear liquids on the second day, and full liquids on the third day. Starting on the fourth day, soft and easily digested solid foods chosen from stage III of the progressive bland diet are gradually introduced. As the patient improves, six small feedings of soft, low-fiber foods are given, keeping the carbohydrate intake relatively low. Mineral and vitamin supplements are needed because of impaired absorption.

Gastritis. During the acute stage, food is restricted for 24 to 48 hours to rest the stomach. For relief of thirst, small amounts of water or bits of crushed ice may be given. Food is progressed until the patient can take a soft diet. In chronic gastritis, stage IV of the progressive bland diet given in small, frequent feedings may be used initially, with progression to greater amounts and wider variety of foods as tolerated by the patient. Some restrictions in fat intake may be beneficial, as fat depresses gastric acid production and motility. Alcohol is to be avoided.

Glomerulonephritis. Sufficient calories must be supplied by carbohydrate and fat to spare protein and reduce breakdown of endogenous or body protein. Salt intake is restricted to 500 to 1000 mg in the presence of edema and high blood pressure, and fluid intake is restricted to 500 to 700 ml when there is oliguria. Protein restriction is indicated only when there is nitrogen retention. Allow 0.2 to 0.3 g/kg body weight (about 15 to 20 g protein) of high quality protein supplied chiefly by egg and milk protein. As the condition improves, protein intake is gradually increased until a normal allowance is taken. In chronic glomerulonephritis, normal protein intake of 0.9 to 1.0 g/kg body weight

is sufficient to maintain nitrogen balance. There is no sufficient evidence that a high-protein diet is useful and will make up for losses in the urine. Sodium intake is restricted in the presence of edema.

Gluten (gliadin)-induced enteropathy. Elimination of wheat, oat, rye, barley, and buckwheat from the diet.

Glycinuria. Protein restriction with arginine and pyridoxine supplementation may be beneficial. The exact dietary treatment is not known.

Glycogen storage disease. A high-protein diet given in small, frequent feedings. The use of corticosteroids in the control of hypoglycemia may require mild sodium restriction.

Gout. Weight reduction for the obese is beneficial. The diet should be high in carbohydrate, to increase urate excretion, and low in fat, since fat inhibits excretion of uric acid. For acute gouty attacks some physicians prescribe a diet restricted in purine. Alcoholic drinks should be avoided. Therapy by drugs has largely replaced rigid purine restriction in the diet. Patients with increased plasma triglyceride concentrations may benefit from the type IV diet for hyperlipoproteinemia.

Hartnup disease. A liberal protein intake (90 to 120 g per day) with niacin and pyridoxine supplementation has been recommended.

Heartburn. A soft diet given in six small meals. Avoid excessive intake of alcohol. Also avoid spices, gas-forming vegetables, rapid eating, and large meals.

Hemorrhoids. A low-fiber diet is indicated to provide comfort for the patient. A high fluid intake (8 to 10 glasses) is also desirable to avoid constipation and to reduce possible irritation from too much roughage. Irritants such as highly seasoned foods, relishes, and harsh laxatives should be avoided. After hemorrhoidectomy, progress the diet from clear liquids to full liquids without milk and then to the low-residue and soft diets until the patient is fully recovered.

Hepatic coma. The basic principle of the diet is to avoid tissue protein catabolism and to reduce ammonia production. It is not always necessary to reduce protein intake. Initial treatment may be directed at reducing the intestinal production of ammonia by bacteria. When antibiotic therapy is not sufficient or effective, it may be necessary to restrict dietary protein. The level of protein restriction may range from 0 (protein-free) to between 0.2 and 0.3 g/kg body weight. Protein restriction should be used for as short a time as possible, because it is important in healing the liver tissue. As the condition improves, increase the protein intake by 10 to 20 g daily until a normal allowance is consumed. Provide sufficient calories from carbohydrate and fat (1800 kcal or more) to keep body tissue breakdown to a minimum.

Hepatitis. A high calorie, liberal protein, high carbohydrate, and moderate fat intake. The objectives of the diet are to aid in the regeneration of liver tissue and to avoid further injury to the liver. A high calorie intake of 3000 to 4000 kcal will counteract weight loss and assist in maximum utilization of protein. A liberal protein intake of 90 to 110 g per day or an allowance of 1.5 to 2 g/kg is sufficient for regeneration and maintenance of liver tissue. A carbohydrate intake of 300 to 400 g daily will protect the liver against injury, ensure a large glycogen reserve for liver function, and spare protein. Recent investigations reveal that fat intake may be liberalized as long as carbohydrate and protein intakes are adequate. Give a liquid or semiliquid diet during the acute phase of the disease, gradually progressing the diet to a soft and eventually a regular diet as the condition improves. Frequent small feedings are better tolerated than three large meals.

Hiatus hernia. Small, frequent feedings to prevent gastric distention. Avoid eating 2 hours before retiring.

Hypercholesterolemia. Weight reduction for the obese, reduction in cholesterol intake to 300 mg or less, moderate restriction in fat, and replacement of saturated fats with those containing polyunsaturated fatty acids. See the discussion of the hyperlipoproteinemia type II diet.

Hyperinsulinism. Carbohydrate in the diet should be drastically reduced (75 to 125 g per day) to minimize the production of insulin. A high protein intake (120 g or more) is recommended; fat furnishes the remaining calories. The diet is calculated by using the food exchange lists, and the day's food allowance is divided into three meals with equal distribution of carbohydrate, protein, and fat. In planning meals, bread and starchy carbohydrates are ordinarily omitted. Milk, fruits, and vegetables supply the prescribed carbohydrate. Artificial sweeteners may be used.

Hyperlipoproteinemia. Five types of diets have been recommended by the National Institutes of Health, depending on the particular lipoprotein fraction that is elevated in the blood. These diets are summarized below.

Type I. The diet is aimed at restricting the intake of dietary fat to a minimum level (35 g or less daily) to keep blood triglycerides low and prevent abdominal pain associated with the ingestion of dietary fat. The intakes of carbohydrate, protein, and cholesterol are not restricted. Alcohol is not recommended. All separable fats and oils are eliminated, and only lean, trimmed meat is used. Meat is restricted to 5 ounces cooked weight per day. Additional protein should come from skim milk, fruits, and vegetables. To increase fat intake, 30 to 40 g of medium-chain triglycerides may be prescribed. The medium-chain triglycerides are absorbed directly into the portal system and transported to the liver without chylomicron formation.

Type IIa. The diet involves lowering the intake of cholesterol to 300 mg or less per day, restricting the intake of saturated fats, and increasing the use of vegetable oils and margarines high in polyunsaturated fatty acids to give a P/S ratio of about 2. All foods high in cholesterol are eliminated, and the desired P/S ratio may be achieved by consuming 2 teaspoons polyunsaturated fat or oil per ounce of cooked meat. Calories, carbohydrate, and protein are not restricted. Alcohol may be used with discretion.

Types IIb and III. Initially a weight reduction diet is given if necessary and then maintenance of desirable weight. Carbohydrate and fat intake are controlled to contribute 40% of kilocalories from each. Protein intake is high at 20% of kilocalories. Sugars and concentrated sweets are to be avoided, and polyunsaturated fats are preferred to saturated fats, although the P/S ratio is not emphasized. Cholesterol is restricted to 300 mg or less per day. Alcohol is limited to two servings per day in exchange for a serving from the bread or cereal group.

Type IV. Weight reduction to attain desirable body weight is needed, followed by a maintenance diet restricted in carbohydrate and alcohol (excess of either tends to increase endogenous triglyceride concentrations). Protein and fat intakes are not limited, although saturated fats should be restricted and replaced with polyunsaturated fats. Cholesterol is only moderately restricted to 300 to 500 mg per day, with an allowance of 3 egg yolks per week or the substitution of 2 ounces of organ meats or cheddar cheese for an egg. Because of its caloric content and its effect on blood triglycerides, the total amount of alcohol is limited to two servings per day, which should be taken as a substitute for bread.

Type V. After weight reduction, a maintenance diet is prescribed with the following modifications: restricted and modified fat, controlled carbohydrate, and moderately restricted cholesterol (300 to 500 mg per day). Alcohol is not recommended. Fat is computed at 25% to 30% of total kilocalories (50 to 85 g per day). It is best to keep the level of fat in the diet as low as possible. A fat allowance of 1 g/kg body weight is a safe intake. The P/S ratio is not emphasized. However, polyunsaturated fats are recommended in preference to saturated fats. Carbohydrate is about 50% of total kilocalories. Because of restricted fat and carbohydrate intakes, the protein intake is higher than the normal intake (20% to 25% of kilocalories or an allowance of 1.5 g or more per kilogram body weight).

Hypertension. Weight reduction for the overweight is desirable. Strict sodium restriction (200 to 250 mg per day) is the best dietary regimen for lowering blood pressure. The diet, however, is unpalatable, difficult to follow, and requires about a month or longer before noticeable improvement may be seen. The use of antihypertensive drugs combined with mild sodium restriction (1500 to 2000 mg per day) has become the cornerstone of therapy.

Hyperthyroidism. A high-calorie, liberal-protein and carbohydrate diet with calcium, phosphorus, and vitamin D and B complex supplementation. The basic aim of the diet is to compensate for the increase in basal metabolic rate (3500 to 4000 kcal) and nitrogen metabolism (90 to 120 g protein). A high carbohydrate intake will replenish depleted liver glycogen storage. Vitamin D is essential for the utilization of calcium and phosphorus, and the B complex vitamins are needed for the increased caloric intake and high basal metabolic rate.

Hypoglycemia. Mild hypoglycemic reactions to insulin disappear following ingestion of fruit juice or candy. In the fasting type of hypoglycemia as seen in Addison's disease, liver disease, and hypopituitarism, a high carbohydrate intake with between-meal feedings is recommended. Restrict carbohydrate intake in stimulative or functional hyperinsulinism. Insulin secretion by the pancreas is stimulated by carbohydrate foods.

Hypokalemia. Dietary supplementation with natural foods may suffice in mild cases. Food sources rich in potassium include bananas, tomato juice, citrus fruits and juices, prunes, and potatoes.

Hypothyroidism. Reduce caloric intake because of reduction in basal metabolic rate (30% to 40% below normal). Dietary aim is to control increase in weight.

Ileitis. In the acute stage prescribe a defined-formula diet or the minimal residue diet with mineral and vitamin supplementation. Progress the diet to one low in residue and then to a low-fiber, high-protein diet as the condition improves. Resume the normal diet as soon as tolerated.

Indigestion. Eat slowly and find time to relax after meals. Avoid overeating, especially foods that are bulky and difficult to digest.

Irritable colon. A soft diet with high fluid intake is suitable. Sometimes it is necessary to begin the dietary treatment with a bland, low-residue diet. A defined-formula diet may be used during the acute stage. Gradually introduce fiber but select those foods that are soft and nonirritating to the mucous membrane of the intestinal tract. The use of bulking agents may be necessary to avoid constipation. Emphasize high fluid intake, good habits of personal hygiene, relaxation, and freedom from nervous upsets.

Jaundice. A high-calorie, high-protein, low-fat diet with mineral and vitamin supplementation (especially calcium, iron, and vitamin K). Fortification of the diet with bile salts will help correct poor fat absorption.

Kwashiorkor. Protein in the form of skimmed milk is commonly prescribed. An initial allowance of 2 to 5 g protein per kilogram body weight is necessary. Sufficient carbohydrate and calories are needed to spare protein and correct weight loss. After a week a mixed diet may be given in addition to milk. Mineral and vitamin supplementation should correct the other nutritional deficiencies.

Lactose intolerance. Omit lactose and all sources of lactose. For infants give Nutramigen, Sobee, or Mullsoy and gradually introduce foods that do not contain milk and added lactose.

Leucine-induced hypoglycemia. Restrict leucine to 150 to 230 mg/kg body weight. Protein-rich foods are restricted, particularly milk and eggs, until tolerance to these foods is established. Sugars and other readily absorbable carbohydrates should be avoided. Ingestion of small amounts of carbohydrate (about 10 g) 30 to 40 minutes after each meal will help counteract the hypoglycemic effect of leucine.

Liver diseases. A diet high in protein, carbohydrate, and calories with vitamin supplementation, particularly fat-soluble vitamins. Alcohol is not allowed. Sodium intake should be restricted in ascites, and protein is curtailed in hepatic coma. Foods should be soft and low in fiber in the presence of bleeding esophageal varices. See the recommended diets for ascites, cirrhosis, hepatitis, and hepatic coma.

Malabsorption syndrome. Feeding of medium-chain triglycerides is effective in alleviating the steatorrhea associated with a variety of malabsorption syndromes such as cystic fibrosis, pancreatitis, sprue, and gastrectomy. During the initial phase of the treatment, patients are usually maintained on a liquid formula emulsion containing 45% carbohydrate, 15% protein, and 40% fat of the medium-chain triglyceride type. Intake of dietary fats is restricted to the amount found in 1 egg and 4 ounces of lean meat, fish, or poultry. For additional protein, use skim milk, egg white, legumes, and cereal products. A product made with sodium caseinate and MCT is available commercially (Portagen). Medium-chain triglycerides may be mixed with salad dressings, fruit juices, and fried and sautéed foods.

Malaria. A high calorie, high protein and high fluid intake with vitamin supplementation. During an acute attack with chills and fever the diet outlined for acute febrile condition is suitable. Frequently the liver is enlarged and liver function is impaired. Diet indicated for liver disease is beneficial.

Maple syrup urine disease. A diet restricted in leucine, isoleucine, and valine. A preparation with reduced levels of these amino acids may be made from acid hydrolyzed casein. Give small amounts of milk to aid growth.

Marasmus. Dietary management depends on the presence of complications such as dehydration, electrolyte imbalance, vitamin deficiencies, and infections. Fluid and electrolyte imbalance should be corrected promptly. Oral or parenteral administration of glucose solution provides immediate energy. After a day or two, give skim milk as the basic food and gradually add solid foods as tolerated. Provide sufficient protein of good quality and adequate calories to bring about greater nitrogen utilization. Vitamin and mineral supplements are needed.

Mental illness. Dietary management must be individualized. The basic dietary aim is to maintained good nutitional status while providing security and pleasurable satisfaction from food. Among the feeding problems encountered one will find (1) a depressed patient loses interest in food; (2) an overactive patient will not sit long enough to eat; (3) the delusional patient may develop fears and suspicions about his food; (4) an emotionally insecure patient may indulge in overeating for personal satisfaction; (5) patients with anorexia nervosa are difficult to feed; and (6)

patients undergoing shock therapy may need a high caloric intake.

Myocardial infarction. Restrict sodium intake (1000 to 2000 mg per day) and initially give a liquid diet. As the patient improves, progress the diet to a soft and eventually a regular diet.

Nephritis. Basic dietary objective is to reduce the work of the kidneys by minimizing the rate of excretion of waste products, especially urea and salt. The diet also is intended to prevent edema caused by retention of water and salt, prevent uremia caused by retention of nitrogen, and adjust body electrolytes, especially sodium, potassium, and chloride. Fluid intake should approximate measured output plus 600 ml for insensible loss. Sodium restriction is necessary (1000 to 2000 mg per day) during the acute phase of edema formation and hypertension. Protein intake need not be restricted unless renal failure develops. Give high quality protein and adequate calories to ensure positive nitrogen balance.

Nephrosclerosis. Weight reduction is recommended for the obese to lessen the work of the circulatory system. Dietary considerations in the management of atherosclerosis should also be noted. Unless there is nitrogen retention, allowance for protein is generally normal.

Nephrotic syndrome. The basic dietary objective is to replace protein (albumin) lost from the plasma into the urine. High-protein foods of good biological value are provided (about 120 to 150 g per day). Calorie and carbohydrate intake should be high to ensure efficient utilization of protein. Sodium is restricted to 1000 to 2000 mg per day in the presence of edema. A more severe sodium restriction would present problems in planning a diet high in animal protein foods, especially if the patient does not like low-sodium milk.

Obesity. Reduce caloric intake below the total energy requirement and permit a rate of weight loss satisfactory to both the physician and the patient. Protein allowance must be normal or slightly higher to keep the patient in nitrogen equilibrium and to enhance water elimination. Dividing the total food allowance into small portions at frequent intervals (six to eight meals a day) gives better results than planning a diet around three meals a day. Reduction in salt intake may be necessary for patients who are not losing weight because of water retention. For the resistant obese patients, some physicians recommend a few days of fasting before starting on a reducing regimen. The ketosis and anorexia resulting from fasting precipitate the weight loss. The application of behavior therapy or behavior modification to promote changes in dietary eating habits has been tried with some degree of success. The key to a successful weight reduction program is patient education. The patient must change basic eating habits and learn to maintain desirable weight through the years.

Pancreatic insufficiency. The condition is generally relieved by pancreatic enzyme preparation. The diet should be low in fat with the bulk of the calories coming from concentrated forms of carbohydrate such as sugars, jellies, and sweets. Use of medium-chain triglycerides (about 3 to 4 tbsp per day) will increase fat and calorie intake. Provide adequate amounts of tender meats and restrict fruits and vegetables to the ones low in fiber content.

Pancreatitis. The basic dietary aim is to rest the pancreas by restricting foods that will stimulate it to action. In the acute stage, nothing is given orally. Then the diet is progressed from a clear to a full liquid diet, and eventually to a bland, low-fat diet as the condition improves. Medium-chain triglycerides are usually well tolerated. Divide the meals into six small feedings per day.

Parkinson's disease. A low protein intake of good quality protein (0.5 g/kg or about 35 g per day) tends to potentiate and stabilize the therapeutic effects of levodopa. High protein intakes tend to cancel the therapeutic effects of levodopa and lower the capacity to work. Pyridoxine (vitamin B_6) also reverses the therapeutic effect of levodopa. Doses as small as 10 to 25 mg of pyridoxine may be sufficient to produce this effect.

Peptic ulcer. Dietary restriction in the treatment of gastric or duodenal ulcer is now minimal. The current emphasis is on size and frequency of feeding and liberalization of choice of foods. Only those foods known to cause distress are avoided. Except for alcohol, caffeine, pepper, and chili, most foods can be tolerated. The conservative and traditional dietary regimen is planned on a progressive five-stage diet, starting with the hourly feeding of milk and gradually adding soft and smooth foods that are considered to be chemically, mechanically, and thermally nonirritating.

Pernicious vomiting. In severe cases, give nothing orally for 24 to 48 hours. Glucose solution is generally administered intravenously. As vomiting becomes less severe, toast, crackers, jelly, and other simple carbohydrate foods may be given as tolerated. Give fluids between meals and avoid or limit fluid intake with meals. Gradually resume the normal diet, but restrict fat if not tolerated.

Phenylketonuria. The only treatment is restriction of the phenylalanine content of the diet. Since phenylalanine is required for normal growth and protein synthesis, management of the disease consists of supplying just the required amount so that there is no excessive accumulation in the blood. The daily phenylalanine requirement ranges from 15 to 25 mg/kg body weight, with children over 5 years requiring the lower value, infants the upper value, and 2- to 5-year-old children the medium value. The initial phenylalanine prescription serves only to assess phenylalanine tolerance. Dietary management must be individualized and adjusted as required. Since phenylalanine naturally occurs in protein foods (average of 5% phenylalanine), the diet calls for a special proprietary milk formula containing small amounts of phenylalanine (Lofenalac). This may constitute 85% to 100% of the diet, depending on the age of the child. For the newborn a small amount of milk is mixed with the formula to furnish the phenylalanine requirement. Solid foods are introduced at the usual ages and in the usual texture. Subtract the phenylalanine allotment in the special milk formula from the total phenylalanine requirement. The difference is the amount of phenylalanine to be given in solid foods.

Poliomyelitis. During the acute febrile stage the same dietary considerations as in any acute febrile condition are indicated. A high-calorie, high-protein, and high-vitamin liquid or semi-solid diet is needed to compensat for the rapid tissue destruction. Difficult dietary management is met in bulbar poliomyelitis where there is failure or difficulty in swallowing food and the possibility of choking or aspiration. This often necessitates initial feeding by the parenteral route, followed by tube feeding. When the patient is able to swallow, give small amounts of clear liquids. Milk and cream are not well tolerated, as they produce mucus. As the patient improves, supplement the liquid diet with small amounts of soft, easily digested foods. The tube feeding is decreased proportionately as the oral intake is increased.

Psoriasis. A diet restricted in the amino acid taurine has been tried. Several investigations point out that animal protein foods, particularly seafoods, influence the course of the disease and that psoriasis seems to be an error in taurine metabolism.

Pyelonephritis. An acid-ash diet may be beneficial to increase the acidity of the urine and inhibit bacterial growth. Cereals and animal protein foods give an acidic residue. The intake of basic-forming foods such as milk, fruits, and vegetables should be limited.

Refsum's syndrome. A diet restricted in phytanic acid has been recommended.

Regional enteritis. Nutritional deficiencies may be present because of malabsorption. Weight loss may be helped by a diet containing medium-chain triglycerides, which are more readily absorbed. Hypoproteinemia due to loss of protein from the gut requires a high-protein diet. Vitamin supplementation, particularly vitamin B_{12}, is necessary.

Renal calculi. See the discussion of dietary management of calculi.

Renal failure. Dietary management in acute renal failure includes the following: (1) restriction of fluid intake to a volume equivalent to urine output plus extrarenal losses, including an allowance of 600 ml per day for insensible water loss; (2) sodium restriction (500 mg per day) to improve edema and hypertension; (3) potassium restriction because of limited ability to excrete potassium; (4) restriction of protein to 20 g per day to reduce urea nitrogen retention; and (5) provision of sufficient calories (1800 kcal or more) to prevent breakdown of body tissues. The protein in the diet should be of high biological value and preferably supplied by egg and milk. Special proprietary products such as Controlyte, Cal-Power, Hycal, Polycose, and low-protein wheat starch are good sources of calories low in protein. In chronic renal failure, dietary protein intake is determined by the degree of renal impairment and function. This may range from 20 to 40 g per day. After hemodialysis has been started, the daily protein intake may be increased to 60 to 65 g, or a normal allowance of 0.8 g/kg body weight. Protein restriction may not be necessary after successful renal transplant. The sodium and potassium restrictions vary with individual patients. These may range from 1000 to 2000 mg per day.

Rheumatic fever. The full liquid diet is suitable during the acute phase. The diet is increased gradually to a soft diet and eventually to a regular diet high in vitamin C, protein, and calories to recover weight loss. Restrict sodium if there is fluid retention.

Sprue syndrome. A high protein intake (120 g per day) with elimination of gliadin from wheat, oat, rye, and barley. Carbohydrate and fat are given as tolerated. Substitution of medium-chain triglycerides for dietary fats greatly improves the steatorrhea associated with sprue. Minerals (especially calcium and iron) and vitamins (especially folic acid and vitamin B_{12}) are needed to correct nutritional deficiencies that accompany the disorder. Use low-fiber foods during the initial stage of the disorder.

Surgical conditions. The objectives of dietary management are to improve the nutritional state of the patient in preparation for the stresses of surgery, to help hasten recovery, and to maintain good nutrition in the postoperative period.

Preoperative diet. Prescribe a high protein and high calorie intake. Since obesity is a hazard in surgery, a low-calorie diet is indicated for the overweight with a moderate intake of carbohydrate to build up glycogen reserves needed during surgery. The night before surgery all foods are withheld after supper through the following morning to empty the stomach.

Postoperative diet. Immediately after surgery nothing is given by mouth for several hours; glucose solution is given intravenously. Depending on the patient's condition, the diet is progressed from the clear liquid to the full liquid, to the soft, and finally to the regular diet. In surgery of the colon a low-residue diet or defined-formula diet is initially given. Soft and low-fiber foods are gradually added as tolerated. For patients who cannot be fed orally, nourishment is given by tube feeding or by parenteral means. Gastric intubation is indicated for those who are unable to swallow because of extensive mouth, head, neck, or esophageal surgery. As soon as the patient regains an appetite, a high-calorie, high-protein diet with plenty of fluids will hasten replacement of protein and glycogen stores, correct electrolyte and water imbalance, restore losses from bleeding, and shorten the time required for wound healing.

Tonsillectomy. After surgery give cold liquids such as bland fruit juices, plain sherbet, and ginger ale. Milk and ice cream are not well tolerated because they produce mucus. On the second or third day, soft and smooth foods such as soft cooked eggs, strained cereals, and plain puddings may be given. Resume the regular diet as soon as tolerated by the patient.

Tuberculosis. The diet should supply liberal amounts of protein (90 to 100 g per day), minerals, and vitamins. Maintenance of desirable body weight is also important. Calcium is necessary for calcification of tuberculous lesions, and iron is needed if there has been hemorrhage from the lungs. Important vitamins to consider are vitamin C for wound healing, vitamin D for efficient utilization of calcium, B complex vitamins to stimulate appetite, and vitamin B_6 to counteract the polyneuritis associated with INH therapy.

Typhoid fever. Give a high-calorie, high-protein liquid diet during the acute stage. Gradually add soft foods low in fiber content to prevent intestinal irritation. Frequent small feedings are recommended to avoid overloading the stomach.

Tyrosinemia. A diet restricted in phenylalanine and tyrosine is recommended.

Ulcerative colitis. A diet high in protein and calories with vitamin and mineral supplementation. In the acute stages, use a defined-formula diet or the minimal-residue diet to avoid undue irritation to the colon. As soon as tolerated, give a bland diet high in protein, preferably in six small feedings. Only heavy roughage need be avoided.

Undernutrition. It is dangerous to force-feed se-verely undernourished individuals. Skim milk fed in small amounts is probably the best food at the start. As the person begins to recover, give small amounts of easily digested foods. Gradually increase the amount until a full meal can be eaten.

Underweight. The basic dietary aim is to increase body weight. Theoretically, an excess of 500 kcal per day results in a weekly gain of 0.45 kg (1 lb). Give a high-calorie, high-protein diet with snacks between meals. Supplement with B complex vitamins to stimulate the appetite.

Uremia. Protein is restricted to 15 to 20 g per day supplied mainly by 1 egg and 120 to 180 ml (4 to 6 oz) of milk. Provide sufficient calories to prevent breakdown of body tissues. Calories should come from fats, sugars, low-protein fruits and vegetables, and special low-protein, high-calorie proprietary products.

Wilson's disease. Restrict the intake of copper to 1 mg per day or less.

Index